The Texture of Life

The Texture of Life

Purposeful Activities
in Occupational Therapy
2nd Edition

Jim Hinojosa, PhD, OT, FAOTA
Marie-Louise Blount, AM, OT, FAOTA
Editors

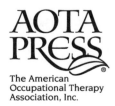

The American
Occupational Therapy
Association, Inc.

Mission Statement

The American Occupational Therapy Association advances the quality, availability, use, and support of occupational therapy through standard-setting, advocacy, education, and research on behalf of its members and the public.

Karen C. Carey, CAE, Associate Executive Director, Membership,
   Marketing, and Communications
Audrey Rothstein, CAE, Group Leader, Communications

Chris Davis, Managing Editor, AOTA Press
Rick Ludwick, Project Manager
Barbara Dickson, Production Editor

Sarah E. Ely, Cover Designer

Marge Wasson, Marketing Manager

The American Occupational Therapy Association, Inc.
4720 Montgomery Lane
Bethesda, MD 20814
Phone: 301-652-AOTA (2682)
TDD: 800-377-8555
Fax: 301-652-7711
www.aota.org
To order: 1-877-404-AOTA (2682)

Disclaimers

This publication is designed to provide accurate and authoritative information in regard to the subject matter covered. It is sold or distributed with the understanding that the publisher is not engaged in rendering legal, accounting, or other professional service. If legal advice or other expert assistance is required, the services of a competent professional person should be sought.
—*From the Declaration of Principles jointly adopted by the American Bar Association and a Committee of Publishers and Associations*

It is the objective of The American Occupational Therapy Association to be a forum for free expression and interchange of ideas. The opinions expressed by the contributors to this work are their own and not necessarily those of either the editors or The American Occupational Therapy Association.

ISBN: 1-56900-193-6

Library of Congress Control Number: 2004105886

Composition by Grammarians, Inc.
Printed by Boyd Printing Company, Albany, NY

Contents

Foreword

Writing the foreword to a book is a new activity in the texture of my life. Where to start? What to say? Who will read it? How to end? Why me? My colleagues in the Writing Center at the Medical University of South Carolina always coach me to begin responding to an invitation to write by answering the question, Why did they ask me? In this instance, I believe the editors were looking for a person whose philosophy and outlook would complement the work they've crafted together. Writing this foreword provides me with yet another opportunity to look beneath the surface of what appears to be a deceptively normal task and to examine its underpinnings. Whenever we try to describe explicitly what is implicitly self-evident in ordinary, everyday activities, we become tongue tied and lose the thread of what holds the profession of occupational therapy together. The second edition of *The Texture of Life* helps us unravel the complexities that are intertwined in everyday life and develop a new appreciation for the richness and the subtlety of our profession.

Occupational therapy is a health profession predicated on the basic tenet that engagement in occupations and their inherent activities is a powerful health determinant. How does our knowledge base about occupation and activities make the world a healthier place? How are people's lives changed after an encounter with occupational therapy? How much does the public know about and appreciate what we do? What would happen if our profession went away? The answers to these types of questions lie in our understanding of activity and how it is interpreted from the inside and from outsider perspectives. In occupational therapy, we place our focus on the rhythm of living and the way life plays out, not only on a daily basis but also throughout the life span. Life as it is viewed through an occupational lens lets us explore how we engage our time and energy in doing the daily round of activities that makes up all our lives. However, for those whose lives come into contact with health care, educational, and community-based systems, occupational therapy practitioners are increasingly challenged to embrace health-promoting approaches and provide interventions that are personally meaningful, socially satisfying, and culturally relevant for our clients: Interventions that third-party payers understand and are willing to reimburse, no matter the system in which we work or the country in which we live. To keep occupational therapy at the forefront of societal changes, we need to know and thoroughly understand all the dimensions and expressions of activities and the ways they are enfolded into human occupation.

Throughout the second edition of *The Texture of Life,* authors use language and expression to broaden our understanding of human activity and the idiosyncratic way in which people orchestrate the activities in their lives. The authors further help us see the ways in which we can apply new understanding in real and practical ways and become more artful in the practice of occupational therapy. For students new to the field, this book lays down a blueprint to guide professional preparation and entry into the practice milieu. Once there, readers will find this book helpful in reinforcing what they know and what they do, thereby enabling them to further broker their knowledge in ways that enhance the dreams and well-being of their clients.

The challenge for occupational therapy in the years ahead is to ensure that the ordinary becomes extraordinary. We are surely aware of the changing face of all societies in the world. When we look closely, we see a new picture emerging in which people with chronic conditions are living longer, people with disabilities are making up larger percentages of subpopulations, and minority populations are no longer minorities. In most countries, needs far outweigh the resources available to eradicate the ever-burgeoning number of health disparities. When occupational therapy practitioners embrace the core of their profession and use activities enfolded in occupation with increasing skill and sophistication, they become agents of change and facilitators of growth and development. Sadly though, we often relegate our activity core and occupational perspective to the commonplace. I believe passionately that activities enfolded in occupation have the power to recraft lives that, of necessity, are different. Likewise, activities have the strength to create new meaning for those whose lives are impoverished. Furthermore, as we move forward in our professional lives, let us not become like the poor old centipede that couldn't walk any further after a toad asked her which leg moved next:

> The centipede was happy quite.
> Until the toad in fun,
> Said, "Pray which leg goes after which?"
> And worked her mind to such a pitch
> She lay distracted in the ditch
> Considering how to run.

—Maralynne D. Mitcham, PhD, OTR/L, FAOTA
Professor, Medical University of South Carolina
Charleston

Reference

Palmer, G. H. (2003). *The nature of goodness.* Whitefish, MT: Kessinger.

Acknowledgments

For all of their joint and individual efforts in the preparation of this book, the editors sincerely thank the faculty and staff of the Department of Occupational Therapy, Steinhardt School of Education, New York University. Special thanks are extended to the authors and contributors to this work, both those who are faculty and graduate students at New York University and to those colleagues who work at other universities and sites. When the faculty and the department first considered this project, Deborah R. Labovitz was the department chair. We would like to recognize her contributions to the book and her 20 years of service as chair. Among those who contributed mightily to the book, but whose names do not appear elsewhere, is Shan Li, who prepared many of the final manuscripts and figures and checked references. The editors are in her debt. Jayson Garcia helped to coordinate and process all of the photographs that appear in the text. We are also in his debt. We also wish to thank Christina A. Davis who, as managing editor of AOTA Press, encouraged and supported all of our efforts.

Marie-Louise Blount profoundly appreciates the love and support of Elena and Wesley Blount and family members Barry Levinson and Meyer Levinson-Blount, who have made all of her endeavors worthwhile. Jim Hinojosa thanks both his parents, who instilled in him a love for engagement in purposeful, meaningful activity. Additionally, he thanks Dr. Anne C. Mosey, who provided the insight that would refine his thinking about activity and occupational therapy.

To our clients, we are indebted to them because they reaffirmed our beliefs about the value of active engagement and the meaningfulness of occupational therapy. Finally, we are indebted to our students, current and former, who provided the reason for writing this book. We continually learn from them the value of what we do.

Contributors

Fran Babiss, PhD, OTR/L
Associate Service Director
South Oaks Partial Hospital
Amityville, NY

Paulette Bell, MA, OTR
Occupational Therapist
Rehabilitation Results Group
DeKalb Medical Center
Decatur, GA

Marie-Louise Blount, AM, OT, FAOTA
Clinical Professor
Department of Occupational Therapy
Steinhardt School of Education
New York University
New York

Wesley Blount, BS
Editor
New York

Karen Buckley, MA, OT/L
Clinical Assistant Professor
Department of Occupational Therapy
Steinhardt School of Education
New York University
New York

Ann Burkhardt, OTD, OTR/L, BCN, FAOTA
Director of Occupational Therapy
New York Presbyterian
University Hospital of Columbia and
Cornell

Associate Clinical Instructor
Columbia University
and
Clinical Associate
Mercy College
Dobbs Ferry, NY

Shu-Hwa Chen, MA, OTR
Doctoral Candidate
Department of Occupational Therapy
Steinhardt School of Education
New York University
New York

Lisa E. Cyzner, PhD, OTR
Pediatric Private Practitioner
Co-founder, Therapeutic Children's Center
Charlotte, NC

Mary Donohue, PhD, OT, FAOTA
Clinical Professor
Department of Occupational Therapy
Steinhardt School of Education
New York University
New York

Ellen Greer, PhD, OT, CPSYA
Assistant Professor
Long Island University
Brooklyn, NY

Prudence Heisler, MA, OTR
Special Programs in Occupational Therapy
Services
New York

Jim Hinojosa, PhD, OT, FAOTA
Professor and Chair
Department of Occupational Therapy
Steinhardt School of Education
New York University
New York

Paula Kramer, PhD, OTR, FAOTA
Professor and Chair
Department of Occupational Therapy
College of Health Sciences
University of the Sciences in Philadelphia

Deborah R. Labovitz, PhD, OTR/L, FAOTA
Professor
Department of Occupational Therapy
Steinhardt School of Education
New York University
New York

Paula McCreedy, MEd, OTR
Clinical Assistant Professor
Department of Occupational Therapy
Steinhardt School of Education
New York University
New York
and
Special Programs in Occupational Therapy Services
New York

Jane Miller, MA, OT
Director of Post Professional Admissions
Department of Occupational Therapy
Steinhardt School of Education
New York University
New York

Laurette Olson, PhD, OTR
Assistant Professor
Graduate Program in Occupational Therapy
Mercy College
Dobbs Ferry, NY

Anita Perr, MA, OT, ATP, FAOTA
Clinical Assistant Professor
Department of Occupational Therapy
Steinhardt School of Education
New York University
New York

Sally Poole, MA, OT, CHT
Clinical Assistant Professor
Department of Occupational Therapy
Steinhardt School of Education
New York University
New York
and
Co-owner
Hands-On Rehab
Valhalla, NY

Elizabeth Roarty O'Herron, MS, OTR
Senior Occupational Therapist
South Oaks Hospital
Amityville, NY
and
Professional Associate
Mercy College
Dobbs Ferry, NY

Joyce Shapero Sabari, PhD, OTR, BCN, FAOTA
Associate Professor and Chair
Occupational Therapy Program
State University of New York
Downstate Medical Center
Brooklyn, NY

Dalia Sachs, PhD, OT
Senior Lecturer
Department of Occupational Therapy
Haifa University
Haifa, Israel

Ruth Segal, PhD, OT
Assistant Professor
Steinhardt School of Education
Department of Occupational Therapy
New York University
New York

Judy Urban Wilson, MA, OT
Assistant Director
Department of Occupational Therapy
Belleview Hospital Center
New York

1

Purposeful Activities Within the Context of Occupational Therapy

Jim Hinojosa, PhD, OT, FAOTA
Marie-Louise Blount, AM, OT, FAOTA

Activities, what we do, the foundation of much of our routine, enterprise, and art in the world, have a unique place in the context of occupational therapy. The import of activities in occupational therapy is, in fact, a varied landscape, one with multiple meanings.

We address in this chapter some of the more fundamental of these meanings and establish that occupational therapy's application of these meanings is the core of the profession and an integral part of practice. We discuss how occupational therapy practitioners apply the varying ideas to be analyzed in Chapter 2 to describe their reasoning and create their practice. The labels used are not always the same, and the ideas behind the labels are not necessarily uniform. It is our position that the varying labels and ideas represent important ferment in our thinking as well as a richness in the methods that we use, and we should, therefore, take stock of these ideas and develop our understanding of their potential for our practice. In occupational therapy, we use the term *purposeful activity* rather than *activity* to highlight that we use activities that have a purpose and are goal-directed therapeutically.

Today, occupational therapy practitioners strive to have an unambiguous personal definition of *occupation* and *activity*. Although the use and distinction between the two words may be clear to many, for others the two terms describe similar phenomena. That is, they describe the person's participation in daily life pursuits (American Occupational Therapy Association [AOTA], 2002). Occupation, meaningful personal tasks, and purposeful activities that a person engages in are composed of purposeful activities. When a person participates in an action to realize a goal, and this activity is personally important, the person is engaged in what is called a purposeful activity. When a person engages in purposeful activities out of personal choice and they are valued, these clusters of purposeful activities form occupations (Hinojosa,

Kramer, Royeen, & Luebben, 2003). Thus, occupations are unique to each individual and provide personal satisfaction and fulfillment as a result of engaging in them (AOTA, 2002; Pierce, 2001).

If purposeful activity refers to portions of occupations and encompasses a variety of behaviors and performances (AOTA, 1993), the need still exists to discuss, delimit, and understand the behaviors and tasks that are part of the activity and at the same time appreciate the occupations under which it is subsumed. That is, having a definition does not necessarily simplify one's understanding of a phenomenon or of the issues that it raises.

We suggest, therefore, an approach to these questions recommended by Mosey (1985), that is, the adoption of a "pluralistic approach" to these questions, and continued attention to questions raised by Henderson et al. (1991), who dissected some of the dilemmas raised by our uses of and preferences for ideas surrounding purposeful activity. These authors also have suggested that we embrace a multidimensional view of purposeful activity both as an entity and as a therapeutic modality.

Because purposeful activity is fundamental to occupational therapy practice, we need to understand the many modes in which we use the term. As Henderson et al. (1991) pointed out, both purposefulness and the varied meanings invested in the term are "attributes of persons and not of activities" (p. 370). To agree further with these same authors, we support their belief that occupational therapy services can and do include approaches and methods other than purposeful activity.

As noted in Chapter 2, a number of different approaches exist in occupational therapy to the use of the term *purposeful activity* and to the uses of other terms that often are substituted for it. Henderson et al. (1991) also noted that occupational therapy practitioners use a wide range of types and levels of activities in practice. One dimension of these ranges that they described is from low level (e.g., reaching for an object) to high level (e.g., a simulated work activity). There are other dimensions, however, in ranges of activities from simple to complex that might include (a) a continuum from gross (e.g., an assembly toy in which a smaller plastic ring is placed on top of a larger plastic ring) to fine (e.g., attaching a small nut to a bolt, screwing it in place) and (b) a continuum from very brief (performing a very time-limited activity once) to more lengthy (demanding work or leisure activity is carried out in a concentrated fashion for an hour or more). The reader should consider other aspects of activities that range from simple to complex, identifying not only polar ends of a given continuum but also various stages of complexity that exist along the continuum.

Henderson et al. (1991) were rightly concerned that occupational therapy practitioners realize that the *meaning* (purposefulness) of an activity is invested in it by the person performing the activity or, sometimes, by the occupational therapy practitioner, often with the collaboration of the client, in order to accomplish or move toward a legitimate therapeutic goal. These authors identified the fact that, in acute care settings and in any situation in which remediation of disability is the goal of intervention, activities or segments of activities may be a means to attain a purpose or goal. Their view, which we share, is that all activities have the potential to be meaningful and purposeful. A number of variables, such as the person performing the activity, the context within which it is used, and when in the course of a program or series of activities it is introduced, affect the activity's meaningfulness and purposefulness. Other techniques (e.g., performing an activity in a group or stabilizing a joint while an activity is being performed), as noted by Henderson et al., contribute to the effectiveness of an activity and, although not being a purposeful activity per se, are legitimate methods that the occupational therapy practitioner uses to facilitate or enhance the activity.

Henderson et al. (1991) identified another dimension of activity that relates to occupational therapy: the history of the use of activity in the profession, which leads to certain historical and traditional applications of activity as well as to more contemporary expressions of choices or applications of activity. Chapter 2 delves into some of these issues. The same authors were concerned not only with the ways in which occupational therapy practitioners view and use activities but also with the ways in which we investigate activity's therapeutic aspects. The key point in this discussion is the multiple and varied meanings that occupational therapy practitioners apply to this concept, purposeful activity. For everyone, activities represent the core and the texture of our daily lives. For occupational therapy practitioners, purposeful activities have additional manifestations.

Occupational Therapy: The Profession's Mandate

Before examining the tools that a profession uses, it is important that we consider the purpose and focus of a profession. Professions exist to apply knowledge for the benefit of the members of society (Kielhofner, 1992; Mosey, 1981, 1996). Although each profession has a unique purpose, professions often overlap in the services they provide and the tools they use as part of their interventions to benefit members of a society. A profession's practice is grounded in the society within which it exists. Therefore, a profession's practice may vary depending on the region of the country, the city, or the culture where it is practiced. These differences in a profession's practices often create tension for the members of the profession who would like to believe that all members of the profession practice in the same manner with the same goals (Strauss, 2001).

All members of a distinct profession share a specialized training and a unique expertise. They also share a common philosophy and a code of ethics. The philosophical beliefs of occupational therapy outline how we view the person, society, and individuals within the context of their environments. The tools we use to intervene with clients as occupational therapy practitioners are heavily influenced by occupational therapy's philosophical orientation. Chapter 2 discusses the foundational beliefs of occupational therapy as they relate to one of occupational therapy's most important tools—purposeful activity. No profession, however, is unique in owning a philosophical orientation or the tools that its practitioners use.

In 1979, the AOTA Representative Assembly approved an association policy related to the philosophical base of occupational therapy (AOTA, 1979). In this statement, AOTA articulated the profession's basic beliefs about human nature and adaptation. Further, it stated that occupational therapy practitioners believe in the importance of purposeful activity to facilitate the adaptive process. Adoption of this statement highlights the importance of purposeful activity, which was considered to be synonymous with occupation. This relationship between purposeful activities and occupation has been a major philosophical discussion within the profession. The following definitions are intended to delineate the terms as they will be used in this book.

Occupation

"Occupations are the ordinary and familiar things that people do every day" (AOTA, 1995, p. 1015). The meaningful groupings of activities that people engage in as part of their daily lives are occupations. These occupations give life meaning and have been broadly categorized by occupational therapy practitioners as work, self-care, and play or leisure. The range of activities included in any one occupation is defined by the individual who is engaging in the activity and the circumstances around which the activity is performed. For example, eating can be work or pleasure at a state fair, work at a business lunch, and self-care at home.

Many important dimensions to an occupation make it a unique classification for occupational therapy practitioners. First, and most important, occupations have personal, specific meaning to the individual. This personal meaning is variable and determined by contextual, temporal, psychological, social, symbolic, cultural, ethnic, and spiritual dimensions. Second, occupations involve mental abilities and skills. They may or may not have an observable physical dimension. Third, the occupations that a person engages in define him or her. Fourth, as the person interacts with his or her environment, matures, or responds to life conditions, the person's preferred occupations are likely to change (AOTA, 1997).

Purposeful Activity

"Purposeful activity refers to goal-directed behaviors or tasks. . .that the individual considers meaningful" (AOTA, 1993, p. 1081). People engage in purposeful activities as part of their daily life routines. Purposeful activities are tasks or experiences in which the person actively participates. While engaged in a purposeful activity, the person directs his or her attention to the task (AOTA, 1993). Purposeful activities are one of the foundational elements of an occupation. Unique combinations of purposeful activities link together with the individual's personal meanings to form a person's occupations. Purposeful activities are goal-directed in that they involve active participation and require coordination among a person's physical, emotional, and cognitive systems. Goal-directed means that the person actively engages in actions to meet a personal purpose or need; it does not mean that the end-product must be a physical outcome. In occupational therapy, purposeful activities are an important therapeutic tool. They are used alone to address a specific need, or they are used in patterns or groups to help a person develop meaningful occupations (AOTA, 1997).

Linking Purposeful Activity and Occupation

The principal concern of occupational therapy is to maintain, restore, or facilitate a person's ability to function within his or her daily occupations. We have broadly defined daily occupations to include active participation in self-maintenance, work, leisure, and play activities. The ability to engage in these occupations requires that the person be able to complete many purposeful activities.

Occupational therapy practitioners use a wide variety of strategies and tools in their practice. These therapeutic tools are selected to be consistent with well-defined theoretical bases or rationales. It should be noted that there is not one universally accepted way that occupational therapy practitioners conceptualize practice. Some view practice as based on a model, others suggest paradigms, and others use frames of reference. In this book, we are not going to address the issue of how practice is conceptualized. We are going to accept that many scholars use different organizational structures and view practice differently. What is important is that each of the models, paradigms, or frames of reference provides the guidelines for the selection and use of therapeutic tools. Each occupational therapy practitioner selects from a wide assortment of tools in which he or she is both knowledgeable and competent for practice. Specialization of practice has resulted in some occupational therapy practitioners using different tools than do other practitioners. Whatever tools an occupational therapy practitioner chooses to use, we all share a common goal: The person will be able to engage in daily living, work, or play or leisure activities.

Tools of the Profession

With advancement of knowledge and technology, the practices and concerns of a profession change over time. Thus, a profession changes its priorities and practices in response to changes in society. This continuous change ensures that a profession remains viable and is responsive to the needs of the society that it serves. Occupational therapy's evolution in response to changes in society, knowledge, and technology has contributed to a viable, dynamic profession that continues to meet its mandate from society. These changes have been difficult for some occupational therapy practitioners. For example, the early extensive use of crafts has been replaced with new modalities such as manual manipulation, computer adaptation, or physical activity. Changes in the importance and use of a modality are sometimes seen as not consistent with the philosophical base of the profession. Using the previous example, some occupational therapy practitioners continue to believe that "true" occupational therapy must involve active engagement in an activity.

Figure 1.1
Lesson: Personal Hierarchy of Needs

An important concern of educators is what motivates humans and how this interrelates with the development of human potential. Abraham Maslow, the founder of humanistic psychology, proposed that a person's gratification of needs is the most important single principle underlying development. He proposed seven hierarchical levels of needs: physiological, safety, love and belongingness, esteem, self-actualization, knowing and understanding, and aesthetics. The way people fill these needs is by engaging in meaningful activities. Reflect on the past two days and how you satisfied your personal needs in the categories identified in Maslow's hierarchy:

■ Physiological needs (food, drink, sleep, survival)

■ Safety (avoidance of danger and anxiety, desire for security)

■ Love and belongingness (affection, feeling wanted, roots in a family or peer group)

■ Esteem (self-respect, feelings of adequacy, competence, mastery)

■ Self-actualization (striving for or using talents, capacities, potentialities)

■ Knowing and understanding (curiosity, learning about the world)

■ Aesthetics (experience and understand beauty for its own sake).

After completing the list, consider:

■ What needs were being met, not met?

■ What activities contributed to the satisfaction of your needs?

■ What does the list suggest about your health status?

Note. This exercise is adapted from Glover, Bruning, and Filbeck (1983).

Occupational therapy's mandate has always been to enable people to engage and participate in their own daily life activities. Occupational therapy, a health care profession, has been influenced by the trends and concerns of medicine (Christiansen & Baum, 1991). Although medicine continues to affect the evolution of the profession, other more recent changes in society seem to be having a greater influence. Responsive to societal change, occupational therapy has moved into education and community-based service delivery models. This change in society's priorities has led to an increase in the number of practitioners working in education-based practices and a change in the site of practice to schools and community settings (Kramer & Hinojosa, 1999). This shift in the site of practice and service delivery models also is evident in other areas of practice. In the 1990s, we saw a shift from "clinic" settings to more integrated community, classroom, and home settings. These changes have been in response to numerous internal influences (e.g., growth in knowledge, advances in technology) and external influences (e.g., social and government policy, payment practices).

This chapter presents views of purposeful activities as they relate to occupational therapy practice today. It defines and outlines the relationship among the major constructs of the profession: occupation, purposeful activity, and occupational performance. Further, it provides the framework for the rest of the book.

Occupational Therapy's Intervention Tools

The application of any frame of reference (model, practice guidelines, paradigm) involves the use of a variety of intervention strategies and tools. Tools are those items, actions, means, modalities, methods, or instruments that are used in practice in a theoretically prescribed manner to bring about change. Items, actions, means, modalities, methods, or instruments become the legitimate tools of a profession when the profession's members have expertise in their use (Mosey, 1996). A profession's tools change with evolving knowledge, technological advances, and the changing needs of clients. Occupational therapy practitioners use a variety of tools, depending on the particular frame of reference (Mosey, 1986). Beyond purposeful activities, other legitimate tools discussed in the literature are nonhuman environment, conscious use of self, activity analysis and adaptation, activity groups, teaching–learning processes, stimulus–response interactions, atmospheric elements, physical agent modalities, and technology (Luebben, Hinojosa, & Kramer, 1999; Mosey, 1986, 1996). In addition to these tools, the profession has others that are very specialized and often specific to one frame of reference (Luebben et al., 1999).

One of the major issues related to tools is that many practitioners consider the tools of the profession to be exceptionally significant. Some may even consider the tools to be symbolic of the profession as a whole (Luebben et al., 1999). This significance may be a result of the tangible aspects of the legitimate tools and because practitioners use them daily as they interact with clients (Mosey, 1986). In addition, many practitioners view the tools of their profession as unique. In reality, however, the legitimate tools are not unique and are shared by many professions. What is unique is the way that a specific profession applies them. In occupational therapy, this uniqueness lies in how they are used together in the application of the specific frame of reference or guideline for intervention.

Activities

Each day, we engage in numerous activities as part of our lives. Some of these activities we perform to meet our self-care needs. Some we do because we enjoy them. Others result from our responses to others' expectations or to circumstances that require us to do them. Thus, activities are the things that we do. They are the building blocks that we use to construct our lives. Occupational therapy evolved from the realized importance of how we occupy our time as human beings. This concern with occupations is central to our beliefs about what we do and believe in as occupational therapy practitioners. From our perspective as occupational therapy practitioners, activities are the actions that people do to accomplish a goal or function. Activities consist of groupings of actions or tasks that a person does as part of accomplishing a goal or fulfilling an expected or required function. Activities are purposeful when they are goal-directed and meaningful to the person who is completing the task or action. Tasks are the component parts of some activities. One or more tasks also can be combined to become one activity. When we view a pattern of daily activities together that have personal meaning to the person, we categorize them as occupations. Thus, occupations are fundamentally based on activities (Hinojosa et al., 2003; Kramer & Hinojosa, 1995).

From this perspective, both activities and the consequent occupations are fundamental and an essential aspect of life. Our daily activities and occupations define who and what we are. Engagement in purposeful activities gives our lives meaning. In defining our domain of concern, we as occupational therapy practitioners typically view activities as part of occupations (e.g., we divide activities into activities of daily living, work or productive activities, or play or leisure activities). By viewing activities in this manner, we think about activities related to the end-result for the person who engages in the particular purposeful activities. Thus, the same activities may fit into several occupations, depending on the goal of the activity, the person's developmental status, and the specific circumstances and context in which the person performs the activity. The following example of writing illustrates this point. For a school-age child at camp who has to write a letter to his parents, it may be work. For a young person, writing a letter to a girlfriend may be a leisure activity. For an adult, writing a shopping list may be an activity of daily living. In these examples, note that the activity is writing. The occupations for which writing is an activity component include work, leisure, and activities of daily living. For the professional author, writing is an occupation in both the job and the occupational therapy senses, the essential core of his work. In this scenario, the professional author engages in a number of writing activities that together are viewed as an occupation. The following discussion outlines the unique view we share related to purposeful activities and occupations.

ACTIVITIES OF DAILY LIVING

Each day, all humans engage in a variety of daily living occupations. These occupations are composed of self-care activities, which are the means that we use to interact and respond to our life demands and needs. Not all self-care activities are interesting or enjoyable. In fact, many basic self-care activities of our lives are boring, routine, and unexciting. These ordinary daily self-care activities, however, are basic to our surviving as social human beings. We should not minimize the importance and significance of our ability to engage in these activities. Our ability to take care of ourselves and meet our daily needs is vital to our existence. The ability to feed ourselves, dress ourselves, or take care of our own toileting needs provides valued independence. As mundane as many self-care activities can be, they are crucially important to self-esteem and self-worth. The multitude of purposeful activities categorized as self-care are determined by a wide range of factors, including individual attributes and abilities, culture, context, developmental status, and socioeconomic status.

Work or Productive Activities

The occupations of work or productive activities are composed of the numerous activities that people engage in to support themselves and their families, to fill time in a socially acceptable fashion, to give expression to their interests, to apply their education and training, to maintain important social status, to alleviate stress, to mitigate loneliness, or to avoid doubts about life's purposes, to name just a few possibilities. Work is an obligation for many people, but in our society, it is not usually a requirement for children, some students, some people with disabilities, and most retirees. Much of our time is devoted to work and productive activities. In addition to time spent working, time often is devoted to preparing for work and traveling to and from work. Many people have more than one job. Activities involved in work are extremely varied. Many American workers must adjust to the demands of large, formal organizations and complex technology. Work activities are central to the lives of most adult men and women and become a key focus to what makes many people's lives meaningful.

Play or Leisure Activities

Play or leisure occupations include a wide range of activities that one engages in for intrinsic pleasure because they are fun. They can range from solitary activities, such as reading a book, to physically demanding sports. An important characteristic of play or leisure activities is that people engage in them because they want to. As with self-care activities, a wide range of factors, including individual attributes and abilities, culture, context, developmental status, and socioeconomic status, determines play and leisure purposeful activities.

As occupational therapy practitioners, we are concerned with the wide range of activities that people engage in. Activities are fundamental and normal for all humans. For everyone, purposeful activities and the associated occupations define what and who we are. They allow us to express feelings and have personal and social meaning. We learn from engaging in purposeful activities and get satisfaction from them. From a purposeful activity, a person can explore interests, satisfy needs, determine and assess capacity and limitations, meet personal and interpersonal needs, and cope with life. Most important, from participating in purposeful activities a person acquires and participates in his or her own occupations.

Purposeful Activities as a Tool of Intervention

Occupational therapy practitioners use purposeful activities as a tool of intervention. Therefore, it is crucial that we have more than just an appreciation for them. We must have in-depth knowledge of purposeful activities as the foundation to occupation, which is a core concept in our profession. We also must understand the value and benefit of purposeful activities as therapeutic media. Part of using purposeful activities as therapeutic tools is an understanding of the component elements of purposeful activities. In addition, because of the characteristics of purposeful activities, we take a broader view of them within the context of the person's life, abilities, and life circumstances. When using purposeful activities, we must always keep in mind the person's occupations.

Why do we use purposeful activities? Occupational therapy practitioners have always used activities as part of their interventions with clients. Although specific activities have changed and will continue to change, the basic reasons that we choose to use purposeful activities are relatively constant. The following are six reasons for using purposeful activities:

1. *Purposeful activity builds upon the person's abilities and leads to achievement of personal and functional goals.* For an activity to be purposeful, it must have four qualities. First, the activity must be directed toward a goal that the participant considers important. Second, the participant must be actively engaged in it because he or she wants to. Third, the activity must have personal meaning to the participant (Evans, 1987; Gilfoyle, 1984; Mosey, 1986; Nelson, 1988). The purposefulness of an activity is always grounded in the person who is doing the activity and the situational context in which it is done (Henderson et al., 1991). Fourth, the participant must be capable and have the knowledge, skills, and abilities to engage in the activity. Therefore, we select purposeful activities because they are meaningful to the person and build upon his or her capacities to bring about change. The person's ability to complete purposeful activities provides the foundation for his or her occupations. When a person engages in purposeful activities out of personal choice because they are meaningful and significant, these purposeful activities form occupations.

2. *Purposeful activity offers the person opportunities for effective action.* Activity means doing something to achieve an end-goal. Therefore, it is necessary to be an active participant. The completion of the activity results in something. The something may be a physical outcome, such as finishing a chore, or an intellectual achievement, such as acquiring information from reading a book. An important factor is that the person is personally involved in actively doing it. We believe that successful accomplishment will lead to the person's development of abilities and skills. With these improved skills and abilities, we believe that the person will begin or continue to engage in occupations.

3. *Purposeful activities provide opportunities for the person to achieve mastery of the environment, and successful performance promotes feelings of personal competence.* By skillfully selecting the appropriate activity, we can make the match among the person's capabilities, potential and desires, and the particular tasks. The appropriate purposeful activity provides an opportunity for a person to master skills, accomplish something, and build self-confidence. Accomplishment of the various tasks leads to the person's having successful experiences and ultimately to the accomplishment of purposeful activities. These accomplishments, when grouped together, develop into achievement of occupations. A person

who can master washing his or her face (purposeful activity) and then bathing (purposeful activity) gradually may become capable of independently completing his or her own self-care (occupation). This person's feelings about and mastery of the environment are realized as he or she engages in purposeful activities (washing, bathing) as part of the intervention plan.

4. *When engaged in a purposeful activity, the person directs his or her attention to the goal rather than to the processes required for achievement of the goal.* One major value of engagement in a purposeful activity is that the person's attention is not on the specific tasks but on the accomplishment of the activity and the end-goal. For example, a child who is playing with a doll is less likely to attend to the increased upper-extremity range of motion, cognitive challenges, or psychosocial interaction sought by the practitioner. The child's goal is to have fun while engaging in an imaginary activity. If an adult concentrates on making a sandwich, he or she may not focus on the pain or limited range of motion associated with arthritis.

5. *Engagement in purposeful activity within the context of interpersonal, cultural, physical, and other environmental conditions requires and elicits coordination among the individual's sensory, perceptual, motor, and cognitive systems and his or her emotions.* The nature of being involved in an activity, which has a goal, has anticipated outcomes and involves several tasks, leads to engagement in a purposeful activity and occurs in complex interactions between the individual and his or her environment. Although a practitioner can control the degree of each factor to some extent, the nature of selecting an activity that is meaningful requires multiple levels of processing. The therapeutic value of purposeful activities is enhanced by the complex interaction of factors that stem from involvement in a specific purposeful activity.

6. *Engagement in purposeful activity provides direct and objective feedback about performance to both the occupational therapy practitioner and the client.* Occupational therapy practitioners use purposeful activities because by actively engaging a person in the activity, the practitioner and that individual receive feedback about the person's own action. Feedback is gained during the doing of the activity and as a result of the actions. Because the purposeful activities are part of real-life occupations, they provide additional insight into the individual's potential to engage in occupations successfully. Feedback from real-life, meaningful activities provides valuable information that we cannot obtain from simulated or fabricated tasks.

These reasons provide a rationale that occupational therapy practitioners have always used to justify their use of purposeful activities. Although the types of activities have continually changed, occupational therapy practitioners are committed to using meaningful, real-life purposeful activities as the best tool for evaluation and intervention.

Occupational Therapy Practitioners' Examination and Use of Purposeful Activities

To use purposeful activities as part of our intervention, we examine their use from a number of perspectives. The following discussion outlines some of the general characteristics of purposeful activities that we consider as we use them as evaluation and therapeutic tools.

GOAL OF THE ACTIVITY TO THE PERSON

Each person has his or her personal goals for engaging in an activity. These goals may be immediate or long term. The goals also vary depending on the person's purpose for doing the activity and the time the person has to do it. For the occupational therapy practitioner, the person's goal for engaging in the activity is an important factor to consider when judging performance. We often assume that when the goal for engaging in the activity comes from the person, the person has greater investment and values the activity. Likewise, we often assume that if the person is completing the activity for someone else, he or she may not put forth the same effort or have the same investment in the activity. These assumptions, however, may not be true. When analyzing performance of a task or completion of an activity, one factor a practitioner must consider carefully is the person's motivation to perform. We must consider what we know about the person's occupations and select purposeful activities that will support these occupations.

MEANING AND VALUE OF THE ACTIVITY TO THE PERSON

As occupational therapy practitioners, we use activities in evaluation and intervention that have personal value and meaning for the person. When we select activities to use with a person, we choose those that are important to that person based on such factors as his or her personal attributes, culture, lifestyle, and life situation. For example, when working with children, we frequently choose play activities that are meaningful and appropriate to the child. If the child has a physical limitation, comes from a Hispanic background, and lives in a large metropolitan area, we carefully consider each of these factors when selecting a specific activity.

REQUIRED KNOWLEDGE, ABILITIES, AND SKILLS TO ENGAGE IN THE ACTIVITY

Every purposeful activity has requirements of knowledge, abilities, and skills to produce an effective outcome. As practitioners, we use our understanding of activity and task analysis to determine what is required to engage in the activity. Based on this analysis, we select activities that match the individual's capacities.

OBJECTS, ARTICLES, OR PARAPHERNALIA THE ACTIVITY REQUIRES

Most purposeful activities involve the use of objects, articles, or paraphernalia in the accomplishment of the various tasks. As practitioners, we examine the materials that are essential to the task. At times, we modify, adapt, or change the materials required, but we try to maintain the integrity of the purposeful activity. A key point of an activity analysis is to determine what materials are actually required and to what extent they are required.

ACTIONS REQUIRED TO ENGAGE IN THE ACTIVITY

Although many activities usually are done in specific ways, often they can be modified, adapted, or changed if needed. The actions required of an activity are the structure, rules, organization features, and timing that each task in the activity requires. Additionally, actions may have to be done in a specific way (order) in a set amount of time. Occupational therapy practitioners examine activities related to the actions required to engage in and complete them. Such examination requires adept activity analysis skills.

LEVEL OF ENGAGEMENT WITH THE HUMAN ENVIRONMENT REQUIRED BY THE ACTIVITY

Whereas all purposeful activities require that the person who is engaged in the activity participate, many necessitate the participation of other humans. Depending on the activity, it can be a specific person (e.g., mother, spouse, family member, friend), an acquaintance (e.g., peers, colleagues, health care providers), or a stranger. Sometimes the activity demands that the people involved have particular knowledge or skills. The specific activity and the context in which it is done also may influence the degree of participation of all the participants. Practitioners carefully examine the degree and quality of participation required for the whole activity and its component tasks.

LEVEL OF ENGAGEMENT WITH THE NONHUMAN ENVIRONMENT REQUIRED BY THE ACTIVITY

As discussed previously, most purposeful activities involve the use of objects, articles, or paraphernalia. Beyond these, the nonhuman environment includes pets and other animals that may be crucial to the activity. Purposeful activities that involve interaction between the nonhuman elements of the environment and the people included in the activity also vary in terms of the degree of involvement. Again, as with the human environment, practitioners carefully examine the degree and quality of participation required for the whole activity and its component tasks.

CONTEXT IN WHICH THE ACTIVITY IS PERFORMED

Performance of a task or an activity can be context dependent. The context within which an activity is done includes physical, social, cultural, and temporal factors.

Purposeful Activities in Evaluation and Intervention

The person's actual performance in purposeful activities is used with other assessment data to develop a comprehensive intervention plan. The person's actual performance in purposeful activities provides insight into ability to engage in occupations and function in his or her real world.

By definition, prescription of purposeful activity is client specific. Thus, activities are selected on the basis of the person's needs, the person's abilities and disabilities, and the inherent characteristics of the activity. Once the activity has been selected, the occupational therapy practitioner grades or adapts the chosen activity to promote successful performance or elicit a particular response.

Purposeful activities have the potential to facilitate a client's mastery of a new skill, restore a deficient ability, provide a means for compensating for a functional disability, maintain health, and prevent dysfunction. During intervention, we select activities or modify them in response to the crucial changes in the person and to provide opportunities for gradual development of skill and related therapeutic benefits. Aspects of the purposeful activity that we manipulate as part of the intervention include sequence; duration; procedures of the task; the person's position; the position of the tools and materials; the size, shape, weight, or texture of materials; the nature and degree of interpersonal contact; the extent of physical handling by the practitioner during the performance; and the environment in which the activity is attempted. All of these are discussed in detail in later chapters.

Summary

As occupational therapy practitioners, we use purposeful activities to restore function and compensate for functional deficits (AOTA, 1993). Before using a purposeful activity as part of an intervention plan, we complete an analysis of the activity based on the client and the context. This process is called activity analysis, which includes identifying the essential information, abilities, skills, and proficiencies necessary to complete each task. We also consider the person's age, occupational roles, cultural background, gender, interests, and preferences. Scrutinizing the context and circumstances encompassing the performance of the activity, we skillfully select purposeful activities within the conditions of the frame of reference that has been selected to guide our intervention. Using activity synthesis, we implement purposeful activities that are appropriate. ■

References

American Occupational Therapy Association. (1979). Philosophical base of occupational therapy, Resolution #531-79. *American Journal of Occupational Therapy, 33,* 785.

American Occupational Therapy Association. (1993). Position paper: Purposeful activity. *American Journal of Occupational Therapy, 47,* 1081–1082.

American Occupational Therapy Association. (1995). Position paper: Occupation. *American Journal of Occupational Therapy, 49,* 1015–1018.

American Occupational Therapy Association. (1997). Statement: Fundamental concepts of occupational therapy: Occupation, purposeful activity, and function. *American Journal of Occupational Therapy, 51,* 864–866.

American Occupational Therapy Association. (2002). Occupational therapy practice framework: Domain and process. *American Journal of Occupational Therapy, 56,* 609–639.

Christiansen, C., & Baum, C. (1991). Occupational therapy intervention for life performance. In C. Christiansen & C. Baum (Eds.), *Occupational therapy: Overcoming human performance deficits* (pp. 3–43). Thorofare, NJ: Slack.

Evans, K. A. (1987). Definition of occupation as the core concept of occupational therapy. *American Journal of Occupational Therapy, 41,* 627–628.

Gilfoyle, E. M. (1984). Transformation of a profession, 1984 Eleanor Clarke Slagle Lecture. *American Journal of Occupational Therapy, 38,* 575–584.

Glover, J. A., Bruning, R. H., & Filbeck, R. W. (1983). *Educational psychology: Principles and applications.* Boston: Little, Brown.

Henderson, A., Cermak, S., Coster, W., Murray, E., Trombly, C., & Tickle-Degnen, L. (1991). The Issue Is—Occupational science is multidimensional. *American Journal of Occupational Therapy, 45,* 370–372.

Hinojosa, J., Kramer, P., Royeen, C. B., & Luebben, A. (2003). The core concept of occupation. In P. Kramer, J. Hinojosa, & C. B. Royeen (Eds.), *Perspectives in human occupation: Participation in life* (pp. 1–17). Philadelphia: Lippincott, Williams & Wilkins.

Kielhofner, G. (1992). *Conceptual foundations of occupational therapy.* Philadelphia: F. A. Davis.

Kramer, P., & Hinojosa, J. (1995). Epiphany of human occupation. In C. B. Royeen (Ed.), *AOTA self-study series: Lesson 8: Human occupation.* Bethesda, MD: American Occupational Therapy Association.

Kramer, P., & Hinojosa, J. (1999). Domain of concern of occupational therapy relevance to pediatric practice. In P. Kramer & J. Hinojosa (Eds.), *Frames of reference for pediatric occupational therapy* (2nd ed., pp. 9–26). Baltimore: Lippincott, Williams & Wilkins.

Luebben, A. J., Hinojosa, J., & Kramer, P. (1999). Legitimate tools of pediatric occupational therapy. In P. Kramer & J. Hinojosa (Eds.), *Frames of reference for pediatric occupational therapy* (2nd ed., pp. 27–40). Baltimore: Lippincott, Williams & Wilkins.

Mosey, A. C. (1981). *Occupational therapy: Configuration of a profession.* New York: Raven.

Mosey, A. C. (1985). A monistic or a pluralistic approach to professional identity? 1985 Eleanor Clarke Slagle Lecture. *American Journal of Occupational Therapy, 39,* 504–509.

Mosey, A. C. (1986). *Psychosocial components of occupational therapy.* New York: Raven.

Mosey, A. C. (1996). *Applied scientific inquiry in the health professions: An epistemological orientation* (2nd ed.). Bethesda, MD: American Occupational Therapy Association.

Nelson, D. L. (1988). Occupation: Form and performance. *American Journal of Occupational Therapy, 42,* 633–641.

Pierce, D. (2001). Untangling occupation and activity. *American Journal of Occupational Therapy, 55,* 138–146.

Strauss, A. L. (2001). *Professions, work, and careers.* New Brunswick, NJ: Transaction.

2

Perspectives

Marie-Louise Blount, AM, OT, FAOTA
Wesley Blount, BS
Jim Hinojosa, PhD, OT, FAOTA

As much as occupational therapy has always been defined by the use of purposeful activity and occupation, very little has been done to pull together the philosophical concepts about purposeful activities that theorists use to define the profession. Needless to say, many differing theoretical approaches have grown and transformed as the profession has grown and changed over the years. And although each theorist has added to the body of knowledge from differing perspectives, these differing approaches have led to multiple realities in the ways in which occupational therapy is seen, with each relevant term taking on a different meaning with each new theorist. At the same time, to carve out unique vantage points, frequently one theorist will ignore the definitions of others or subtly redefine the scope of others' work.

With the broadening range of occupational therapy's areas of practice, there has been a continual need for expanding the definitions that make up the very notion of the profession. What began as a limited range of arts-and-crafts activities has taken in the rehabilitation of soldiers; pediatric therapy and the role of play; examination of self-care; and, recently, spirituality and nonactive occupations of different kinds. Each expansion brought with it a reexamination of the very notion of what constitutes purposeful activities and occupation and nuances as separate terms that often seem as similar as *occupation* and *purposeful activities*.

It would be difficult under any circumstances to give an overview of the development of theoretical terms in occupational therapy, which may explain why there are few attempts to bring the various contributions of the important theorists in the profession together and examine them one upon another. Since the publication of the first edition of this book, however, several books and articles have similarly laid out historically based approaches to developing theories or practice models. A number of new theorists have entered the fray with new conceptual approaches to the profession, how it is defined, and the theoretical approaches underpinning the therapeutic models. Some of the theorists we originally discussed have refined their approaches, and occupational science has grown in ways that may often be beyond the scope of occupational therapy. What has become clearer in the years since the first edition is that "theory" in occupational therapy has become in many ways a synthesis of ideas relating to activity and performance.

There is no one "right" answer to the question of "which theory," which is why we still believe that nothing substitutes for reading each of these distinguished contributors in their original works. Each theorist has, in some way, attempted to respectfully draw on earlier work to ground their approach, and each definition of activity is in some way a refinement of past work. What we present here is an overview of the major theorists, with summaries of their important contributions to concepts of purposeful activities and occupation. We believe that in understanding these differing approaches comes perspective and awareness of the important work already done in laying a theoretical basis for the profession.

There is no one "right way" to look at these issues of purposeful activities and occupation. What we are attempting to develop is a taxonomy that will afford a consistency in referencing and will add to the body of knowledge regarding occupational therapy. The profession is a dynamic entity, growing and changing even as these ideas are gathered together. Any attempt at defining terms must reflect this dynamic change and the constant synthesis that continues in developing theoretical approaches.

Activities and Lifestyle Performance: Gail Fidler

As an occupational therapist, an association leader, an educator, and a scholar, Gail Fidler has had a powerful influence on the profession's knowledge and understanding of purposeful activities. Fidler's views and opinions about purposeful activities come from her convictions that doing activities is vitally important and therefore meaningful to people. For occupational therapy, they have powerful therapeutic merit. Purposeful activities are at the core of occupational therapy practice. From her perspective, *purposeful activities* and *occupation* are synonymous terms for the same construct (Fidler, 1996).

Fidler recognized that if society is to value occupational therapy and the use of activities as authentic therapeutic modalities, occupational therapists need a conceptual rationale for using activities. Further, occupational therapists need to develop methods for empirically examining activities and their value. In 1948, observing that the occupational therapy literature discussed only the appeal, interest factors, and popularity of activities, Fidler argued that occupational therapists needed a scientific method of analyzing activities. She proposed an activity analysis as one approach to learning more about activities. Activity analysis gives therapists a means to examine activities by dividing them into component parts. Understanding the component parts of an activity provides the information that a therapist needs to match a specific activity to a client's needs. Thus, therapists can match the activity to the needs of the client and the objectives of treatment (Fidler, 1948). This original activity analysis is the foundation for many activity analyses used today.

After proposing a structure for examining activities and emphasizing the importance of matching the activity to the client's needs and the objectives of treatment, Fidler turned her attention to the therapeutic value of active involvement in doing activities in task groups (Fidler, 1969). In 1954, with her husband, Jay Fidler, she published a book titled *Introduction to Psychiatric Occupational Therapy*. This text included extensive discussion of the use of activities in psychiatric settings. It also provided a conceptual rationale for using purposeful activities for all occupational therapists. Analyzing the component parts of an activity provides the information that therapists require to correlate the client's needs, interests, and abilities. Further, occupational therapy impels the person to develop skills through an action-oriented learning experience (Fidler & Fidler, 1954). Fidler and Fidler introduced occupational therapists to the psychodynamic properties of activities. Some aspects of the activity to be examined were related to then-contemporary psychodynamic beliefs and included motion, procedures, materials, creativity, symbols, hostile and aggressive components, control, predictability, narcissism, sexual identification, dependence, reality testing, and group relatedness. They also stressed the importance of human and nonhuman environments in understanding and performing activities.

In a 1978 article, "Doing and Becoming: Purposeful Action and Self-Actualization," Fidler and Fidler provided a theoretical rationale for purposeful activities. They selected the word *doing*, saying, "Doing is viewed as enabling the development and integration of the sensory, motor, cognitive, and psychological systems, serving as a socializing agent, and verifying one's efficacy as a competent, contributing member of one's society" (p. 305).

Knowledge about activities provides the basis on which an occupational therapy practitioner selects a particular activity that matches the client's therapeutic needs, learning readiness, intact functions, and values. The practitioner then plans and implements an action-learning experience to allow the client to develop skills (Fidler & Fidler, 1978). Purposeful activities provide opportunities and means for a person to achieve mastery and competence because all activities have social relevance; each person has individual activity interests, which have personal meaning as well as a place in the social construct; these activities can remediate dysfunction and have therapeutic value (Fidler, 1981). In the introduction to *Activities: Reality and Symbol*, Fidler and Velde (1999) summarized the elements that define activity:

- *Structure and form*: the required rules, procedures, time element, and standards

- *Physical properties*: the essential objects, materials, and setting

- *Action processes*: the psychomotor behaviors required in relation to the use of form and properties

- *Outcome*: the discernable results or end-product of the activity

■   *The realistic and symbolic dimensions of the activities' social, cultural, and personal meanings*: of the total activity or occupation as well as each of its parts (structure, properties, action, outcome).

Recently, Fidler and coauthor Beth Velde put forward the Life Style Performance Model (Velde & Fidler, 2002) to provide a comprehensive picture of a person's activities, abilities, needs, interests, capacities, and self-expectation with his or her human and nonhuman world. This model highlights the interrelatedness of person, environment, activity profile, and quality of life. The model describes four activity domains: (a) activities concerned with self-care and self-maintenance, (b) personally referenced pleasure and intrinsic gratification, (c) societal contribution, and (d) interpersonal engagement. The role of an occupational therapy practitioner is to work with a client toward a healthy activity pattern. Quality of life is considered extremely important, and the occupational therapy practitioner needs to have a holistic view of practice (i.e., getting direction from the client). In this respect, Velde and Fidler's model closely resembles the work of Mary Law and the person–environment–occupation model that developed out of the client-centered approach as presented in the first edition of this book. As with Law (see next section), the client interview is paramount, the client's needs are foremost, and the measures for successful intervention are on the personal rather than the scientific level. Velde and Fidler (2002) acknowledged

> There are no standards of right or wrong, of normal–not normal, no statistical or other measures against which to compare the data. Evaluations are based on an emic perspective. In maintaining this perspective, the practitioner attempts to understand the individual's perspective of reality. This emphasizes the person's capacities, interests and needs. (p. 5)

Thus, the role of purposeful activity is, in many ways, individual and personalized. This approach focuses on the benefits of therapeutic intervention for the person, which is obviously an important part of practice. The difficulty of objective study of the roles and effectiveness of different activities within these client-centered performance models also needs to be recognized, however.

Person–Environment–Occupation Model: Mary Law

In conjunction with a variety of different collaborators, Mary Law has focused on the relationship between the practitioner and the "person receiving services," or client, to develop an approach to occupational therapy. In developing *Client-Centered Occupational Therapy*, Law and her Canadian colleagues have continued to refine their theories developed in the person–environment–occupation model (Law, 1998). The model defines the interrelationship of the person to his or her environment as well as both of these elements in relation to the role of occupation. In defining each element, Law and colleagues differentiate among activity, task, and occupation:

> *Activity* is considered to be the basic unit of a task. It is defined as a singular pursuit in which a person engages as part of his/her daily occupational experience. An example of an activity is the act of writing.

Task is defined as a set of purposeful activities in which a person engages. An example of a task is the obligation to write a report.

Occupation is defined as groups of activities in which a person engages over the lifespan….Occupations are defined as those clusters of activities and tasks in which the person engages in order to meet his/her intrinsic needs for self-maintenance, expression, and fulfillment. These are carried out within the context of individual roles and multiple environments (Law et al., 1996).

Using the model, the Canadian team has looked across the literature to validate its approach (Peachey-Hill & Law, 2000), and worked to turn the model into a practical application for occupational therapy (Strong et al., 1999). In its application, the person–environment–occupation model becomes a way for the therapist to take into account the multiplicity of factors affecting the client's performance, and a treatment plan is developed that takes into account not only the impact of different activities on the client, but also how those activities are appropriate for the environment where the client will make use of them.

All of this work is informed by the client-centered approach that Law and her team have developed alongside the model. This approach to occupational therapy brings together several strands of observation and research from occupational therapy and other disciplines. As an early basis for the client-centered approach, Law and Mills (1998) cited psychologist Carl Rogers, who emphasized the need for therapists to work with clients in developing solutions to problems rather than "direct" the course of therapy. Law and Mills also took into account the views of people with disabilities and their feelings regarding treatment.

The client-centered approach developed in Canada has a series of guidelines for practice produced by the Canadian Association of Occupational Therapists (1991). Law et al. (1994) produced the Canadian Occupational Performance Measure, an assessment that measures "a client's self-perception of occupational performance" (p. 191). Although the authors subsequently referred to the pilot testing as covering a "broad spectrum" of clients and environments, the study participants were mostly people older than age 60 in inpatient geriatric facilities. Thus, the participants' ability to assess their own conditions and treatment needs may have been better facilitated by the client-centered approach than a population less able to indicate self-awareness or occupational needs, such as children with developmental disabilities. In fact, contributors to *Client-Centered Occupational Therapy* discussed in several chapters the various ways of interpreting the term *client*. The client comes to be seen as not only the person receiving therapy but also as "someone who wishes to make a change through the process of therapy" (Pollock & McColl, 1998, p. 91) (i.e., possibly the caregiver or the parent). A frequent example used in the works of these authors and Law is that of the Alzheimer's patient who may be unable to communicate needs. The client is considered to be the spouse (and the term *spouse* is the one most often used in this example) giving care because, in the client-centered approach, it is the caregiver's role that is to change.

In the client-centered approach, then, the activity and occupation that provide therapeutic benefit are defined by the client, and the client's needs are foremost in the development of *interventions* created in partnership between the client and the therapist. The client-centered approach may seem somewhat reflexive because an assessment model would seem to always require that the client's needs are part of the determination of appropriate therapy. What is important to Law and her colleagues, however, is that the assessment comes from the client and that the value of the therapy is always evaluated best by the client; the therapist serves as a *facilitator* who aids the client in identifying areas of concern and assists in developing a plan to address these areas (and, in theory, those areas alone). One of the central concepts of client-centered practice is that occupational therapy service delivery is flexible and individualized, and the very flexibility and mutability of using occupation and activity make it difficult to determine a specific approach to using occupation as a means of therapy in the client-centered practice. Law and Mills (1998) acknowledged the lack of specific methodologies in client-centered therapy.

The focus of client-centered occupational therapy is on changing an overall approach to therapy from a medical model. In the medical model, therapists are perceived as all-knowing, and treatment is evaluated on generalized goals, such as "independence at all costs" (Law, 1998, p. 71; see also Baum & Law, 1997). In the client-centered approach, the focus is on the client's finding meaning in everyday occupations and the development of active collaboration between the occupational therapy practitioner and client to resolve occupational performance problems (Baum & Law, 1997). Specific assessments and treatment plans are not spelled out because the client-centered approach makes those determinations part of the larger client–therapist development of a relationship. As with Fidler, the approach makes scientific and comparative evaluation of treatment methods challenging but refocuses the role of therapy on the benefits to the individual.

Occupation: Charles Christiansen and Carolyn Baum

The Canadian models also inform Charles Christiansen and Carolyn Baum's attempts to bring together differing theories of activity and occupation to lay a theoretical framework for teaching practice. In *Occupational Therapy: Overcoming Human Performance Deficits* (Christiansen & Baum, 1991), they proposed an occupational performance hierarchy, which centers on "*the activity*, which consists of specific goal-oriented behaviors...directed toward the performance of a task" (p. 28). The emphasis on activities as related to the performance of tasks creates the theoretical basis for occupational therapy as a way to treat dysfunction or disability. The work of previous authors serves in this context as a way to take ideas about activity and apply them to the practice of occupational therapy. By contrast, in *Occupational Therapy: Enabling Function and Well-Being* (Christiansen & Baum, 1997), the second edition, they focus much more on the development of a definition of occupation, moving away from both activity and the notion of disability. The revisions to the text allowed for the incorporation of newer ideas from different theorists but also underscored the difficulty of taking the differing approaches and blending them into a coherent whole. Like Kielhofner (see discussion later in this chapter), Christiansen and Baum developed a model in the second edition that is referred to at the start of each chapter, attempting to encompass all possible facets of human performance in an arrow-shaped form that points to "well-being," and each chapter within the text is meant to present a part of this triangular model. Using the ideas developed by Law and colleagues, the "client-centered" approach is emphasized, with a resulting deemphasis on specific practice solutions to problems and greater emphasis on the client's needs and perceptions. This deemphasis of specific treatments for dysfunction also incorporates the occupational science model's focus on wellness and healthy occupational performance.

The two volumes exemplify the contemporary dilemmas facing practicing therapists in bridging and balancing the differing theoretical expectations expressed within the profession. Placing occupation into a sociocultural context that emphasizes the role of the person in society is an important concept, but without practical methods of addressing dysfunction, students may not completely understand the role of the occupational therapy practitioner in aiding the achievement of wellness.

Occupational Behavior: Mary Reilly

A seminal and critical writer and thinker in occupational therapy is Mary Reilly. Although she has not devoted all of her attention to issues of activity and occupation, her ideas, eventually subsumed under the title of *occupational behavior* (Reilly, 1966), give attention to these issues of activity and occupation, making concerns about these issues an underlying theme.

Among Reilly's concerns is the impetus to study and investigate the profession in order to establish clearly its contributions to science. She therefore suggested that a major area for occupational therapy research should be the nature and meaning of activity (Reilly, 1960). The presumption that people require activity in order to attain and maintain health is fundamental to the profession's beliefs, in Reilly's opinion: "We are becoming more aware of the fact that the interests of man [*sic*] emerge in the gratification of his senses" (Reilly, 1960, p. 208). Indeed, she stressed that investigation of the need to engage in activity should move beyond traditional occupational therapy reliance on arts and crafts and into analysis of such activities as the appropriate level for the investigation (Reilly, 1960). She emphasized the physical, sensory, and psychic rewards inherent in activity and spoke against the idea that various approaches to the use of activity (e.g., subdividing dance from recreation from crafts) serves as the best approach to the application of therapeutic activity.

In her Eleanor Clarke Slagle Lecture (Reilly, 1962), she further affirmed the centrality of work to human existence. Her thesis in this presentation was that human productivity provides most life satisfaction and that occupational therapy applies this principle to the maintenance and restoration of health. Occupational therapy intervention ("treatment" in her words) requires that the therapist investigate and address problems people have in coping with "play, work, and school" (Reilly, 1962, p. 7). Reilly also expressed in this presentation her rejection of the word *activity* to describe how occupational therapists engage patients because she had become wary of the increasing use of terms like *activity therapy* in treatment settings, which moved occupational therapy away from seeking to enhance individual human productivity.

As Reilly's approach to the study of occupational therapy came to be called *occupational behavior* (Reilly, 1966), she referred back to the core ideas of early occupational therapy thinkers: that a satisfying life required a balanced approach to work, rest, and play. Occupational therapy, appropriately applied, would establish a setting in which all of these aspects of life could be addressed. In describing a model program that did address all of these aspects, she included exercise programs, required work activities, learning recreational skills, some group activities, social skills, and others.

Reilly's interest in occupation and related activities later developed into a special concentration on the occupation of play as it applies to both children and adults (Reilly, 1974). She, along with her students, investigated the development of occupational behaviors during play and their relationship to humans' exploration of their environments, their development of competence, and their fulfillment of the drive to achieve.

Her striving to understand the nature and functions of human occupation and to apply this knowledge to occupational therapy intervention led to the development of the model of human occupation and eventually to the school of thought called *occupational science*.

Model of Human Occupation: Gary Kielhofner

As students of Reilly, Gary Kielhofner and Janice Posatery Burke have taken theories on occupational behavior and expanded both the theory's external framework and its organizing principles. Kielhofner has continued to refine this theoretical approach, a model of human occupation (Forsyth & Kielhofner, 2003; Kielhofner, 1995, 2002; Kielhofner & Burke, 1980), and uses the model to observe and explain most aspects of theory related to occupational therapy. Indeed, one of the central tenets of the model is that human occupation can be used for therapeutic benefit, which also advocates a balanced lifestyle that includes both work and leisure (thus expanding on Reilly's notion of play).

In Kielhofner's view, "occupation is a multifaceted phenomenon that involves the simultaneous operation of biological, psychological, social, and ecological factors" (Kielhofner, 1985, p. xvii). Like most of his definitions, his notion of occupation relies on multiple levels of explanation to allow for as many aspects within a framework as are needed to explain the multitude of possibilities inherent in human behavior.

Kielhofner begins his model by developing historical perspectives on human behavior within the context of systems theory. From this, he posits that human beings are an example of an *open system*, that is, that human activity involves taking in information (or *input*), synthesizing the information, and then creating *output*. The important quality of an open system, he has argued, is the opportunity for *feedback*, responses to the output that allow the individual to make changes, and with the same input, create a different output (Kielhofner, 1995).

Within the person, Kielhofner (and Janice Posatery Burke) sees several components and determinants that affect human behavior. These include *volition, habituation,* and *performance*. Volition refers to the impulses that cause the person to value certain types of occupation, including *personal causation* (the knowledge of self), *values* (images of what is good, right, and important), and *interests* (the disposition to find particular occupations pleasurable). Habituation, in turn, refers to the normative definitions the individual places on occupation, encompassing *roles* (publicly recognized positions or society's input) and *habits* (the private regulation of behavior). Performance deals with the *skills* of the individual in performing occupations, containing *communication, process,* and *perceptual motor skills* (Kielhofner, 1995; Kielhofner & Burke, 1980).

After laying down the internal structures that make up individual behavior, Kielhofner then deals with the external aspects of human occupation, including determining whether the person is *functional* or *dysfunctional* and thus in need of therapeutic intervention. Just as function in his view has three levels of *exploration, competence,* and *achievement*, Kielhofner sees dysfunction as having three corresponding levels of *inefficiency, incompetence*, and *helplessness*. He emphasizes that both function and dysfunction should be seen as processes, not static states. For there to be occupational dysfunction, he explains that the person in his or her social group does not meet expectations for productive and playful participation. Further, the individual "does not fulfill the urge to explore and master" (Kielhofner, 1985, p. 64) his or her environment.

Using this model, Kielhofner has developed ideas about the optimal use of therapy in treating dysfunction and has worked to fit the model into larger contexts, such as the *Conceptual Foundations of Occupational Therapy* (Kielhofner, 1992). Indeed, the model was initiated with the specific goal of developing resources to guide and enhance practice (Forsyth & Kielhofner, 2003), and his recent collaborations have focused on the application of the model into practice. Kielhofner does not engage in the debate regarding terms like *activity* or *occupation* as much as he ignores the debate altogether. Occupation is the central concept he uses in developing theories regarding occupational therapy, but more fundamentally, the person's role in the complex process of human occupation defines what people and, following his model, practitioners will do to improve human function. Kielhofner's detailed model, with its emphasis on human behavior, goes a long way toward establishing a psychological framework for the human need for occupation in daily life.

Activities Health: Simme Cynkin

Simme Cynkin has provided perspective on the fundamental nature of activity as a therapeutic response to dysfunction (Cynkin, 1979; Cynkin & Robinson, 1990). In this perspective, the value of activities as fundamental to humans is the basis for occupational therapy. Activities are part of our human existence; Cynkin believes that activity's very presence in our daily lives promotes our physical and mental well-being. This belief is discussed in four assumptions about activities:

1.   Activities of many kinds are the essence of human existence based on the interactions of individual and environment. Activities are centered on survival, subsistence, and coexistence.

2.   Activities are a culmination of acceptable norms of behaviors that are defined by a sociocultural system of values and beliefs.

3.   Acceptable and unacceptable variations exist in individual activities.

4.   An individual's engaging in meaningful activities leads to a satisfying way of life and personal fulfillment (Cynkin, 1979; Cynkin & Robinson, 1990).

Cynkin and Anne Mazur Robinson's assumptions are derived from a historical perspective: Activity has always defined human existence, and activities are basic to human survival. Drawing on the works of Piaget and Reilly, they centralized human nature and a person's humanity around the performance of a variety of activities, both personal and interpersonal. On this foundation the authors added the notion of differing sociocultural norms and differing values placed by various societies on particular activities.

Building on the notion that people can change, Cynkin and Robinson further argued that behavior related to activity can be changed and that behavioral changes can improve functioning in the individual. Further, the person can learn to improve function, and the learning process can take place in a variety of ways, both direct and indirect.

The importance of the assumptions and the framework Cynkin and Robinson developed from them is the laying of a foundation for the teaching of ideas behind occupational therapy. "Early occupational therapy was founded on the belief that being engaged in activities promotes mental and physical well-being and that, conversely, absence of activity leads. . .at worst to deterioration or loss of mental and physical functioning" (Cynkin & Robinson, 1990, p. 4). Whereas theorists like Fidler developed ways of analyzing activity, Cynkin provided an important link: that placing activity in a context of overall human behavior provides greater understanding of its therapeutic importance. Cynkin has offered the strongest method possible to give the occupational therapy student not just the tools to assist in restoring function but also the philosophical structure that underlies the importance of activity in everyday life.

Occupational Form and Occupational Performance: David Nelson

David Nelson (1994) is particularly interested in the term *occupation* and its meaning for occupational therapy practitioners. In his 1996 Eleanor Clarke Slagle Lecture, he proclaimed this interest as part of a historical tradition and set of beliefs of occupational therapists: "The human being can attain enhanced health and quality of life by actively doing things that are personally meaningful and purposeful, in other words, through occupation" (Nelson, 1997, p. 11). His principal contribution to this perspective has been semantic and includes developing a nomenclature to delimit the use of the term *occupation* by occupational therapy practitioners. The nomenclature Nelson developed describes his essential terms for the therapeutic discipline of occupational therapy.

Nelson (1994) divided the term *occupation* into his terms for its essential aspects: *form* and *performance*. The form has to do with the objects and circumstances that make the occupation possible. Forms can be a game, a building where an occupation takes place, a piece of equipment, a piece of music, or another person, to name just a few. Forms are essential to the way in which the specific occupation takes place. Performance, on the other hand, is what the person does to accomplish the occupation. Nelson stated that performance, in this sense, must be voluntary. "The 'doing' is the occupational performance, and the 'something' to be done is the occupational form" (Nelson, 1994, p. 11). Performance, then, is playing the game, constructing the building, lifting the weight for exercise, playing the music, or teaching something to the other person. Again, multiple performances are possible, depending on the relevant occupations.

Nelson (1994) viewed occupation as the relationship between an occupational form and an occupational performance. Occupations may be as variable as the people who are performing the occupation. If the occupation is eating a meal, the occupational forms, at a simple level, may be breakfast, lunch, or dinner. The occupational performances may be as divergent as that of a baby eating some oatmeal and "feeding" the rest to the high chair tray and the floor or a diet-conscious 20-year-old woman picking carefully at the low-fat foods on her plate. Many variables come into play, including duration, certainty of outcome, and intricacy.

Nelson (1994) subdivided the term *occupational form* into a *physical dimension* and a *sociocultural dimension*. The physical dimensions are measurable factors. They include objects, other physical characteristics of the occupation, and the temporal aspects of the occupation. In this sense, the form of a piece of music, for example, might include the musical composition itself, the piano, the concert hall, and the length of time required to play the piece. The sociocultural dimension includes social and cultural practices, expectations, and settings. For the occupation just described, a contemporary, atonal classical piece may be played on an electronic keyboard in a museum in Bucharest, Romania. These aspects would help define the piece's sociocultural dimension.

Nelson and Jepson-Thomas (2003) also discussed aspects of this sociocultural dimension. They divided these into *symbols, norms, roles, variations,* and *language*. For the person playing the keyboard, some of the symbols are the notes on the musical score. A norm might be the loudness or softness at which the piece is usually played. The pianist is enacting a role that has expected parameters. The variations are the "alternatives and options" (p. 95) present in almost every occupation. The language, perhaps Romanian in this case, may not be as relevant as the musical sounds in the example. Recently, Nelson and Jepson-Thomas incorporated concepts of change into the system as well as into social hierarchies (stratification) and organizations. Overall, they see the occupational form as a very complex entity, with all of the variables mentioned previously interacting with each other.

The person brings his or her "developmental structure" to the occupational performance (Nelson & Jepson-Thomas, 2003). The structure is all of the "abilities and characteristics" (p. 99) that the person conveys to this performance. Nelson particularly uses terms that occupational therapy practitioners use—*sensorimotor, cognitive,* and *psychosocial*—to describe the developmental structure. For the pianist, hearing, memory, and appreciation of the music are some of these structural elements. The capacities inherent in this structure arise from body systems.

Meaning also is brought to the occupation by the person performing it. If the performer in the music example actually disliked atonal music, his concert might be very divergent from one in which he had selected his favorite piece.

According to Nelson (1994), purpose is the desire for a certain "outcome," embodied in an occupational performance. Purpose is the reason for the actions a performer takes and, according to Nelson, provides the "energy" to act. As is true with *meanings,* any given occupation may have more than one purpose. Not only may a given person have more than one purpose for performing an occupation, but also others may each have different purposes for performing the same occupation. Nelson subdivided purpose into several dimensions. One subdivision is that of the *intrinsic or extrinsic purpose:* "Intrinsic purpose involves doing something for its own sake, as in wanting to explore the situation or wanting to master the situation" (Nelson, 1994, p. 24). Reading a novel for enjoyment is an example of an intrinsic motivation. Extrinsic, on the other hand, is a purpose or motivation found outside of the occupation itself. Reading a textbook for the purpose of passing an exam is an example of an extrinsic purpose. Another subdivision of the term *purpose,* for Nelson and for other occupational therapy practitioners, is that of *conscious and unconscious purposes.* Unconscious purposes are those of which we are not aware. The best example, according to Nelson, are purposes involved with habitual occupations that we perform routinely with little thought. If we purposely set out to brush our teeth in a certain way, the task develops a conscious purpose.

By viewing occupations as a series of steps, Nelson (1994) applied the term *impact* to describe the effect that completion of one step has on the performance of the next step. For example, purchasing fabric and using a pattern to cut out a jacket are steps that have an effect on the actual construction of the jacket. Nelson introduced the term *adaptation* to describe changes in the person performing an occupation caused by carrying out that very occupational performance. Referring back to the example of making the jacket, having completed the construction of the jacket, the person who accomplished this may have satisfaction and a garment to wear. For Nelson, the effect of adaptation is on the person's "developmental structure" (p. 99).

Nelson and Jepson-Thomas (2003) define activities as the building blocks of adaptation. They designated these portions of occupations as *sub-occupations* or even *sub-sub-occupations*. The determiners for what are occupations and what are their components are the person performing the occupation and the "sociocultural norms" that apply.

Understanding therapeutic occupations, according to Nelson (1994), requires the same set of ideas about occupational performance delineated previously. The occupational therapy practitioner and the occupational therapy student must have a structure and process in which to perceive occupation to move onto therapeutic application. Nelson termed that process *occupational synthesis*, which is the designing of an occupational experience that will have therapeutic impact. The recipient of service is a collaborator in the therapeutic process. A person recuperating from a serious leg fracture might work with the occupational therapy practitioner to incorporate progressively longer periods of standing, walking, and bending at the hip while playing his favorite game, billiards. In addition, Nelson and Jepson-Thomas (2003) stated that occupational synthesis is the job of the occupational therapy practitioner. Currently, Nelson and Jepson-Thomas have devoted much attention to models of practice (Kielhofner), frames of reference (Mosey), and other theoretical directions for conceptualizing therapeutic occupation and choices of occupational forms for therapy.

Nelson deliberately avoids the word *activity*. In his view and in the view of others, the term is not specific enough because it is sometimes applied to other than human enterprises and because it is not always purposeful. He pointed out that terms like *molecular activity* and *solar activity* (Nelson, 1994, p. 42) clearly do not refer to human enterprises and that *activity* can refer to any kind of liveliness (see also Darnell & Heater, 1994). Nelson and Jepson-Thomas's (2003) more recent writing offers somewhat greater attention to the person performing the occupation but generally gives most attention to the occupation itself. Their most recent work terms the approach a conceptual framework for therapeutic occupation.

Ecology of Human Performance: Winnie Dunn

Drawing on the interest in developing a comprehensive framework, Winnie Dunn, along with Catana Brown and Ann McGuigan, constructed the ecology of human performance (Dunn, Brown, & McGuigan, 1994). Similar to the Canadian person–environment–occupation model, the central focus of this group from the University of Kansas is on the *environment*, and how the individual fits into it. Drawing on Mosey's (see discussion later in this chapter) notion of *frame of reference* and Nelson's *occupational forms*, the Kansas group developed a framework of *context* to explain the way a person and the *tasks* the person does fit into an environment. Tasks are defined as objective sets of behaviors necessary to accomplish a goal (Dunn et al., 1994; Dunn, Brown, & Youngstrom, 2003).

Drawing on the work of environmental psychologists, the ecology of human performance thus makes context the center of the therapeutic evaluation and intervention. In this way, it is similar to the notion of "lifestyle" advanced by Fidler and the holistic approach envisioned in the Canadian client-centered approach. A key difference, however, is the change in emphasis to "environment." As with Kielhofner, Dunn's group is less interested in the questions of defining activity versus occupation and, instead, focuses more on the external framework in which the person and the therapeutic intervention fit in various situations.

Using the ecology of human performance framework, the Kansas group described five different potential relationships for therapeutic intervention as it relates to the person. Therapeutic intervention can *establish or restore (remediate)* the person's skills and abilities. Intervention also can *alter* the context in which a person performs, selecting a context that enables the person to perform with current skills and abilities. The practitioner also can *adapt* the contextual features and task demands to design a more supportive context for a person's performance. Another alternative is to *prevent* the occurrence or evolution of maladaptive performance in context. Finally, the practitioner can *create* circumstances that promote more adaptable or complex performance in context. Using these five therapeutic choices, the therapist can evaluate the person in the appropriate context and design an intervention best suited to the person's needs within that context (Dunn et al., 1994).

By emphasizing the role of context and environment in making therapeutic assessments, the ecology of human performance takes a different look at familiar concepts. In so doing, the framework exemplifies the value of synthesis within the profession, taking familiar, existing ideas and thinking about them in new and different ways. The ecology of human performance takes many things as given—the role of tasks in a person's life, the use of tasks to provide therapeutic benefit—ideas that other theorists continue to debate. But clearly, the importance of making careful, individualized assessments has become a key part of the theoretical approach to practice, and the ecology of human performance offers yet another way to look at the notion of the environmental factors that can affect treatment.

Occupational Adaptation: Janette Schkade and Sally Schultz

Also synthesizing much of the work that had come before them, Janette Schkade and Sally Schultz of Texas Woman's University developed the model of occupational adaptation as a holistic approach for contemporary practice (Schkade & Schultz, 1992). Occupational adaptation focuses on the interaction between the person and the occupational environment, which are contexts in which occupations occur. Occupations, in their approach, are activities characterized by three properties: active participation, meaning to the person, and a product that is the output of a process (Schkade & Schultz, 1992). In their model, the individual's *desire for mastery* will cause a person to develop an *adaptive response* to an *occupational challenge*. At the same time, a *demand for mastery* comes from within the occupational environment. In the interaction between the desire and the demand, the person will develop adaptive responses in order to gain mastery of the occupational challenge.

Schultz and Schkade (1992) then applied this model to occupational therapy practice. In practice, occupational adaptation is focused on occupational function (i.e., the ability of the person to function in the environment) rather than on the acquisition of particular functional skills. In practice, the practitioner works in a *therapeutic climate* with the client to determine the goal of therapy. The therapist then uses *occupational activities* (discrete activities that can promote occupational adaptation) as well as *occupational readiness* (skill-based activities and interventions to prepare for occupational activities [e.g., resistive exercise or assistive devices]) to allow the client to develop *relative mastery*. In many cases these activities are related to *occupations of daily living*, the unique patterns of occupations in which the person regularly engages.

In attempting to make universal the model of occupational adaptation, Schkade and Schultz (2003) synthesized many of the theoretical notions of activity and occupation that have come before to draw together a common perspective. The focus is on synthesizing ideas, not developing altogether new ones, and occupational adaptation as a theory adapts the material that has come before to develop a holistic methodology. Though their focus on the adaptive process and the desire for mastery is differentiated from others, the notion of activity and occupation (as well as the client-centered approach) for therapeutic benefit fits comfortably into the theoretical underpinnings of the profession as it continues to develop.

Occupational Science: University of Southern California, Department of Occupational Science and Occupational Therapy

Occupational science is literally the study of occupation and its role in human experience. Clark et al. (1991) defined *occupation* as "chunks of culturally and personally meaningful activity in which humans engage that can be named in the lexicon of culture" (p. 301). The study of occupation is grounded in a model of human subsystems that influence occupation. Similar to Kielhofner's model of human occupation, it is based on an open systems model that includes feedback, which allows the person to make changes in occupational behavior. It should be noted that occupational science as a discipline at present encompasses the studies of human and nonhuman occupation and occupational behavior, with noted zoologist Jane Goodall serving as a member of the University of Southern California Occupational Science faculty.

Because of the focus on generalized concepts regarding occupation and not on specific uses of purposeful activities in therapeutic settings, occupational science writings deal with the theoretical issues developed here principally in tangential ways to larger questions. Interest in occupational science as a field of study related to occupational therapy has continued to grow, leading to additional graduate programs around the world, a scholarly journal, and many meetings to share new work. These works range from broad studies of occupations in different societies to looking at occupational roles and their therapeutic benefit.

Yet purposeful activities are embedded within the occupational science definition of occupation. A person's participation in meaningful and socially valued activities is emphasized as a core to the moral philosophy of occupational therapy (Zemke & Clark, 1996). This belief is generated from the fact that as occupational therapy practitioners we focus on the everyday things that people need to do. Some occupational scientists have felt the need to immerse themselves in the study of these occupations of daily living that we engage in during our lifetime. Henderson (1996) stated that confusion exists between occupation and purposeful activity. She described occupation similarly to Clark et al. (1991) as chunks or units of culturally and personally meaningful activity within the stream of human behavior. Each level of occupation is further subdivided into smaller ones. The vocabulary used has not been agreed on, and the terms are interchangeable. Henderson believes that these terms are equated in the field of occupational therapy, and therefore, we must seek to understand further the interrelationships to distinguish the levels of occupations we engage in.

Purposeful activities are defined in relation to the particular activities and accepted with the notion that adaptations can occur in our activities. Human beings have a self-reinforcing power to challenge themselves in an array of adaptive strategies to improve quality of life. These strategies are most relevant post disability when occupations we engaged in at a prior time require adaptation to participate in again (Frank, 1996).

An important milestone for human beings discussed in occupational science is play. Play is a purposeful vehicle for change, one that truly encompasses the traditional definition of purposeful activity. The literature on play and purposeful activity go hand in hand and are the root of much of what we talk about in the therapeutic process. Play, as a purposeful activity, encompasses much of what occupational science is centered on. Through childhood play exploration, the act of doing is created in the activities that a child carries out daily. Play is an important occupation beginning at childhood and continuing through the life span. Play has its importance in the ability to interact with our environment and, thus, children use it to cope when changes occur (Burke, 1996).

Occupational science writings often attempt to take theories of occupation and broaden their context to create enhanced possibilities for study and application. Concepts such as adaptation, work, and play (following on theories developed by Reilly) are all examined for their value as parts of human culture, not in areas of specific application. The very expansiveness of the scope of occupational science suggests a substantial philosophical difference in method and application from occupational therapy as it has come to be understood. Mosey has gone so far as to suggest that the field should be "partitioned" from occupational therapy because such a separation would serve to clarify the role of the discipline from that of the profession (Mosey, 1993). Although the two areas of study may not benefit from a total separation, the ideas of occupational science, developed in the years that have followed its genesis, are clearly far broader than the use of occupation for therapeutic benefit. At the graduate level of study, an occupational therapy student may find a text like *Occupational Science: The Evolving Discipline* (Zemke & Clark, 1996) a useful set of readings for contemplating the larger cultural implications of activity and occupation. Because they contain few practical strategies, practitioners may not find these writings directly applicable to practice.

Legitimate Tool: Anne Cronin Mosey

In 1968, Anne Cronin Mosey proposed that occupational therapists should develop and use frames of reference to guide their evaluation and interventions. Frames of reference provided therapists with an organized theoretical knowledge base for practice. Occupational therapy practitioners use a variety of means to carry out or implement their theoretically based interventions, which she labeled as the profession's legitimate tools. Legitimate tools are the means that a professional uses to accomplish a goal and include activities, actions, instruments, modalities, methods, and processes (Mosey, 1981). This perspective of a profession having legitimate tools acknowledges that, although many different professions use the same therapeutic modalities, no one profession "owns" them. Although professions share tools, each profession uses them in unique ways that are authorized by society. This dynamic view of a profession's legitimate tools means that a profession's tools change as the profession evolves. Further, this view recognizes that the use of a tool is directed by the theoretical perspective that the therapist has selected to address the client's needs.

Before her classification of legitimate tools, Mosey identified the unique therapeutic value of activities to assist people with mental illness to become part of their communities and to engage in their daily lives (Mosey, 1973). In this text, *Activities Therapy*, she described the power of doing an activity as a means for a person to learn new skills and behaviors. She underscored the potential of learning through doing: Purposeful "activities are used to provide familiar life situations in which participants are assisted in identifying faulty patterns of behavior and the ideas, feelings, and values that support these faulty patterns" (p. 2). Activities provide practitioners with a means to understand the person and a method to assist the person to participate in the tasks at hand. Important aspects of using activities therapeutically are, among others, that they involve the here and now, they are action-oriented, and they involve learning through doing. Mosey also emphasized the notions of satisfaction and enjoyment of the activity and the therapeutic benefit to the client.

In 1986, Mosey proposed that practitioners have six primary legitimate tools: nonhuman environment, conscious use of self, the teaching–learning process, purposeful activities, activity groups, and activity analysis and synthesis. In her extensive discussion of purposeful activities as a legitimate tool in 1986, she described the characteristics important for occupational therapy for evaluation and intervention. Therapists develop expertise and skills in using these therapeutic tools as part of their basic professional education and ongoing postprofessional education (Mosey, 1986, 1996).

Mosey (1986) defined *purposeful activities* as a "doing process that requires the use of thought and energy and are directed toward an intended or desired end result" (p. 227). The characteristics of purposeful activities as she proposed are as follows:

■ People who are engaged in purposeful activities are aware of the reason for doing the activities.

■ People participate in purposeful activities at their own free will and are not being coerced.

■ Purposeful activities have a planned end-result that is not necessarily a material product.

■ Purposeful activities have the potential to be symbolic.

■ Purposeful activities are universal in that they exist as part of the human experience of interacting with our environments.

■ People participate in purposeful activities throughout their daily lives.

■ Purposeful activities are ordinary in nature.

■ Purposeful activities are essential to the development of humans in all aspects of their development.

■ Purposeful activities are

> made up of elements that can be identified, holistic, able to be manipulated, promoting differential responses, able to be graded, facilitating communication, having a focusing organizing effect, emphasizing doing, frequently involving the nonhuuman environment, varying on a continuum from conscious to not conscious/unconscious, varying on a continuum from simulated to natural. (Mosey, 1986, p. 241)

Mosey included purposeful activities as one of occupational therapy's major legitimate tools until 1996, when she proposed a different categorization of a profession's legitimate tools, assuming purposeful activities within subcategories of a revised taxonomy. This new taxonomy of occupational therapy's legitimate tools consisted of (a) interpersonal process, (b) activity process, and (c) physical modalities (Mosey, 1996). The revised taxonomy did not include purposeful activity itself as a separate legitimate tool, instead including activity as a subcomponent of other tools. This categorization may reflect the trend in occupational therapy of not using specific purposeful activities and instead focusing on the foundation for participation in occupations.

Recently, Mosey has revised her list of legitimate tools to include seven (A. C. Mosey, personal communication, 2001):

1. *Conscious use of self:* preplanned verbal and nonverbal responses to an individual

2. *Activities:* tasks and interactions that people typically engage in

3. *Activity groups:* types of primary groups that involve participation in activities and discussion of anticipated or current involvement in activities

4. *Stimulus–response interactions:* specific sensory input with a predictable motor response

5. *Atmospheric elements:* aspects of the physical environment that can be modified

6. *Assistive technology:* devices, equipment, or systems specifically designed or adapted to prevent or remediate dysfunction and to maintain or improve function

7. *Physical agent modalities:* properties of temperature, light, sound, water, and electricity that produce selected effects on soft tissue.

This taxonomy continues to recognize that occupational therapy practitioners may use frames of reference or other theoretically based guidelines for intervention that do not emphasize the importance of purposeful activities. Many guidelines for intervention address a specific component deficit. Other guidelines for intervention may use activities but are less concerned with the purposefulness of the activity to the client. In these situations, the purpose is defined by the therapist who has explicit outcomes identified for the client.

Summary

The nature of purposeful activities and occupation as a concept for study and theory presents inherent difficulties, and always has, in that, unlike other treatment modes, the cause and effect in treatment is less easy to quantify and measure. Theories of activity and occupation must take in the broadest possible range of human possibilities and experience but, at the same time, may be applied in incredibly small and specific ways, always remaining as practical and applicable in real situations as possible. That these theorists have taken on such a daunting task and developed a variety of thoughtful, considered approaches to the questions at the heart of occupational therapy is to be respected and acknowledged. As we said in the beginning of this chapter, nothing can really substitute for reading the works of these authors in their own words.

Some concepts that have been raised continue like a running thread through the works of theorists whose conclusions can vary widely from one another. Clearly, theorists are moving toward a more personal, individualized approach to therapeutic intervention, one that in many cases may be hard to quantify but, nevertheless, makes the person receiving treatment and respect for the person's environment paramount in a way that treats the client with dignity. And although the nomenclature may differ, the role of purposeful activities—be they activities, tasks, or occupations—in therapeutic interventions remains a central focus of the theoretical writings.

At the same time, important, unique ideas set these theorists apart from one another. For the practicing therapist, one strategy for processing and incorporating the work of various theorists is to study more than one but to find the one that best matches one's own area of practice. Reilly's focus on pediatrics, Law's on gerontological issues, and Kielhofner's on mental health all offer ways to take theoretical concepts into specific areas of practice. We think that Fidler, in defining ways to think about activity; Nelson, in deriving a nomenclature; and Cynkin, in developing a notion of how to teach activity theory, stand as important guideposts in how theorists in occupational therapy approach writing and thinking about these issues.

The terms presented here and the ways that they are defined deal with important theoretical issues, but the questions that are raised are provocative and open to debate. One of the most central is thinking about who is doing the defining of these concepts: Who determines what is a meaningful outcome? What constitutes a purposeful activity? Whose purpose should it serve?

Most importantly, occupational therapy continues to grow and evolve, bringing out new ideas in a rapidly changing field. There is room for a variety of perspectives and a need to continually reexamine established thought in the face of newly developed concepts and theories. In dealing with the complexities of human occupation and purposeful activities, occupational therapy takes on tremendous challenges and offers substantial rewards. The search for understanding the role of occupation and purposeful activities in human existence remains ongoing. ■

References

Baum, C., & Law, M. (1997). Occupational therapy practice: Focusing on occupational performance. *American Journal of Occupational Therapy, 51,* 277–288.

Burke, J. (1996). Variations in childhood: Play in the presence of chronic disability. In R. Zemke & F. Clark (Eds.), *Occupational science: The evolving discipline* (pp. 413–418). Philadelphia: F. A. Davis.

Canadian Association of Occupational Therapists. (1991). *Occupational therapy guidelines for client-centred practice.* Ottawa, ON: CAOT Publications.

Christiansen, C., & Baum, C. (Eds.). (1991). *Occupational therapy: Overcoming human performance deficits.* Thorofare, NJ: Slack.

Christiansen, C., & Baum, C. (Eds.). (1997). *Occupational therapy: Enabling function and well-being* (2nd ed.). Thorofare, NJ: Slack.

Clark, F., Parham, D., Carlson, M., Frank, G., Jackson, J., Pierce, D., et al. (1991). Occupational science: Academic innovation in the service of occupational therapy's future. *American Journal of Occupational Therapy, 45,* 300–310.

Cynkin, S. (1979). *Occupational therapy: Toward health through activities.* Boston: Little, Brown.

Cynkin, S., & Robinson, A. (1990). *Occupational therapy and activities health: Toward health through activities.* Boston: Little, Brown.

Darnell, J. L., & Heater, S. L. (1994). Occupational therapist or activity therapist: Which do you choose to be? *American Journal of Occupational Therapy, 48,* 467–468.

Dunn, W., Brown, C., & McGuigan, A. (1994). The ecology of human performance: A framework for considering the effect of context. *American Journal of Occupational Therapy, 48,* 595–607.

Dunn, W., Brown, C., & Youngstrom, M. J. (2003). Ecological model of occupation. In P. Kramer, J. Hinojosa, & C. B. Royeen (Eds.), *Perspectives in human occupation: Participation in life* (pp. 222–263). Philadelphia: Lippincott, Williams & Wilkins.

Fidler, G. S. (1948). Psychological evaluation of occupational therapy activities. *American Journal of Occupational Therapy, 2,* 284–287.

Fidler, G. S. (1969). The task-oriented group as a context for treatment. *American Journal of Occupational Therapy, 23,* 43–48.

Fidler, G. S. (1981). From crafts to competence. *American Journal of Occupational Therapy, 35,* 567–573.

Fidler, G. S. (1996). Lifestyle performance: From profile to conceptual model. *American Journal of Occupational Therapy, 50,* 139–147.

Fidler, G. S., & Fidler, J. W. (1954). *Introduction to psychiatric occupational therapy.* New York: Macmillan.

Fidler, G. S., & Fidler, J. W. (1978). Doing and becoming: Purposeful action and self-actualization. *American Journal of Occupational Therapy, 32,* 305–310.

Fidler, G. S., & Velde, B. (1999). *Activity: Reality and symbol.* Thorofare, NJ: Slack.

Forsyth, K., & Kielhofner, G. (2003). Model of human occupation. In P. Kramer, J. Hinojosa, & C. B. Royeen (Eds.), *Perspectives in human occupation: Participation in life* (pp. 45–86). Philadelphia: Lippincott, Williams & Wilkins.

Frank, G. (1996). The concept of adaptation as a foundation for occupational science research. In R. Zemke & F. Clark (Eds.), *Occupational science: The evolving discipline* (pp. 47–55). Philadelphia: F. A. Davis.

Henderson, A. (1996). The scope of occupational science. In R. Zemke & F. Clark (Eds.), *Occupational science: The evolving discipline* (pp. 419–424). Philadelphia: F. A. Davis.

Kielhofner, G. (Ed.). (1985). *A model of human occupation: Theory and application.* Baltimore: Williams & Wilkins.

Kielhofner, G. (1992). *Conceptual foundations of occupational therapy.* Philadelphia: F. A. Davis.

Kielhofner, G. (Ed.). (1995). *A model of human occupation: Theory and application* (2nd ed.). Baltimore: Williams & Wilkins.

Kielhofner, G. (Ed.). (2002). *A model of human occupation: Theory and application* (3rd ed.). Baltimore: Lippincott, Williams & Wilkins.

Kielhofner, G., & Burke, J. (1980). A model of human occupation, part one: Conceptual framework and content. *American Journal of Occupational Therapy, 34,* 572–581.

Law, M. (Ed.). (1998). *Client-centered occupational therapy.* Thorofare, NJ: Slack.

Law, M., Baptiste, S., Carswell, A., McColl, M. A., Polatajko, H., & Pollock, N. (1994). *Canadian Occupational Performance Measure* (2nd ed.). Toronto, ON: Canadian Association of Occupational Therapists.

Law, M., Cooper, B. A., Strong, S., Stewart, D., Rigby, P., & Letts, L. (1996). The person–environment–occupation model: A transactive approach to occupational performance. *Canadian Journal of Occupational Therapy, 63,* 9–23.

Law, M., & Mills, J. (1998). Client-centered occupational therapy. In M. Law (Ed.), *Client-centered occupational therapy* (pp. 1–18). Thorofare, NJ: Slack.

Mosey, A. C. (1968). Recapitulation of ontogenesis: A theory for practice of occupational therapy. *American Journal of Occupational Therapy, 22,* 426–432.

Mosey, A. C. (1973). *Activities therapy.* New York: Raven.

Mosey, A. C. (1981). *Occupational therapy: Configuration of a profession.* New York: Raven.

Mosey, A. C. (1986). *Psychosocial components of occupational therapy.* New York: Raven.

Mosey, A. C. (1993). Partition of occupational science and occupational therapy: Sorting out some issues. *American Journal of Occupational Therapy, 47,* 751–754.

Mosey, A. C. (1996). *Applied scientific inquiry in the health professions: An epistemological orientation* (2nd ed.). Bethesda, MD: American Occupational Therapy Association.

Nelson, D. L. (1994). Form and function. In C. B. Royeen (Ed.), *AOTA self-study series: The practice of the future: Putting occupation back into therapy* (Lesson 2). Bethesda, MD: American Occupational Therapy Association.

Nelson, D. L. (1997). Why the profession of occupational therapy will flourish in the 21st century, 1996 Eleanor Clarke Slagle Lecture. *American Journal of Occupational Therapy, 51,* 11–24.

Nelson, D. L., & Jepson-Thomas, J. (2003). Occupational form, occupational performance, and a conceptual framework for therapeutic occupation. In P. Kramer, J. Hinojosa, & C. B. Royeen (Eds.), *Perspectives in human occupation: Participation in life* (pp. 87–155). Philadelphia: Lippincott, Williams & Wilkins.

Peachey-Hill, C., & Law, M. (2000). Impact of environmental sensitivity on occupational performance. *Canadian Journal of Occupational Therapy, 67,* 304–313.

Pollock, N., & McColl, M. (1998). Assessment in client-entered occupational therapy. In M. Law (Ed.), *Client-centered occupational therapy* (pp. 89–106). Thorofare, NJ: Slack.

Reilly, M. (1960). Research potentiality of occupational therapy. *American Journal of Occupational Therapy, 14,* 206–209.

Reilly, M. (1962). Occupational therapy can be one of the great ideas of 20th-century medicine, 1961 Eleanor Clarke Slagle Lecture. *American Journal of Occupational Therapy, 16,* 1–9.

Reilly, M. (1966). A psychiatric occupational therapy program as a teaching model. *American Journal of Occupational Therapy, 22,* 61–67.

Reilly, M. (Ed.). (1974). *Play as exploratory learning.* Beverly Hills, CA: Sage.

Schkade, J. K., & Schultz, S. (1992). Occupational adaptation: Toward a holistic approach to contemporary practice: Part 1. *American Journal of Occupational Therapy, 46,* 829–837.

Schkade, J. K., & Schultz, S. (2003). Occupational adaptation. In P. Kramer, J. Hinojosa, & C. B. Royeen (Eds.), *Perspectives in human occupation: Participation in life* (pp. 181–221). Philadelphia: Lippincott, Williams & Wilkins.

Schultz, S., & Schkade, J. K. (1992). Occupational adaptation: Toward a holistic approach to contemporary practice: Part 2. *American Journal of Occupational Therapy, 46,* 917–926.

Strong, S., Rigby, P., Stewart, D., Law, M., Letts, L., & Cooper, B. (1999). Application of the person–environment–occupation model: A practical tool. *Canadian Journal of Occupational Therapy, 66,* 122–133.

Velde, B. P., & Fidler, G. S. (2002). *Lifestyle performance: A model for engaging the power of occupation.* Thorofare, NJ: Slack.

Zemke, R., & Clark, F. (Eds.). (1996). *Occupational science: The evolving discipline.* Philadelphia: F. A. Davis.

3

Occupation Across the Life Span

Ruth Segal, PhD, OT

Occupation is a concept that reemerged in importance in occupational therapy in the late 1970s with the work of Mary Reilly and her students (Wilcock, 2003). This group believed that the profession needed to reaffirm and commit to the use of the term *occupation*. Further, they believed that the use of occupation would move the profession beyond the confines of the medical model. Reilly's commitment to the development of the construct of occupation resulted in the development of occupational science. The development of occupational science, focusing on human occupation, occurred as the profession recognized the need to develop its own body of knowledge.

The 1970s were a time of social unrest in the United States. Occupational therapy, like other professions, was dissatisfied with the existing social institutions and cultural values, and while society responded to changes in civil rights, women's liberation, and the antiwar movement, occupational therapy examined its existing norms, beliefs, and practices. This examination resulted in a commitment by many to the importance of occupation to life support and supported the further development of occupational therapy as a profession.

Having an independent status for the profession required that occupational therapy establish itself as an autonomous profession. The sociologist Andrew Abbott (1988) identified several characteristics that differentiate a technology, a profession, and a discipline. The existence of a unique body of knowledge is one feature that identifies a *profession* (e.g., engineering) from a *technology* (e.g., auto mechanics). The development of this unique body of knowledge in occupational therapy has been the focus of discussion and research over the past two decades. One of these discussions was about whether the nature of occupational therapy's unique body of knowledge should be the kind that develops best from applied or basic research (see Clark et al.,

1993; Mosey, 1992, 1993). Another discussion centered on concepts and terminology: Should the profession embrace the term *occupation* as its core concept, or should the more commonly used term *activity* be the core concept of the profession's knowledge? Each term has its strengths and limitations. The strengths of using the term *occupation* lie in its being part of our profession's name, and the difficulties lie in its common use to denote vocation rather than the way we define it in our profession. Activities, on the other hand, are commonly used and understood to mean things people do to fill time. Activities, however, often are understood to refer only to the physical aspect of the actions needed to do them, therefore omitting the aspects of experiences and meanings that are important to occupational therapy practitioners.

In writing this chapter, I take for granted that purposeful activities are different from occupations. Additionally, I assume that the most important aspect of occupation is the meaning attached to it. In this chapter, I discuss the sources of meanings of occupations across the life span. To make this discussion richer, I use the purposeful activity of intake of nutrients (eating) and demonstrate the variety and versatility of occupations related to it. I hope that the reader will be able to look at other people with a fresh understanding of the richness of the person as an occupational human being.

An Approach to Meaning

In Chapter 1, Hinojosa and Blount suggested that meaning lies within the individual. The meanings that people assign to occupations, however, occur within "temporal, psychological, social, symbolic, cultural, ethnic, and spiritual" contexts. Meaning is the sense in which something is understood (*Merriam-Webster's Concise Dictionary*, 2002). It is assigned by people who must engage in interpretation of the "something" in order to do so (Strauss & Quinn, 1997). Such interpretations are the subject of study of academic disciplines, such as philosophy, psychology, sociology, and anthropology.

Strauss and Quinn (1997) proposed a theory in *A Cognitive Theory of Cultural Meaning* that explains cultural patterns of meaning. They defined a cultural meaning as "the typical (frequently recurring and widely shared aspects of the) interpretation of some type of object or event evoked in people as a result of their similar life experiences" (p. 82). In this definition, cultural meanings occur within people rather than apart from them, highlighting the authors' view that culture does not exist apart from people. At the individual level, one aspect to be considered is how and where meanings are located within the person, what the qualities of these meanings are, and what the sources of the meanings are. In addition, at the societal level, one needs to consider how meanings become cultural and historical.

The Construction of Meaning

Meanings are located within the person. The process by which meanings are constructed or embedded within the person requires that the person participate in and interact with various environments. Using connectionist models of cognition, Strauss and Quinn (1997) suggested that all forms of experiences evoke neural responses in the brain in the forms of networks or maps. Similar experiences evoke the responses of the same or closely related networks. The more often these networks respond, the more ingrained those experiences and their meanings are. The more tightly connected a network is, the more stable and hard to change it becomes and vice versa. Varied experiences establish more networks and with it, people's ability to interpret more objects and events. Thus, participation in life creates mapping in the brain that, in turn, is used as schemas for interpreting and assigning meanings to events, practices, and experiences. Schemas are the organization of experience in the brain. They are used as templates for the interpretation of new events and situations into individually familiar and meaningful events and situations.

The nature of neural connections can be used to explain both the stability and the adaptability of cultural meanings (Strauss & Quinn, 1997). Strauss and Quinn suggested the following characteristics of cultural meanings to explain their stability:

- *Meanings can be relatively stable in individuals.* When a particular life experience is repeated many times, the neural connections related to this experience are more ingrained than connections constructed from relatively sparse experiences. When strong emotions are part of an experience, the related neural connections are more ingrained (e.g., responses related to survival). The more ingrained the neural connection, the harder it is to change. Additionally, when information on a situation or event is incomplete, a person will tend to fill in the gap in a way that will accommodate his or her existing schema.

- *Cultural understandings can have emotional and motivational force, prompting those who hold them to act on them.* For example, a person who has experienced relief when sharing a burden with a friend will tend to talk with this friend whenever he or she needs such relief. Alternatively, stereotypes direct people to behave in ways that will minimize the possibilities of disconfirming experiences. A person who was raised with the assumption that street people are dangerous will tend to avoid interactions with these people. Lack of interactions with them, in turn, will prevent them from experiencing disconfirming interactions. Therefore, that assumption remains unchallenged.

- *Meanings can be relatively durable historically, being reproduced from generation to generation.* For example, when parents continue with family traditions they socialize their children into these traditions. Further, if they make sure that their children's experiences of these traditions are positive ones, the children will tend to repeat them as described previously, carrying the tradition from generation to generation.

- *Meanings can be more or less widely shared in a social group.* When meanings are shared in a social group, the groups tend to participate in activities that reinforce these meanings. For example, religious holidays such as Easter, Yom Kippur, Ramadan, or the Chinese New Year are celebrated by people who share beliefs. The celebration of these holidays, in turn, constructs shared experiences in people that lead to shared meanings that are embedded within them. That is, the stability of neural connection related to cultural meanings can be explained by the stability of cultural meanings.

Despite all these factors that support the stability of cultural meanings and practices, the nature of neural connections also explains the flexibility of schemas and, thus, changes that occur in culture. An important aspect of neural connections is that an existing schema does not elicit a uniform response. Thus, the neural connections that compose the schema of our survival need for food do not dictate a single uniform behavior when we encounter food. Our responses depend on the context in which we encounter food. Additionally, the qualities of neural connections that contribute to flexibility are as follows: (a) current information tends to override old associations; (b) situations that cannot be interpreted by existing schemas are particularly noticeable and emotionally distressing, thus leading to the increased likelihood of new neural connections; and (c) schemas can be changed by conscious efforts to do so.

Societal Aspects That Contribute to the Stability of Cultural Meanings

The nature of the neural connections themselves cannot explain how the meanings that people assign are shared. The development of neural connections in the brain depends on people's life experiences. Therefore, living in the same society, social group, and family will tend to construct shared experiences and, therefore, neural connections that construct similar interpretive schema.

The most immediate practices that lead to the development of socially desired schema are the various methods of socialization and education of children. One example is processes in which rewards and punishments are used to elicit socially desired behaviors and experiences. Such rewards and punishments can be tangible (e.g., paying children to do their chores) or ideational (e.g., moral judgments of the goodness and badness of behaviors). Humans tend to internalize both such evaluations and adopt them so that they can believe they are good (i.e., they pass judgment on themselves). At another level, social practices and policies shape behaviors and experiences, thus supporting particular neural connections. For example, policies about retirement age and parental leave shape when people retire and who gets to have a parental leave after the birth of a child.

Cultural meanings have historical durability; that is, meanings are maintained across generations. This durability typically is the result of interpersonal and social forces rather than of intrapersonal ones. For example, religious education and participation in relevant ceremonies are means for reproducing religious meanings and practices across generations. Not all cultural meanings and practices are durable across generations. For example, the definition of healthy food changes in Western society with advancing knowledge in the biological sciences and keeps changing as knowledge changes and grows.

——— ▣ ———

Exercise 3.1—Cultural Meaning

Think about your family. What is your cultural background? What are some of your family traditions?

———————

The Nature of Shared Cultural Meanings

Meanings are considered to be cultural meanings when they are shared within a social group. For example, the consumption of a whole turkey during Thanksgiving dinner is a shared practice of food consumption that is attached to the value of giving thanks (a meaning). The experiences of people participating in Thanksgiving dinner may differ based on the roles they play (e.g., cook, carver, guest), the nature of interactions during the dinner, and many other aspects relating to the immediate and historical past. Such individual experiences may be positive (e.g., happiness to be with relatives) or negative (e.g., arguments with relatives); however, such a variety of experiences does not negate the fact that Thanksgiving dinner has meanings that are shared by many people in the United States and Canada. This sharing of meanings occurs because the similar practices of celebrating Thanksgiving and its meanings evoke in the brains of people neural connections presenting this phenomenon and, thus, constructing the shared cultural meaning through its intrapersonal location.

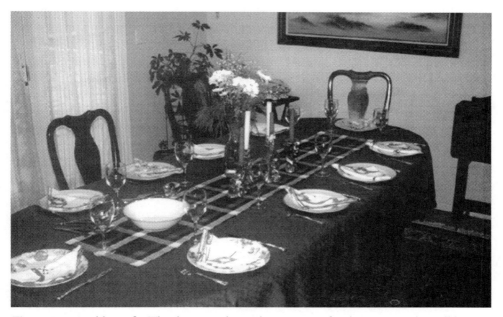

Figure 3.1. A table set for Thanksgiving dinner has meaning for the persons who will be participating.

In summary, Strauss and Quinn (1997) suggested interactions between people and their environment that result in brain connections or mapping that create the schema we use to interpret events and practices and guide our actions that are shared among people, thus creating cultural meanings. This theory of cultural meanings suggests that although we can study cultural meanings using scientific methods, when we are faced with people in intervention situations, we must explore cultural meanings with each person because the interactions between people and their culture does not produce a unified system of meaning by which every person abides. Knowledge of shared cultural meanings allows us useful starting points from which to begin our exploration of meanings with people.

Nevertheless, cultural meaning can be studied in the public domain. That is, patterns of meanings can be learned using various scientific methods. Such generalizations identify patterns that may not apply to all people in society. Such phenomena should be familiar to every person who assumed something about another person only to learn that the assumption was wrong. If these experiences occur very often, then the person who makes this assumption will change the assumption. If that assumption is accurate most of the time, then the person has identified or adopted a common pattern in society and learned through experience that it is not accurate all the time but only most of the time.

Occupations Across the Life Span

The evolution of meaning depends on context; therefore, each person's life in its context will influence but not determine the meaning of activities. This assumption makes it impossible to identify a sequence of occupations that is typical across the life span. I suggest that at the present state of knowledge, no sequence can be identified. Social norms and cultural practices limit and afford a person participation in various contexts. These norms and practices are based on age, ethnic background, socioeconomic status, profession, and many other aspects of society. Therefore, a general description of the evolution of occupations and the socially sanctioned activities involved in childhood, adolescence, adulthood, and older adulthood can be given. This description is not sufficient because the ranges of activities within each age category are wide. Hence, in this chapter I briefly outline contexts or socially sanctioned activities and elaborate on an example of food in each category. The examples are based, as much as possible, on research rather than constructed by me. The evolutionary process or development is based mostly on texts on human development, focusing on the social and psychological aspects of human development.

The Evolution of Occupation

For occupations to become part of the repertoire of one's life activities, they must be assigned meanings and must be interpreted in a cultural context. This definition of occupation means that until a child can assign meanings to phenomena or activities,

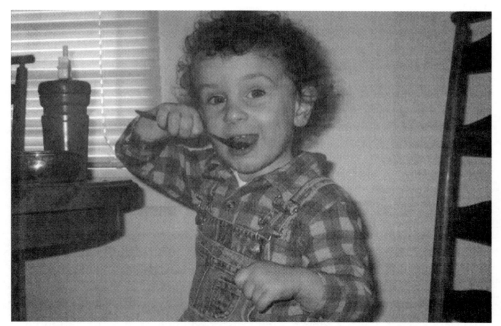

Figure 3.2. A child pretends to feed himself.

a child cannot have occupations. Kramer and Hinojosa (1995) described the early emergence of occupations as follows:

> When children are born, they are purely reflexive beings. Their behavior is dominated by sensory responses to their feeling state and their environment, and occupation is not yet evident. However, as children begin to respond to and interact with people and objects within their environment, they begin to develop rudimentary patterns of behavior. Responses to specific people or stimuli become almost predictable, and they develop into patterns. These patterns involve a variety of actions that have meanings to the children; thus, the children are stimulated to engage in selected activities. For example, infants begin to recognize their parents very early. When a parent walks into the room, the infant follows the parent with his or her eyes and begins to wave his or her arms and legs. This indicates that the child expects there to be some interaction. This initial attachment to the person or object is the first phase of object relations (Spitz, 1965).

> Often, the infant's responses take the form of motor actions. When repeated, these actions become patterns of behavior. In this sense, behavior is used to mean the emotional responses and reactions of the child. The infant first relates to people in the environment and then begins to react and respond to objects. These behaviors often become activities. Activity is used in this context to mean constructive action that enhances development and results in a productive outcome, such as when a child learns to reach out for his or her mother when she walks near the crib. The child's repertoire of behaviors and activities expands and forms a multitude of patterns. As these patterns of behaviors and specific activities are

repeated over time, they develop more and more meaning to the child and become occupations. Thus, occupations are defined in this context as natural patterns of daily activity that are meaningful to the individual. When observing an infant, one can see a particular child enjoying play with a rattle, while another child may ignore the rattle and spend time with a busy box. Personal preference in activities is evident at a very early age, which can then give rise to varying occupational patterns. (pp. 6–8)

Kramer and Hinojosa's overview of the evolution of occupations reflects the typical way in which human development is described. That is, the focus is on the increasing abilities and variety of activities and the different meanings assigned to similar activities (i.e., occupations ascribed to individuals). After the developmental stage that Kramer and Hinojosa described here begins a different aspect of development that commonly is not described: the development of the variety of meanings that each individual attaches to similar activities. These meanings, as also suggested by Hinojosa and Blount in Chapter 1 and Strauss and Quinn (1997), develop as the social world of children enlarges and with it their participation and experiences.

As Kramer and Hinojosa (1995) suggested, occupations do not occur in infancy in general. Food in infancy can be discussed in terms of health and survival only. Although attachment is an important aspect in infancy that has been connected with feeding, it can be discussed in terms of survival rather then in terms of infant occupations, which is consistent with Lowenberg's application of Maslow's hierarchy of needs to food consumption (Lowenberg, 1970, as cited in Kittler & Sucher, 2001). The most basic human need is the physical need for survival. The focus of feeding infants is on their physical survival: They are being measured, and their measurements are compared to existing growth charts that indicate whether their growth is age appropriate and their ratio of length and weight is within normal limits. Having either of these measurements not within normal limits indicates the need for some medical intervention or at least investigation of the infant's health and well-being.

Before I develop the thesis on occupations across the life span, it is important to introduce eating as a social and cultural phenomenon. All humans consume the same type of milk at the beginning of life, but by early childhood, the diets of humankind are greatly diverse (Birch, Fisher, & Grimm-Thomas, 1996), suggesting that food is a vehicle for many nonbiological functions and meanings. Food and eating can be viewed as a system of communication (Douglas, 1982). Meals can demonstrate status differences, social groupings, and relationships. Food also has social and economic symbolic meanings. Finally, giving and receiving foods allow people to exercise their roles correctly. For example, for the young, meals are important socialization tools because they teach what is acceptable and unacceptable behavior. Mealtimes are also good for developing self-image and role control. For sociologists, the underlying parts of food and meal preparation, cookery, and consumption hold the most value (Wood, 1995).

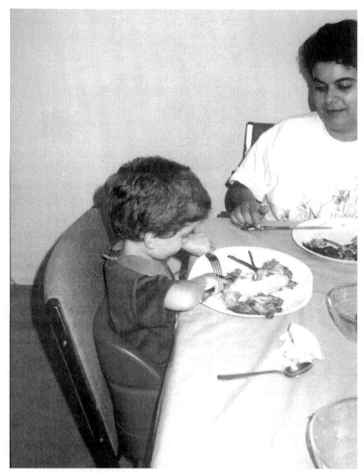

Figure 3.3. Communication between mother and child during lunch.

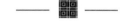

Exercise 3.2—Food

How is food in your life part of a system for communication? What social and economic symbolic meanings does food have for you?

_____

Early Childhood (2–6 Years)

Childhood is a socially constructed status (Lee, 2001). That is, social and cultural values, beliefs, and traditions shape what is considered the appropriate social interactions that children should have, with whom, and doing what. These social and cultural values, beliefs, and traditions have changed with history and still differ among cultures and societies and within society (La Fontaine, 1986; Lee, 2001; Shahar, 1990; Wyness, 2000).

> Childhood is the life period in which children are prepared for adulthood by the adults in society. The social construction of childhood refers to the patterns of activities and participation that are open to children or in which their participation is required. These activities are constructed on the basis of current scientific knowledge about children's physical, cognitive, psychosocial, and emotional development around traditions, beliefs and customs, social status, and ethnic background, to name a few. These activities are time dependent—they change over time with the changes in scientific knowledge and in society (Lee, 2001). The overall structure of childhood in the Western world is that of increasing exposure of children to a greater variety of environments and activities.

In middle-class America, infants tend to be sheltered in modern society, and their environment commonly is limited to their own homes, their mothers, and the rest of the nuclear family. Among families with lower incomes or in families in which both parents work, a paid caregiver or a member from the extended family may be retained to care for infants in their home. In both scenarios, the infant's environments are limited. To a lesser extent in the United States and more so in many other Western countries, infants are cared for in day-care centers. In such cases, the infant's environment is somewhat larger but still very controlled in its nature (Lee, 2001). This sheltering continues until infants are considered old enough to join play groups and eventually graduate to kindergarten. During this period, young children may attend school and have play dates that include ongoing adult supervision.

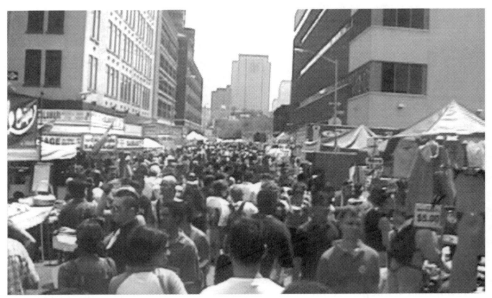

Figure 3.4. Eating at an outdoor celebration.

In early childhood, usually up to 7 years of age or so, children's cognitive, physical, emotional, and psychosocial needs are such that their social status does not include significant social responsibilities for others. During this period, however, their array of social interactions increases in its variety, giving ample opportunities for the development of mapping in the brain. During this period of life, children begin to interact more with other children and adults in a variety of contexts. Therefore, similar activities may be performed in a variety of social and cultural contexts, constructing them as different occupations. Participating in similar activities in different contexts evokes a variety of experiences that are connected with the occupations. For example, play can take the form of playing alone, with a caregiver, with siblings, with friends, at home, in the park, and at school. The variety of play situations and children's experiences create connections in the brain that increase in their versatility and complexity with experiences. Participation in play allows children to develop preferences and assert choices.

During this period, children begin to eat in a variety of contexts. They begin to differentiate between different meanings of food and eating. For example, birthday parties are connected with certain foods, such as the birthday cake, with a particular type of decorations and with party bags that include sweets typically considered unhealthy and not a part of children's regular diet. Birthday parties also include savory food, such as pizza or hot dogs. The context of eating at a birthday party includes singing a birthday song when the birthday cake is brought in with lighted candles on it. By the time children are preschool-age, adults begin to take children to restaurants that serve food appropriate for children and that is consumed in such contexts. Such restaurants include self-service fast food and full-service family dining. Going to school is another context for consuming food. School lunches are either brought from home or served at school. Children socialize around food while eating their lunches. For children in pre-kindergarten through first grade, lunch time is supervised closely by educators or other school employees.

At this phase of life, children are being exposed to a greater variety of foods. Parents provide a variety of food for consumption as a means of promoting and maintaining health. The question of what constitutes a healthy food depends on culture and time. Presently in the United States, healthy diets are commonly believed to lead to health and well-being. Therefore, the U.S. government promotes a "food pyramid" that delineates the amount and type of foods that make up a healthy diet. The food pyramid is believed to be based on scientific data, even though that notion has been challenged (see Nestle, 2002) because of the influence of the food industry on these and many other aspects of food consumption. Such government publications are not unique to the United States and can be found in many Western countries.

Government policies and recommendations such as these are an example of how social organizations affect individual tastes and construct shared meanings. For example, consider the belief that fresh fruit and vegetables are good for one's health. Such a belief seems obvious to us but it has not always been like that; in the Middle Ages, cucumbers and melons were considered dangerous for human health (Albala, 2002).

Another aspect of food and eating habits that begins in early childhood is the socialization of children into the eating habits identified with the family's beliefs, reli-

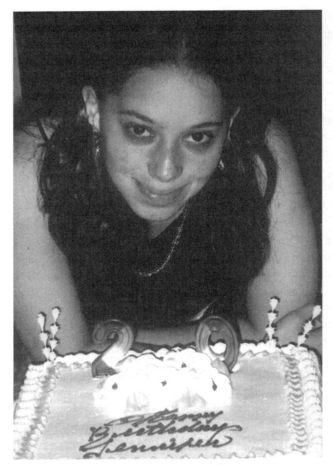

Figure 3.5. Birthday parties involve certain foods, such as birthday cake.

gion, and culture. World religions can be divided into two broad types: prophetic (often called Western) and mystical (often called Eastern). Many food habits stem from religion. Religious groups may use food laws to differentiate themselves from others. Often, religious food restrictions are relaxed or ignored. These restrictions may come from holy books or moral attitudes. *Cultism* is the word used to describe eating patterns that seem bizarre under conventional wisdom. Cultist food practices satisfy the social and psychological needs of followers but often are not nutritious (Fieldhouse, 1986). The following summarizes some of the information about food and beliefs that Fieldhouse (1986) described in greater detail.

PRESTIGE AND STATUS

Some foods confer high status on the eaters; others imply status because of the groups that usually eat these foods. The differences in the meals of medieval nobles and peas-

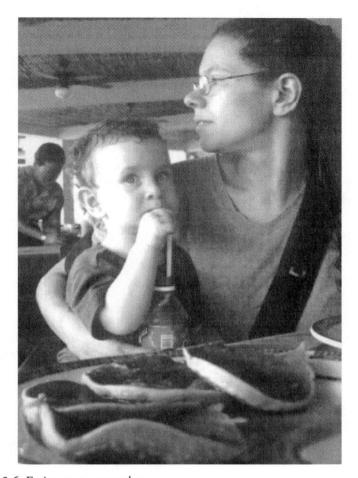

Figure 3.6. Eating matzo pancakes.

ants were a symbolic representation of the power that the nobles held over the food supply and, thus, the peasants. Prestige also can be attached to the circumstances and ways in which food is served. Food can make social distinctions overt or subtly underlined, depending on the situation. The Hindu caste system, which has strict rules of who can eat with whom, has some of the most obvious rules that outline social distinctions.

STATUS AND FOOD BEHAVIOR

Status in food is conveyed three main ways: (a) the freedom to choose rare and costly items to impress others, (b) the freedom to select expensive restaurants for personal gratification, and (c) the freedom to prepare difficult and time-consuming dishes. To be denied any sort of choice in Western society is seen as negative. The ability to choose freely is tied to economic status, which is tied to social status. When food choice is limited, people feel uncomfortable and are more likely to complain. Lack of choice also decreases self-esteem. Exotic, complex, or expensive dishes convey a higher status. It can derive from several aspects: the location, the time, or the skill necessary to prepare the dishes or the distance in preparation between the one who consumes it and the person who prepares it. At dinner parties, the food served can be a sign not only of the host's status but also of the status that the host sees his guests as having.

Food and Fashion

Food may have a high status only because high-status groups consume it. Often, there is a circular process to it, as a food may have a high status but then become widely available to all classes and no longer be seen as high status. Preferences for high-status food may develop without regard to the food's actual taste. Humans are the only group that will shun a nutritious food because of status and replace it with a nutritionally mediocre one of higher status. The importance of prestigious food is how much social recognition it will bring.

Status and Food Ownership

In some places in the world, food ownership has some of the same prestige or status rituals as food consumption. In some parts of Africa, owning cattle conveys tremendous economic status. Cattle are kept as a sign of wealth and rarely killed for food.

Food, Friendship, and Communication

The closeness of people often can be gauged by the foods they share. The act of eating together implies some degree of compatibility—the more elaborate, the greater the closeness. It is common in many places to always keep some sort of food on hand for callers because to not offer food would be to lose social status. One exception to this is the Bemba people of Africa, who send people food to be consumed in private rather than shared together, as a sign of respect.

Peer Acceptance

Food is also an expression of the human need to belong. The wish to eat what others eat may result in altered food patterns that may not be nutritionally sound, with teenagers being especially prone. Food choice in specific cases can be limited by social norms dictated by the choices of others.

Food as Reward and Punishment

Children learn what is acceptable and approved of as food through a system of reward and punishment. These may be explicit or implied and may have accompanying reinforcing messages.

FOOD GIFTS AND SHARING

Shared food is a symbol of social relationships, different from the food's monetary value. Psychologically, those who were raised in an environment where food was in abundance tend to develop a predisposition to sharing, whereas those who were not, do not. As a gift, food can express a wide range of emotions and sentiments. Three basic types of reciprocity for food exchanges exist. First, generalized reciprocity implies no immediate expectation of return, no attempt to determine the gift's value, and no attempt to make gift-giving "balance out." Second, balanced reciprocity between social equals who have a personal relationship takes into account the gift's value and implies some expectation of return. This return may be at a later date. Third, negative reciprocity involves immediate exchange and strict accounting of value in an impersonal exchange. Exchanges also can diffuse the status of the foods. Reciprocity-based food exchanges are common in situations in which environmental resources are limited. If reciprocity is not adopted, then competitive food-giving can result.

FEASTS AND FESTIVALS

Feasts and festivals are held for many reasons and for many types of personal, cultural, or religious observances. Feast foods usually are scarce, high quality, expensive, and difficult and time-consuming to prepare. Festivals are complex, colorful rituals found in nearly every society in some form or another. Four main types of festivals exist: ecofests (astronomical or seasonal events, e.g., May Day), theofests (religious events, e.g., Easter), secular festivals (national holidays, e.g., Independence Day), and personal festivals (major life events, e.g., birthdays).

RITUALS AND SACRIFICE

Many pagan and religious rituals involve food. The need for ritualistic food may have contributed to the spread of some religions. Food offerings in ritual, usually were animals. In many societies, animal sacrifices have fallen out of favor, replaced by prayer or sacrifices involving money. Sacrifices may be given for a variety of reasons, but they always imply an asymmetrical status relationship. The following reasons are the most common: food for the Gods to propitiate an affronted deity or affect communication with a deity by eating of the victim, for maintenance or renewal of life, for divination purposes to confirm a covenant or to ward off evil, and in exchange for favors. The traditional view of sacrifice has been replaced by a recommendation for a moral one instead.

SACRAMENTS

Many cultures, especially ancient ones, have sacred foods (usually animal), which are often embodiments of the Gods. Therefore, sacramental killing and eating of these animals implies that they are too sacred to be eaten and should be spared.

— ⊞ —

Exercise 3.3—Meaning of Food

What meaning does food have in your life? Examine the categories listed above and identify how they relate to your life. How do they relate to your family? How do they relate to others with whom you socialize?

In early childhood, children are beginning to be exposed to a greater variety of social situations in which food is consumed. Additionally, with their increased abilities to perceive and interpret the world, they begin to observe and experience different types of foods and their social and cultural meanings. With these changes and developments, children begin to differentiate between different occupations that involve eating; they know the difference between a birthday party and a daily school lunch; they know the difference between the daily family dinner and a holiday dinner. These differences are not only in the type of food consumed but also in the nature of interactions with others and the experiences. This variety of experiences, in turn, helps to develop a variety of connections in the brain that are related to eating, with their related experiences and meanings unique to each child. These meanings are shared with other children and family members because they participate in the same events.

Middle Childhood (7–11 Years)

In middle childhood, children gain greater exposure to social contexts and decreasing supervision. Lunch time at school is less closely monitored in terms of the interaction among the children. Peer groups become increasingly important, and social interactions, empathy, and other prosocial behaviors are learned. During this period, children become more aware of themselves and others. They learn to control their expression of feelings and become more selective in choosing friends. Children begin to develop empathy. Their self-awareness increases, and self-esteem tends to decrease. Children's peer groups become sensitive to customs and principles in society. Children become more aware of their familial situation compared with that of others. Their well-being continues to depend on the quality of parenting and social setting rather than on the family's constitution (whether the parents are of the same or different gender, whether the family is single- or two-parent, whether the parents are the biological parents).

School-age children are considered more capable and independent, so they are allowed to venture out into the world more. A key part of their development is social cognition—understanding other people and groups. During the school years, this process is complex because children gain a better understanding of human behavior. They can see the origins and future implications of an action, and their understanding of personality traits increases. School-age children begin to learn about customs and principles in societies.

In terms of food consumption, family dinners, if they occur, become a greater social and educational affair because the children's ability to participate in conversations improves. At home, family dinners are an important means of socialization. Dinner conversations are used to convey rules of conversation, conflict resolutions, and establishment and challenges of social roles (Grieshaber, 1997; Ochs, Taylor, Rudolph, & Smith, 1992; Segal, 1999; Vuchinich, 1987). Although the family dinner is considered an important occupation even to the point of making the space and time for family members to become a family (DeVault, 1991), the nature of interactions during family dinner may evoke unpleasant experiences when conflicts occur. These different experiences may lead to different meanings that people attach to this occupation. The following sections summarize a depiction of family dinner in films and the alternatives presented.

THE DINING SPACE

The act of eating together shows the quality of relationships and social interactions. Until the 1950s, the site of this act was almost always the home. Family dining represented family unity. Modern life has seen a shift from dining in the home to dining in restaurants. As depicted in many American films, dining in the home is shown as a source of conflict and distress, whereas the bonding once experienced at home now is shown in fast food establishments and restaurants. These films redefine social order and the boundaries between order (purity) and disorder (pollution) in dining. Technology, advertising, changing family structure, and various other factors have led to the rise of fast food and its place in American society. The films discussed next reveal this new place in American society that often is hard to pin down and the shift in domain from private to public dining.

THE FILMS

In her discussion of the shift from private to public dining, Jane Ferry (2003) used the following examples:

- *Mystic Pizza.* This film follows three young women as they prepare for adulthood—sisters Kat and Daisy and their friend Jojo, who work together at a restaurant called Mystic Pizza. Within the pizzeria the girls bond over meals. The owner, Leona, is a mothering figure to them. No meals are ever shown eaten at home, except for one tense one at the home of Daisy's boyfriend Charlie. The characters seem to eat most of their meals at Mystic Pizza. All bonding between characters in the movie takes place inside the restaurant: Jojo holds her wedding reception there; Kat finds out that Leona has agreed to help with her Yale tuition there; and Daisy reconciles her conflicted relationship with her mother there.

- *Ordinary People.* In this film, home dining is the source of conflict, whereas McDonald's is the only place where the main character can find any nurturing.

The film depicts the lives of Beth and Calvin and their son Conrad after the death of their other son Buck. Buck died in a boating accident while out with Conrad, and the guilt drove Conrad to attempt suicide. Beth finds herself unable to deal with this disorder in her family and responds by behaving coldly toward Conrad, which often is evidenced in dining scenes. The viewer only sees peaceful, communal dining during the McDonald's scenes, when Conrad has a reunion with a girl he met in the hospital there and when he takes another girl on a date there.

- *Better Off Dead.* The family meal scenes in this movie satirize the concept of family mealtime bonding. The mother of the family, Jenny, prepares horrible food that her family does not want to eat. The father, Al, spends meals complaining to or about his teenage son, Lane. The other son, Badger, spends mealtimes cutting coupons from cereal boxes or sitting in his bedroom playing with a Laser Blaster toy. Lane either eats alone, leaves meals early, or is forced into eating with the family by his mother. The film also satirizes the "polluted reality" of fast food restaurants, while also showing them as the only place where Lane can dine with someone and make a connection.

CONSIDERATIONS OF BOUNDARIES AND POLLUTION

The lack of family dining in these movies shows alienation and pollution when it comes to the notion of family dining. According to anthropologist Mary Douglas, the rules of pollution use elements of environment to support social reality (Douglas, 1982). The activity of eating is based on what society classifies as edible (clean) and nonedible (unclean), and the location of eating often is determined by order and disorder. In the three example films, home is shown as a place of disorder whereas restaurants provide order, which provides a unity of experience. These eating scenes reproduce old ideals and update them for modern times.

CONSIDERATIONS OF STRUCTURAL CHANGES AND LANDSCAPE OF POWER

Changes in societal structure may be the cause for the changes in dining because they shape habits and meaning of food. Families integrate the power of these changes into daily life. Capitalism, marketing, giant food conglomerates, fast food chains, and technological advances all have led to the rise of the fast food restaurant in favor of family dining.

CONSIDERATIONS OF FAMILY STRUCTURE

Along with social structure, family structure and daily meaning have changed. With more mothers working, school-age children involved in after-school activities, and teenagers working part-time jobs or playing sports, family dining is harder to coordinate. The cultural importance of family dining has decreased. The three example films are visual representations of these changes (Ferry, 2003).

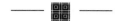

Exercise 3.4—Film

Select a television show or movie that you have seen with a story line that involves a family's daily life. Reflect on how family dining was represented. How have films influenced your thinking about dining?

Adolescence (12–18 Years)

We typically think of adolescence as the time for developing self-identity. This process is related to interactions with family members and friends. It is a time for those relationships to evolve into their adult forms. By late adolescence, teenagers are comfortable with relationships with the other gender; their sexual identity develops; and their communication with same-gender friends and parents matures. With parents, adolescents struggle for independence in term of values, behaviors, and life in general.

One of the issues around food that may begin at this phase of human development is that of eating disorders. There are many psychological explanations behind these disorders. When we talk about eating disorders as an occupation of eating whose meaning lies within the individual (i.e., psychological explanations), we need to address the social and cultural environment that contributes to the meanings of attachment to thinness and the ways to achieve it.

THINNESS IN SOCIOLOGICAL AND HISTORICAL CONTEXT

It is not known whether eating disorders are a modern development or whether they came about over the past 100 years or so. Increased awareness of them in recent decades signals an increase in both medical knowledge of them and an increase in their incidence. Mennell, Murcott, and van Otterloo (1992) suggested that this development is the result of long-term changes in society, civilization, and attitudes toward appetite. In the Middle Ages, nutrition was not distributed evenly among social classes. Abundance of food was a way for the upper class to show its importance. As time went by, abundance of food reached the lower classes as well, and the quality of the food became what set the higher classes apart from the lower ones. Additionally, in the 19th century, the concept of moderation became popular and imposed some restrictions on diets. The 20th century brought an expectation of dietary control that stressed the individual's control over food.

Anorexia nervosa was first diagnosed in the 19th century. Much of the research on eating disorders focuses on the medical and psychological factors and not the social. The fact, however, that anorexia affects particular demographic groups (most typically young, white, affluent women) cannot be ignored. Throughout the 20th century, the ideal body type for a woman has become smaller and smaller. The pressure to be thin and the importance seen in thinness are rooted in the behavior and personality traits associated with it, such as success and power, whereas being overweight carries a negative stigma. The fact that the lower and working classes only acquired the means and abilities to afford enough food to become overweight in the past 100 years may be why the upper classes, who had typically been plump, now find themselves stressing slimness. In light of these beliefs, it is not surprising that women are more obsessed than ever with food and calorie intake and that a majority report that they would like to be thinner (Deunwald, 2003). Correlations between the eating habits that are deemed socially acceptable and those of eating disorders suggest that eating disorders are extreme manifestations of eating habits that are deemed acceptable. Research also notes that this pressure for thinness is felt among women but not nearly as much among men (Mennell et al., 1992). This difference seems to fit into the pattern of female socialization. Modern women are placed in a tough situation, faced with opportunities for success and power but often raised with traditional female values of compliance and passivity. The generation of women in the late 20th century was the first to feel this pressure (Mennell et al., 1992).

Historically, women have tried to change their bodies to meet the cultural standard of beauty. Wiseman, Gray, Mosimann, and Ahrens (1992) analyzed the measurements of *Playboy* magazine centerfolds (1979–1988) and Miss America contestants (1979–1985) as well as the number of weight loss, diet, and exercise articles in *Harper's Bazaar, Vogue, Ladies' Home Journal, Good Housekeeping, Woman's Day,* and *McCall's* from 1959 to 1988. During the period of analysis, Miss America contestants got smaller, in both size and weight, and showed a significant decrease in hip size, whereas *Playboy* centerfolds remained at a steady small size throughout the studied period. During these 10 years, 69% of *Playboy* models and 60% of Miss America candidates were 15% or more below the expected weight for their respective age and height categories, a major symptom of anorexia. This finding suggests that the cultural standard has stayed thin and even has grown thinner. In the *Playboy* analysis, when the body sizes began to level off at a certain low number, it may be because going any lower would prove to be dangerous or fatal. The survey of articles showed an increased emphasis on weight loss over the past 30 years. In recent years, exercise articles have outnumbered diet articles, suggesting a new trend based on health and fitness for weight loss instead of just dieting, although it must be carefully observed because overexercising can be a signifier of bulimia nervosa (Wiseman et al., 1992).

In relation to other aspects of food and eating, adolescents may begin eating in separate social contexts, for example, dating or going out in groups. Typically, considering their budgets, fast food chains and food at the movie theater might be the choice. Adolescents also are left alone at home and may engage in cooking for themselves and younger siblings. That is, at this stage, in addition to refining the skills whose development began in middle childhood around eating and eating right, the aspects of cooking food and providing for one's own nourishment and that of younger siblings may begin.

Adulthood

Adulthood is different from childhood not only because the adult becomes a legally independent member of society, but also because society does not establish a single path for transitioning from early adulthood to older adulthood. In fact, from the late 20th century, adulthood is marked with decreased predictability about the way life will evolve (Lee, 2001). Most texts on human development identify three general foci of adult life: family, career, and friendships and intimacy. The way adults go about attending to these foci is determined by social and cultural aspects (with the exception of childbearing in women). During adulthood, issues such as gender, socioeconomic status, race, ethnicity, religion, and sexual orientation become more apparent in the choices open to and made by people. Although these issues affect children and adolescents as well, the way they encounter and address these issues depends largely on how their parents construct exposures to them. Therefore, I reserved the discussion for adulthood.

FAMILY

For adults, having a family typically means raising children. The family constitution and legal status may vary from marriage to cohabiting to single-parenting. Parents may be from different or the same gender and be the biological or nonbiological parents. In any case, the role of parenting is an important aspect of the lives of many adults. As parents, adults are responsible for the physical, psychological, and social well-being and development of their children. One of these responsibilities is to socialize their children to the different occupations of eating in context. They are responsible for introducing culturally relevant foods to their children as a way of socializing their children into that culture. These things may be fairly simple, such as the kind of breakfast being served, where the choices can be to follow the shared meaning of "breakfast" in terms of the types of food served (see "Food for Breakfast") or to break with these traditions by following new scientific information about foods that are good or bad for one's health (e.g., the consumption of eggs).

FOOD FOR BREAKFAST

> The most flexible versions of breakfast are probably the central and north European buffets of breads, pastries, cheeses, and cold meats or their Middle Eastern equivalents of bread, yoghurt, fruit, and preserves. Really substantial breakfasts include the modern British fry-up and the North American subspecies

of this, with numerous variations on the theme of eggs, plus options of waffles with maple syrup.

> Traditional Indian breakfasts include dal, rice, breads, samosas, and fruit. Comforting bowls of hot cereal mixtures are popular, from the Scottish oatmeal porridge to the rice porridges eaten across much of Asia of which congee is the best known. Minimal approaches to breakfast include croissants and café au lait in France, chocolate and churros in Spain, and many variations of the bowl of muesli theme for those who think that cereal, nuts, and dried fruit are key to good health. (Davidson, 1999, p. 104)

The type of food consumed imparts information and signifies meanings. For example, a television advertisement showing a frying pan with two eggs and bacon while the announcer says, "Breakfast for dinner," suggests that eating eggs in the United States is related to breakfast. In Israel, on the other hand, eggs are a common food for the evening meal, which is supper rather than dinner. Even within the United States, a great variety of foods is consumed by different ethnic groups in various geographic locations, and by many other delineations. The variety is so great that Kittler and Sucher (2001) devoted a whole book to describing it.

To make healthy choices of food, parents must be knowledgeable about what foods are considered healthy. The health-contributing qualities of food are a good example of how meaning is time-dependent, as suggested by Hinojosa and Blount in Chapter 1 of this book. For example, the food pyramid published by the U.S. Department of Agriculture is updated regularly because knowledge about the healthfulness of food and diets keeps changing. In the following sections, I summarize beliefs about healthy foods from the time of the Middle Ages to demonstrate how beliefs have changed.

Food and the Family

Issues of food and family are closely related to those of nutrition and responsibility. Women often deal with balancing diet and health for their families and themselves. Different cultures can have different working understandings of what is healthy. Although knowledge of nutrition among women is high, application of this knowledge is not always consistent. Homemakers' food choices are primarily affected by their desire to be a good spouse and mother, available time, available money, and influences from their environment and their upbringing. The final implication is that nutritional policy and education need to consider culinary value and how it relates to family relationships and power.

Research shows that mass media messages also can influence dietary patterns and decisions, like those about salmonella, mad cow disease, listeria, and botulism. Informal nutritional education can be just as influential and important as formal. In catering to the tastes of everyone else, women often ignore their own tastes and participate less in the domestic dining experience. In times of financial hardships, women are the most likely to go without food. Thus, women are constantly trying to balance the tension between their personal tastes and educational knowledge and those of their families (Wood, 1995).

The role of the midlife adult as a member of the middle generation of their extended family is easier to underestimate. Family ties are strong at this time, and those between middle-aged people and their elderly parents often improve greatly. When adult children have children, a new link between generations is formed. During this stage of life, women tend to be kinkeepers, the ones who keep in touch with family members no longer at home, celebrate achievements, and get the family together. These increased family ties can sometimes be burdensome for middle-aged people because they experience obligations to help both the younger and older members of their families, making them the "sandwich generation."

One way of keeping the extended family together is through a holiday get-together, such as Thanksgiving. The preparation of holiday meals may consist of following traditions and bringing in new traditions. For example, parents who as children did not like certain foods may introduce new ones to make the experience of a festive dinner for their children a better one. These engagements in festive family meals are an important feature of the construction of a family out of its individual members. Without getting together, regardless of the quality of experiences, interactions and attachments would not have occurred (DeVault, 1991; Gillis, 1996; Hasselkus, 2002; Kantor & Lehr, 1975).

Another context of eating that was mentioned earlier is the socialization of children into dining out. Dining out is an experience that has become much more common in the United States and other places with the emergence of fast food and other

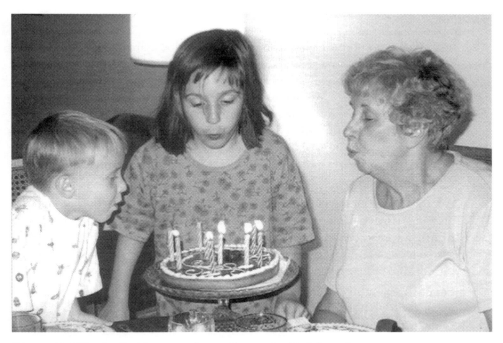

Figure 3.7. The family blows out the candles on the birthday cake.

affordable restaurants. Dining out as a context for eating is large and diversified in every aspect of that context: The cost of a meal can be close to a dollar and up to a few hundred dollars. The type of food served may represent varied tastes and cultural, social, and religious aspects as well as combinations of those. The nature of service can cover the range from self-service to restaurant servers who specialize in different aspects and stages of the service. With all these variations come different behavioral expectations, experiences, and meanings.

Parents are responsible for socializing their children to the dining-out contexts relevant to their social and cultural backgrounds. For example, some cultures whose food is spicy begin introducing spicy food to children around 10 or 11 years of age (Davidson, 1999). Such a socializing aspect of eating in cultures whose food is not spicy may not exist, and people may acquire the taste for it later in their lives. Another aspect of dining out is manners. There are ways to behave in a self-service restaurant, like in the fast food chains, that are different from a self-service restaurant that presents food buffet-style. Eating utensils and their use relate to the type of restaurant one goes to: Chopsticks or knife and fork? One set of knife and fork or several sets? These observable artifacts can give information about the possible ethnic foods served and how expensive they might be. Observing a person holding and using a knife and a fork can give one a broad idea of country of origin; people in the United States do not tend to hold the knife in their right hand and the fork in their left hand simultaneously for eating, whereas people from Europe tend to use that method. These habits and information are what parents impart to their children to support them in their adult life.

CAREER

Career is another important aspect of the life of adults. Career can be a source of income and can be used as a social ladder because of the generation of income and social connections developed. A career often includes its special forms of eating. There is the daily lunch at work that can take the form of bringing lunch from home, buying lunch and eating it in the office, or eating lunch in a restaurant. The variety of restaurants open for lunch affords a differentiation among level of employees or business people who lunch. The type of food consumed and the price are good indicators of the socioeconomic level of the person lunching. Lunch also can be consumed as part of a business meeting.

Another type of eating in the context of career can be in workplace parties and special occasions. These parties may relate to holidays, office events, and personal events such as birthdays, marriages, and childbirths. Each of these events may occur in the office with catered food or potluck or in a restaurant or someone's home. Each event and location is attached to unique behaviors and manners as well as experiences and meanings.

Finally, career also can include business meals—breakfast, lunch, or dinner—and, again, the type of food and location may vary greatly. On these occasions, the focus of the conversation is business rather than social, and the food and location may serve to impress the invited party.

FRIENDSHIPS AND INTIMACY

Adults take on many roles to fulfill the need for intimacy, each of which demands a type of personal sacrifice. Young adults free of overriding commitments find it easy to create broad networks of friends in various settings and among various groups where they can find advice and companionship. After marriage, the wide friendship network shrinks because of the time that establishing a marriage and home takes, on top of other obligations. The focus on raising the family does not exclude an important occupation that is related to maintaining intimacy and friendships, and this is dining out. Dining out, as described as follows, may not be as simple as eating at a different location. The experience of dining out can include that of moving into a different world that may help to maintain and develop relationships.

SOCIAL ASPECT OF DINING OUT

Dining out is not only about the food consumed but also about the experience (Campbell-Smith, 1967). Finkelstein (1989) applied a more sociological, structuralist view to this concept and wrote of her findings in *Dining Out: A Sociology of Modern Manners*. She writes that dining out today has much to do with self-presentation and social relationships.

Restaurants have a cultural reputation as being a site of well-being, excitement, and pleasure, which is why things other than the food are important. For example, the restaurant's décor, cost, and nature of the service may indicate the socioeconomic status of its patrons. Finkelstein (1989) suggested further that cost and status are more important than the nature and quality of the food because both are objective factors that are easier for people to agree on than food.

The objective factors of dining out allow for standardization of the meal experiences; by making these objective factors part of restaurants, the patrons who frequent such restaurants know what the experience should be like and, therefore, go to particular restaurants for the particular experiences they are looking for at particular times (Finkelstein, 1989). For example, when taking children out for dining in the United States, the typical appropriate restaurant (other than the fast food chains) would be not too expensive, relatively casual, and one that has a children's menu. In France on the other hand, it is not uncommon to see children in upscale restaurants that may have a children's menu as well. Another example could be the parents' decision to dine at an expensive restaurant on their anniversary with the hope of having an experience that is different from their typical dining-out experience.

Older Adulthood

Older adulthood is sometimes described in terms of increased frailty and health concerns. In sociological terms, older adulthood often is defined by the changes in the roles and occupations of older people. Some of these changes occur as a result of the biological and physiological changes that occur with aging. Some of them are the result of life circumstances, such as grown children, and some arise from the social organization of society. In general, the way people change their lives with aging greatly depends on their previous lifestyles and their social, cultural, and economic situations. In terms of eating, the changes would be similar and would depend on social status, economic situation, cultural background, and habits of eating. The need to control some aspect of foods may increase as people get older, which accords with the belief that what we consume affects our health. Most of these changes in food intake occur before one reaches older adulthood and depend on one's health considerations, including conditions such as diabetes, high blood pressure, and heart disease. Such changes in diet are dominated by scientific findings and common beliefs about the healthful qualities of different foods.

Occupations That Involve Eating

The previous description and discussion about the different occupations that involve eating was not meant to be exhaustive, but illustrative. My purpose was to demonstrate that the basic human need for food leads all humans to engage in the basic activity of eating. This activity consists of placing food in one's mouth, chewing, swallowing, and digesting. Humans, however, are animals who construct social meanings, and, as such, the activity of eating can be performed and experienced in different contexts and in different formats, thus amounting to multiple occupations that involve eating.

In the process of developing this example, I embedded the activity of eating in the context of human development. I tried, however, to focus more on the social aspects of human development than on biological and psychological ones, assuming that readers are familiar with the others. These aspects, however, are ever present and cannot be divorced from the social and cultural aspects. Of particular interest in the connection among these aspects is the cognitive theory of cultural meaning (Strauss & Quinn, 1997).

Occupations are phenomena that lie within the individual because only the individual can interpret and assign meaning to activities and events. Humans are social animals, and the interpretations and meanings that they assign to occupations are closely related to their life experiences. These life experiences are largely shaped by temporal, psychological, social, symbolic, cultural, ethnic, and spiritual meanings. In the previous description, I used the terms *social* and *cultural* because these are the main academic disciplines that study food in relation to context. Readers, however, are encouraged to explore the literature about food.

In the cognitive theory of cultural meaning, Strauss and Quinn (1997) described how meanings are acquired through life experiences (and therefore are shared among people), while the nature of connections or maps in the brain allows for idiosyncratic variations and change throughout a person's life. In terms of human development, this theory suggests that children's life experiences are the main source of the meanings they attach to activities. Children's life experiences largely are determined by their primary caregivers, typically their parents. In turn, caregivers live in particular temporal, psychological, social, symbolic, cultural, ethnic, and spiritual contexts. These contexts shape their life experiences and their roles as caregivers, and they socialize their children into what they assume will be the children's future life contexts. If they assume that their children's life contexts will be the same as theirs, their children's socialization will reflect their own life experiences; on the other hand, they might correct those experiences that they think need to be changed. If caregivers want their children to have a different array of life contexts, they can socialize their children into making changes. For example, it is not uncommon among first-generation immigrants to encourage their children to become good students and to study for high-paying professions as a way of changing their socioeconomic context. Such encouraging is possible, according to this theory, because people are capable of willful change of their brain mapping.

In addition to parents, society and culture shape children's experiences by sanctioning what environments are appropriate for children and at what ages. With increasing experiences of the same activity in different contexts, the richer the understanding of meanings becomes. That is, eating in various contexts teaches children that hunger can be satisfied with different kinds of food and in different situations. They also learn that there are foods other than the food served at home, and some of the foods they will like better than the ones served regularly (e.g., junk food). Additionally, children learn that different contexts also mean different experiences (e.g., birthday parties, holiday meals).

As children grow up, not only do the environments that they frequent become more numerous, but also they spend their time in environments away from their families and with peers. At this point, activities carried out with peers acquire meanings without the parental ability to shape the experiences. Such experiences and meaning, translated into connections in the brain, contribute to the uniqueness of individuals. Each child or adolescent has fairly similar life contexts to those of his or her parents, yet each one participates in new and different contexts that are shared with peers. All of these lead to shared experiences across generations (with parents) and across cohorts (with peers), allowing the social scientist to study such groups' similarities and differences.

As adults, people are more consciously aware of their contexts and their limitations and how they relate to lifestyle and experiences. As adults, people have the power, as sanctioned by society, to raise and socialize their children as long as they do not violate certain limitations as defined by law (e.g., child abuse and neglect, avoiding schooling, child labor). As adults, parents can shape their children's contexts, thus constructing experiences and meanings for various childhood activities. Examples of such shaping include embracing one's cultural heritages by, among other things, the types of food served at home, thus supporting the development of tastes for ethnic food. Parents also may decide that they want to do just the opposite and not serve ethnic food but what is considered the general culture's food with the hope of assimilating their children into the larger society. Alternatively, parents may serve food that is not related to a particular culture but what is deemed at that time as the healthiest food appropriate for child development and health. In this case, children are socialized into the concept of food as a means to maintain health rather than as a means for cultural identification. In either case, these experiences are mapped in the children's brains, and they learn to identify the foods with the meanings presented at home. These different meanings associated with eating present as different occupations: Eating as cultural identity in which the taste of food, for example, is essential, and eating as a means for health in which the taste of food is not essential.

The sources of parental decisions about how to socialize their children, although coming from within themselves, are influenced by their life experiences. For example, if their social life involves participation in occupations with great cultural emphasis, it is very likely that they would emphasize food as a cultural identity.

In addition to parenting, adults participate in work life, which involves a different set of contexts in which experiences are new to begin with and become more familiar as one's career stabilizes. These experiences contribute to meanings that individuals assign to work. When a person enjoys work and the social environment at work, work will be an enjoyable experience and will be assigned a positive meaning. If the person does not like the work and the social aspect of it, the experience and meaning of work will be negative. In such cases, the person may accept this situation as a given and live with it, or he or she may decide to make a change. In the latter case, the individual decides that the experiences are not acceptable to him or her and embarks on a journey to try and make a change by changing work. That decision to change the experience and meaning of work, although done on an individual basis in which a person tries to change the mapping in his or her brain or the schema of what is work, also is related to the person's knowledge that there are people who enjoy work, a meaning that is part of some peoples' lives, a shared meaning that this person wants to share.

Summary

This chapter is about the commonality and uniqueness of occupations or the meanings that people assign to activities. These meanings typically are shared with one's reference group, which could be based on ethnic and cultural contexts. That is, meaning schemas are a general phenomenon that is shared among a group of people with similar life experiences. For example, when we encounter a person who belongs to a particular category (e.g., a mother of a child with sensory regulation disorder), we immediately surmise what her life experience is like and, therefore, guess at the meanings she attaches to particular activities with her child. We must be open, however, and listen carefully because we may be wrong. It is not enough to know what her experiences are like; we need to know what interpretations she gives to these experiences. These may or may not fit the schema that we developed over a long period of working with mothers like her. ■

Acknowledgment

A special thanks is extended to Kaitlin R. Jessing-Butz, who assisted in the preparation of this manuscript.

References

Abbott, A. D. (1988). *The system of professions: An essay on the division of expert labor.* Chicago: University of Chicago Press.

Albala, K. (2002). *Eating right in the Renaissance.* Berkeley: University of California Press.

Birch, L. L., Fisher, J. O., & Grimm-Thomas, K. (1996). The development of children's eating habits. In H. L. Meiselman & H. J. H. MacFie (Eds.), *Food choice acceptance and consumption* (pp. 161–201). London: Blackie Academic and Professional.

Campbell-Smith, G. (1967). *The marketing of the meal experience.* London: Surrey University Press.

Clark, F., Zemke, R., Frank, G., Parham, D., Neville-Jan, A., Hedricks, C., et al. (1993). The issue is—Dangers inherent in the partition of occupational therapy and occupational science. *American Journal of Occupational Therapy, 47,* 184–186.

Davidson, A. (1999). *The Oxford companion to food.* New York: Oxford University Press.

DeVault, M. J. (1991). *Feeding the family: The social organization of caring as gendered work.* Chicago: University of Chicago Press.

Douglas, M. (1982). *In the active voice.* Boston: Routledge & Kegan Paul

Duenwald, M. (2003, June 22). One size definitely does not fit all. *The New York Times,* Sec. 15, p. 1.

Ferry, J. F. (2003). *Food in film: A culinary performance of communication.* New York: Routledge.

Fieldhouse, P. (1986). *Food and nutrition: Customs and culture.* Dover, NH: Croom Helm.

Finkelstein, J. (1989). *Dining out: A sociology of modern manners.* New York: New York University Press.

Gillis, J. (1996). Making time for family: The invention of family time(s) and the reinvention of family history. *Journal of Family History, 21,* 4–21.

Grieshaber, S. (1997). Mealtime rituals: Power and resistance in the construction of mealtime rules. *British Journal of Sociology, 48,* 649–666.

Hasselkus, B. R. (2002). *The meaning of everyday occupation.* Thorofare, NJ: Slack.

Kantor, D., & Lehr, W. (1975). *Inside the family: Toward a theory of family process.* San Francisco: Jossey-Bass.

Kittler, P. G., & Sucher, K. P. (2001). *Food and culture* (3rd ed.). Belmont, CA: Wadsworth Thompson Learning.

Kramer, P., & Hinojosa, J. (1995). Epiphany of human occupation. In C. B. Royeen (Ed.), *AOTA self-study series: Lesson 8: Human occupation.* Bethesda, MD: American Occupational Therapy Association.

La Fontaine, J. (1986). An anthropological perspective on children in social worlds. In M. Richards & P. Light (Eds.), *Children in social worlds: Development in social context* (pp. 10–30). Cambridge, MA: Harvard University Press.

Lee, N. (2001). *Childhood and society: Growing up in an age of uncertainty.* Philadelphia: Open University Press.

Lewinsohn, P. M., Seeley, J. R., Moerk, K. C., & Striegel-Moore, R. H. (2002). Gender differences in eating disorder symptoms in young adults. *International Journal of Eating Disorders, 32,* 426–440.

Mennell, S., Murcott, A., & van Otterloo, A. H. (1992). *The sociology of food: Eating, diet, and culture.* Thousand Oaks, CA: Sage.

Merriam-Webster's concise dictionary of English usage. (2002). Springfield, MA.: Merriam-Webster.

Mosey, A. C. (1992). The issue is—Partition of occupational science and occupational therapy. *American Journal of Occupational Therapy, 46,* 851–853.

Mosey, A. C. (1993). The issue is—Partition of occupational science and occupational therapy: Sorting out some issues. *American Journal of Occupational Therapy, 47,* 851–854.

Nestle, M. (2002). *Food politics: How the food industry influences nutrition and health.* Berkeley: University of California Press.

Ochs, E., Taylor, C., Rudolph, D., & Smith, R. (1992). Storytelling as a theory-building activity. *Discourse Processes, 15,* 37–72.

Segal, R. (1999). Doing for others: Occupations within families with children with special needs. *Journal of Occupational Science, 6,* 53–60.

Shahar, S. (1990). *Childhood in the Middle Ages.* New York: Routledge.

Strauss, C., & Quinn, N. (1997). *A cognitive theory of cultural meaning.* New York: Cambridge University Press.

Vuchinich, S. (1987). Starting and stopping spontaneous family conflicts. *Journal of Marriage and the Family, 49,* 591–601.

Wilcock, A. A. (2003). Occupational science: The study of humans as occupational beings. In P. Kramer, J. Hinojosa, & C. B. Royeen (Eds.), *Perspectives in human occupation: Participation in life* (pp. 156–180). Philadelphia: Lippincott, Williams & Wilkins.

Wiseman, C. V., Gray, J. J., Mosimann, J. E., & Ahrens, A. H. (1992). Cultural expectations of thinness in women: An update. *International Journal of Eating Disorders, 11,* 85–89.

Wood, R. C. (1995). *The sociology of the meal.* Edinburgh: Edinburgh University Press.

Wyness, M. G. (2000). *Contesting childhood.* New York: Falmer.

4

Activity Analysis

Karen Buckley, MA, OT/L
Sally Poole, MA, OT, CHT

The concept that man must use mind and body to maintain health and well-being was documented as early as 2600 B.C. The ancient Chinese, Persians, and Greeks understood that a mutually dependent relationship existed between physical and mental health and well-being. Egyptians and Greeks saw diversion and recreation as treatment for the sick. Later, the Romans recommended activity for the mentally ill (Hopkins & Smith, 1978).

Many centuries later, in Europe and the United States, the use of activity and occupation was described as treatment modalities for people with mental and physical illness. In 1798, Dr. Benjamin Rush, the first American psychiatrist, advocated for the use of domestic occupations for their therapeutic value. Weaving, spinning, and sewing were occupations that he considered to be therapeutic because of their interest to the patients of the era and because of their social and cultural relevance (Dunton & Licht, 1957). In the 18th and 19th centuries in the United States, the use of occupations was accepted in the care of people with mental illness. In 1892, Dr. Edward N. Bush, superintendent of a psychiatric hospital in Maryland, wrote the following: "The benefits of occupation are manifold. Primarily, even the most simple and routine tasks keep the mind occupied, awaken new trains of thought and interests, and divert the patient from the delusions or hallucinations which harass and annoy him" (as cited by Dunton & Licht, 1957, p. 9).

In addition to the use of occupations in psychiatric treatment in the 18th and 19th centuries, early documentation shows that occupations were used to build muscles and improve joint range. In 1780 in France, Dr. Clément-Joseph Tissot, a physician in the French cavalry, described the beneficial use of arts and crafts and recreational activities to mediate the physical effects of chronic illness (Dunton & Licht, 1957). Tissot cited "shuttlecock, tennis, football, and dancing" (as cited in

Dunton & Licht, 1957, p. 9) as activities to promote range of motion for all joints of the upper and lower extremities. In this early literature about the use of occupations or activities, little description is available about the precise methodology used to select activities that addressed specific problems. Activities appear to have been selected for their cultural, social, recreational, and diversional characteristics.

In the early 1900s, occupational therapists embraced the arts-and-crafts movement that was a backlash to the social ills perceived to have resulted from the industrial revolution (Reed, 1986). The arts-and-crafts movement promoted a simpler life in which activities were performed at a slower pace than required by factory production, where the process was as important as the end-product, where the creative spirit was valued, and where the manual learning was valued rather than the intellectual learning alone (Reed, 1986). Before World War II, little literature indicated that therapists selected activities on anything other than intuition (Creighton, 1992; Reed, 1986).

At the end of World War I, two factors had a strong influence on occupational therapists' use of activities and related occupations. First, the end of the arts-and-crafts movement in the United States and Europe meant that many activities were not valued in the same way. Second, therapists found themselves treating patients who were exhibiting both physical and psychological trauma. Therapists began selecting activities on the basis of the patient's particular deficits and needs. They first carefully analyzed each patient's deficits and, using a problem-solving approach, determined which specific activity would be appropriate to address the deficit. Therapists used activities because of their characteristics, but no formal analysis was part of the therapist's treatment routine. Therapists and physicians, however, began to look beyond the profession of occupational therapy to gain knowledge about activity analysis.

In this early development of the occupational therapy profession, activity selection and subsequent intervention were influenced by at least two men outside the profession: Frank Gilbreth and Jules Amar (Creighton, 1992). Gilbreth, an engineer by training, studied jobs in order to identify the most productive and least fatiguing methods of job performance. His work, which was well accepted by industry, examined the worker, environment, and motion. While visiting hospitals in Europe to study physicians and how they work, he became acquainted with the research of Amar, a French physiologist. Amar had been commissioned by the French government to study how to effectively prepare wounded soldiers for reentry into the workforce, which he did by measuring the physiological requirements of many jobs. His work influenced Gilbreth by making him aware of the possibilities of applying motion studies to the reeducation of returning wounded veterans. Gilbreth presented his work at the 1917 annual meeting of the National Society for the Promotion of Occupational Therapy (NSPOT), leading to the eventual inclusion of this concept of analysis of activity into the field of occupational therapy. In 1919, activity analysis was incorporated into occupational therapy textbooks (Creighton, 1992).

The years between World War I and World War II saw the establishment of the American Occupational Therapy Association (AOTA), formerly NSPOT, and further development of the profession in general. The AOTA encouraged therapists to establish departments and to publish papers to help them do so. In addition, papers were published to assist therapists in the appropriate selection of activities. Crafts were the treatment activities of choice, although "crafts" included work-related and recreational activities (Creighton, 1992). In 1922 and 1928, AOTA published papers promoting the analysis of crafts for psychiatric occupational therapy and for physical restoration.

World War II propelled women out of the home and into the workforce and propelled occupational therapists from traditional roles to new real-life circumstances. Resulting from improvement in medical and surgical care, veterans were surviving severe physical injuries and living with permanent disability. Occupational therapists began to specialize in the practice area of physical disabilities. Again, occupational therapists referred to Gilbreth's work, now being carried on by his wife Lillian, who proposed that engineers and rehabilitation professionals work together to assist soldiers with disabilities (Creighton, 1992). At the same time, the U.S. Army developed its own manual of therapeutic activities (War Department, 1944) that detailed activities to use to improve joint range of motion and strengthening of all extremities. The military, in fact, "divided" the body so that occupational therapists worked with the upper body and physical therapists worked with the lower body (Hinojosa, 1996). Many policies and procedures laid down by the military were and still are followed by the profession.

Immediately after World War II in 1947, Dr. Sidney Licht, who at that time was president of the American Congress of Rehabilitation Medicine and the editor of *Physical Medicine Library*, published a paper advocating the use of a more precise method for analyzing activity for those occupational therapists working in physical disabilities. He believed that craft analysis looked at "psychomotor values, economic factors, tempo, or other inherent characteristics" (Licht, 1947, p. 75). When the tools or activities, however, were to be analyzed for the motions involved, he coined the term *kinetic analysis*. Many of Licht's ideas continue to influence practice in the area of physical disabilities. Contemporary occupational therapists who are concerned about muscle contractions, joint range of motion, precision and accuracy of intervention, ergonomics of body mechanics, and control variants are continuing to use the criteria for examining motion that Licht originally proposed for kinetic analysis.

Occupational therapists in physical medicine appear to have become interested in activity analysis before therapists working in the area of mental health. In 1948, Gail Fidler proposed that occupational therapists working in psychiatric occupational therapy use scientific analysis of activities:

> While the functioning of a personality is certainly not as quantifiable as a muscle, the use of activity for the psychiatric patient should be more scientifically allied with the principles of dynamic psychiatry and treatment objectives than it is at the present. (Fidler, 1948, p. 284)

Fidler also proposed an outline for activity analysis to help occupational therapists meet the goals or aims of treatment so that occupational therapy in psychiatry could, in fact, be elevated from diversion to the level of therapy.

Activity Analysis: Definition and Purpose

Activity analysis is the process of closely examining an activity to distinguish its component parts (Mosey, 1986). A careful examination allows a skilled occupational therapy practitioner to select the most therapeutic and appropriate activity from those activities available. A careful examination ensures that the activities that a practitioner selects are relevant and correspond to the client's needs. Originally in occupational therapy, activity analysis was rudimentary and focused almost exclusively on the product and not the process of analysis. Gradually, the process of analysis has become more important than the end-product. Today, activity analysis is an important tool that practitioners use to analyze activities and to examine the process and outcome of intervention. Activity analysis also plays an important part of deductive reasoning in whatever frame of reference or approach practitioners use with clients.

Activity analysis enables occupational therapy practitioners to determine an activity's therapeutic properties so that they can make an appropriate match between the interests and abilities of the client and the activity that will meet the client's health needs (Mosey, 1986) and established intervention goals. Llorens's (1993) definition of *activity analysis* exemplifies the broadened scope of our current thinking:

> a process by which the properties inherent in a given activity, task or occupation, may be gauged for their ability to elicit individual intrinsic and extrinsic motivation and to fulfill patient needs in occupational performance and performance components. Occupational therapists use activity analysis in activity selection for guiding and evaluating activity use by the patient (p. 199).

Without going through this process, practitioners cannot use activities therapeutically.

When completing an activity analysis, occupational therapy practitioners must keep in mind the total activity and the occupations underlying the activity. There are many approaches to analyzing activities. *Uniform Terminology* (AOTA, 1994) provided a framework for activity analysis that allowed analysis of the small foundational components without losing the whole. This taxonomy proposed that each activity be examined according to its fundamental small aspects under three general categories: performance areas, performance components, and performance context. The recently adopted *Occupational Therapy Practice Framework: Domain and Process* (AOTA, 2002) does not address activity analysis; instead, it focuses on the analysis of occupations.

Activity analysis can be approached from many perspectives, depending on the reason for the analysis and the specific focus of interest. Cynkin and Robinson (1990) proposed that occupational therapy practitioners begin an activity analysis with the performance context. Trombly and Scott (1977) proposed that performance areas be analyzed first. Hinojosa and Kramer (1998) argued that an analysis should begin in the area (performance component, performance area, performance context) that is most appropriate to the client and his or her needs. For example, a therapist who works in a hand therapy practice would begin with an analysis of the activity grounded in the performance components; hence, activities used in the clinic would be selected on the basis of how they address specific performance component deficits. An activity analysis should consider the person's present, past, and future occupations.

Occupational Therapy Perspectives on Activity Analysis

There is extensive literature in our profession on activity analysis. In occupational therapy professional education, much time is spent on activity analysis, that is, learning how to do it and learning the aspects of dividing an activity into its component parts. Traditionally, occupational therapy students learn to analyze an activity by focusing on the performance components that make up the individual tasks. This process of microanalysis often leads the student to not consider the whole activity and the context in which it is usually performed or the important occupation with which the activity is associated. As discussed, many forms related to activity analyses are based on *Uniform Terminology* and follow the outline of performance components, performance areas, or both. Students learning how to do activity analysis need to be able to identify more than just the fact that the component is functional; they need to know to what extent it is functional and the way it is functioning in the context of the activity being performed. The following section outlines such a process with a focus on an analysis that examines activities within the context in which they are performed.

Activity Analysis in Occupational Therapy

Occupational therapy practitioners have an organized conceptual approach to activity analysis. The activity is viewed as a whole, then an analysis is done to break it down into component parts. This section outlines one method of completing an activity analysis and was drawn from various sources within the occupational therapy literature. Many of the ideas presented have become common knowledge within occupational therapy. Hence, it is impossible to determine who originated the idea or concept (Allen, 1987; Ayres, 1983; Kremer, Nelson, & Duncombe, 1984; Llorens, 1973, 1986; Neistadt, McAuley, Zecha, & Shannon, 1993; Nelson, 1996; Pedretti & Wade, 1996).

An activity analysis begins with a description of the activity and each of its fundamental tasks, that is, the steps necessary to complete the activity. The occupational therapy practitioner describes the activity and how people perform it under usual circumstances. The following is a suggested framework for occupational therapy students and practitioners to follow when analyzing the component aspects of activities. Like many other activity analysis forms, this form is based on several documents, including the *Uniform Terminology for Occupational Therapy—Third Edition* (AOTA, 1994), the *Occupational Therapy Practice Framework: Domain and Process* (AOTA, 2002), and the *International Classification of Functioning, Disability, and Health* (ICF; World Health Organization, 2001).

The Activity

The occupational therapy practitioner describes the activity and how a person performs it under usual circumstances. When the analysis is used as part of an intervention, the practitioner should keep the whole person in mind, that is, how and why the activity is relevant to the person. The practitioner also appraises the activity relative to the context in which the client will perform it and the activity's associated performance areas.

In this section (see Appendix 4.A), we name the activity and describe the specific tasks (steps) required to perform it. Each step is identified in the order in which it is performed to complete the full activity and is described in detail. We then list the needed materials, tools, and equipment; their source and availability; and estimated costs. After identifying safety precautions and contraindications, we discuss the time needed to complete the entire activity. In this section we consider the following:

■   Is this an activity that must be completed in one session?

■   Is this an activity that can be performed over time?

■   Can the activity naturally be divided so that it can be performed over time?

■   Do the tasks (steps) in the activity require that it be performed over a period of time?

The Person

The activity is done by a person. Thus, in the activity analysis, the occupational therapy practitioner must consider the person, including his or her values, interests, and goals. In this section of the analysis form, we discuss the personal aspects that define the activity.

VALUES

Identify ideas or beliefs that are important to self and other. Which of the following features potentially influence the person's participation or engagement in the activity?

■   The person's inferred personal value for the activity

■   Presence, dissent, degree, and type

■   The person's underlying meaning associated with the activity

■   The person's perceived purpose of the activity

■   How the activity relates to the person's goal

■   The extent to which the activity is seen as having social relevance and is socially accepted (e.g., family, peers, financial benefit)

- Inherent praise or rewards associated with the activity

- The activity's ability to meet a desired need

- The activity's ability to promote independence or self-reliance

- Whether participation in the activity results in personal qualification or enjoyment

- Whether the activity presents a personal challenge

- Whether participation in the activity will result in a desired personal change

- Whether participation in the activity will assist in attaining a personal long-term goal.

INTERESTS

Identify mental or physical activities that create pleasure and maintain attention.

- How does the activity stimulate the person?

- Is it repetitive?

- Does it offer an appropriate degree of challenge (e.g., cognitive, motor)?

- Is there variety in the activity?

- What are possible attractions for wanting to participate in the activity?

- What are the positive feelings associated with this activity (e.g., physical challenge, fellowship with others, intellectual challenge, demonstration of capacity or creativity)?

We begin by identifying the roles that might be associated with the activity and determine the relevance and meaningfulness to past, present, and future roles. The analysis can be used to identify whether the activity incorporates skills that can be associated with a desired role. The practitioner also appraises the activity relative to the context in which the client will perform it, considering physical, social, and temporal aspects.

Performance Components

The ICF is concerned about people's ability to participate in activities and society. Its taxonomy divides into two broad categories: (a) functioning and disability and (b) contextual factors. According to the ICF, functioning and disability include two components: (a) body function and structures and (b) activities and participation. Contextual factors include personal factors and environmental factors that influence performance of the activity and the level of participation. Using these broad categories, the following activity analysis uses performance components and component elements (AOTA, 1994) and the more global structure of the ICF taxonomy as a framework for analysis. The ICF taxonomy is not used in its entirety but is limited to categories that were determined to be most relevant to the process of activity analysis.

The ICF taxonomy provides a broad structure for the analysis and the basis for identifying basic requirements of the activity. The occupational therapy practitioner identifies whether a specific skill is necessary during the performance of the activity (yes or no). A response of yes indicates that the performance components will need to be focused on the subsequent sections of the analysis form. On the basis of the performance components (AOTA, 1994), the occupational therapy practitioner assesses the level of influence that each component has on the client's ability to do the activity. In other words, what kinds of effects do the performance components have on the activity? Eventually, the practitioner must understand how a deficit in a performance component affects or challenges the client to complete the activity. Another reason for analyzing an activity is so that potential for providing stimulation or opportunities to use the specific performance component element are elicited. A five-point scale is used to rate the influence of each component as follows:

0   The component has no effect or influence on the ability to do the activity.

1   The component has only a minimal effect or influence on the ability to do the activity. The activity would not substantially stimulate or address the performance component element.

2   The component has a moderate effect or influence on the ability to complete the activity. If a client has a deficit, compensation may have to be made for the client to perform the activity. The activity would present a challenge to the performance component element.

3   The component has a significant effect or influence on the ability to complete the activity. The activity would be extremely difficult to complete if the client has a deficit in this performance component. The activity would present a significant stimulation or opportunity to address the performance component element.

4   The component has a major effect or influence on the completion of the activity. A performance component deficit in this area would seriously influence the person's ability to do the activity. Such a person would be very likely not to be able to complete the activity. The activity would present a major stimulation or opportunity to address this performance component element.

The observation section is used to describe special circumstances or concerns and provides a space to include any other comments a practitioner has relative to the influence of the performance component on completion of the activity.

In the following section, each performance component is defined and several questions are provided to help occupational therapy practitioners understand the role the performance component has in completing the activity. The questions should not be considered definitive but rather as a jumpstart when considering each performance component. After considering each question, the occupational therapy practitioner rates the influence and writes observational notes (see Appendix 4.A).

Performance component	
Level of Influence	Observations:
☐ 0 ☐ 1 ☐ 2 ☐ 3 ☐ 4	

LEARNING AND APPLYING KNOWLEDGE

Knowledge is what is learned. Learning is based on thinking, solving problems, and making decisions. Learning also is influenced by sensory experiences. Activities are about applying knowledge for a meaningful outcome. The first step to examining this aspect of the activity is to consider what the activity requires the person to do. This screening gives the occupational therapy practitioner guidance about which components need to be analyzed further. Answering the following questions guides practitioners to the next step of the analysis:

■ Does the activity require *watching* (using the sense of seeing intentionally to experience visual stimuli, such as watching a sporting event or children playing)? The prerequisite performance component to be examined is visual reception.

■ Does the activity require *listening* (using the sense of hearing intentionally to experience auditory stimuli, such as listening to music or a lecture)? The prerequisite performance component to be examined is auditory.

■ Does the activity require *other purposeful sensing* (using the body's other basic senses intentionally to experience stimuli, such as touching and feeling textures, tasting sweets, or smelling flowers)? The prerequisite performance components to be examined are tactile, proprioceptive, vestibular, olfactory, and gustatory.

Occupational therapy practitioners also analyze activities in relation to the *sensory processing demands*. A person's central nervous system processes sensory information and integrates this information so that the person can make an adaptive response. Sensory processing is the internal mechanism a person uses to process and respond to sensory input. It may influence the client's ability to reach a calm state of alertness and, thus, influence his or her ability to engage in and complete the activity. Each activity presents unique sensory processing requirements. Thus, the ability to organize and integrate multiple sensory processes during performance of an activity is critical (adequate response).

Sensory Processing

Using an internal mechanism to process and respond to sensory input.

- Does the activity require the person to make changes based on sensory input?

- Does continuity of performance depend on the ability to proceed based on sensory input?

- Is the ability to cease performance based on sensory processing (e.g., physical discomfort, a problem with the activity)?

- What degree of sensory modulation is required?

- Is response to the sensory input important to activity performance?

- Will an aversive response influence the performance (e.g., defensiveness)?

- Will a diminished response influence the activity?

Visual Reception

Interpreting stimuli through the eyes, including peripheral vision, acuity, and awareness of color and pattern.

- Does the activity require the person to fixate on a stationary object (visual fixation)?

- Does the activity require slow, smooth movements of the eyes in order to maintain fixation on a moving object (visual tracking)?

- Must the person rapidly change fixation from one object in the visual field to another (scanning) (e.g., locating a misplaced utensil during cooking, locating a dropped object while performing a sport)?

- What degree of discrimination of fine detail is required to do the activity?

- What degree of accommodation is required?

- Does the activity require changes in focus as in near to far?

Auditory

Interpreting and localizing sounds and discriminating background sounds.

- Does the activity require the person to listen to sounds and interpret their meaning (e.g., musical notes, verbal instructions, verbal communication, warning sounds [alarm buzzers])? Are there functional sounds that assist the person in monitoring the environment (e.g., water running, frying, opening sounds, traffic, closing sounds)?

- Does the activity produce loud or harsh sounds during performance (e.g., hammering, power tools)? Could these sounds be stressful to a person?

■ Does the activity environment require the person to discriminate or suppress background sounds?

■ Does the activity require attention to soft sounds or low tones (degree of auditory detail and auditory processing) (e.g., instructions, commands, communication)?

■ Does the person use or rely on sound while moving (e.g., search for a source of sound and move toward it)?

Tactile

Interpreting light touch, pressure, temperature, pain, and vibration though skin contact and receptors.

■ Does the activity require the person to hold objects gently?

■ Is the amount of force and pressure important (e.g., Styrofoam cup, plastic cup)?

■ Are the materials used at room temperature, or do they require heat or cooling?

■ Does the activity require the person to appreciate vibration (e.g., electric tools that require control in relation to the vibratory responses)?

■ Does the activity require tactile discrimination?

■ Are body parts always within the visual field? When must a person rely on tactile input?

■ Could the tactile properties of the activity be perceived as noxious (e.g., defensiveness, overload, localization)?

■ Is the ability to localize tactile input part of the task?

Proprioceptive

Interpreting stimuli originating in muscles, joints, and other internal tissues that give information about the position of one body part in relation to another.

■ Does the activity stretch or compress joints and tissues (elongation, shortening, compression)?

■ Is weight bearing part of the activity (lower extremities or upper extremities)?

■ What is the degree of pushing, pulling, or lifting that occurs during the activity (gross or fine)?

■ Do movements and position of the extremities occur outside the visual field (reaching in or out)?

Vestibular Input

Interpreting stimuli from the inner ear receptors with regard to head position. Vestibular input contributes to appropriate righting and equilibrium reactions, automatic postural responses, and maintaining posture and movement during activity performance.

- Does the activity require quick rotational movements of the head or body?

- Does the activity require postural change in relation to gravity (acceleration and deceleration) (e.g., sit to stand, vertical and horizontal changes)?

- Does the activity require co-contraction?

- Does the activity require coordinated eye movements?

- Does the activity require postural background movements (e.g., adequate extension, ability to dissociate head, neck, and arm movements)?

Olfactory

Interpreting odors.

- Does the activity contain odors that might be interpreted as noxious?

- Does the activity involve odors that might be alerting (e.g., burning) or calming?

- How might the scents affect one who is hypersensitive to odors?

Gustatory

Interpreting tastes.

- Does the person need to interpret taste to enhance or contribute to performance?

- Does the taste or texture elicit an aversive response? An alerting and calming influence?

BASIC LEARNING

Basic learning encompasses the skill areas of copying and rehearsing. Answering the following questions guides practitioners to the next step of the analysis:

- Does the activity require *copying* (imitating or mimicking as a basic component of learning, such as copying a gesture, a sound, or the letters of an alphabet)? Prerequisite performance components to be examined are recognition, form constancy, spatial relations, and position in space.

- Does the activity require *rehearsing* (repeating a sequence of events or symbols as a basic component of learning, such as counting by tens or practicing the recitation of a poem)? The prerequisite performance component to be examined is sequencing.

Recognition

Identifying familiar faces, objects, and other previously presented material.

■   Does the person have to recognize people, body parts, and objects to engage in the activity?

Form Constancy

Recognizing forms and objects as the same in various environments, positions, and sizes.

■   Does the activity occur in two dimensions or three dimensions?

■   Does the activity require the person to respond to changing representations of objects?

■   Do the materials change form (e.g., laundry [folded clothes], cooking)?

■   Does the size of the tools, utensils, or letters change?

Spatial Relations

Determining the position of objects relative to one another.

■   Does the activity require the use of spatial concepts (manipulation, take apart, put together)?

■   Does the activity require that the person estimate sizes?

■   Does the activity require that the person judge distances or estimate size?

■   Does the activity require orientation of shapes, sizes, or designs?

■   Does the activity require attention to detail in positioning?

Position in Space

Determining the spatial relationship of figures and objects to self and other forms and objects.

■   Does the activity require the person to determine front, back, top, bottom, beside, behind, under, or over?

■   Does the activity require that the person understand the relationship between action and his or her body?

Sequencing

Placing information, concepts, and actions in order.

■   Does the activity require the person to arrange items in a serial order?

■   Does the activity require that the person perform steps in a serial order?

- Does the activity require an understanding of before and after?

- Does the activity require the person to reverse a sequence (backward) (e.g., don clothing, doff clothing; put a toy together, take it apart)?

- Does the activity allow for the person to have personal choice in the manner of sequencing (e.g., morning care, dressing, showering)?

ACQUIRING SKILLS

Engaging in an activity creates situations in which people gain skills. Skills are the sets of actions that a person has learned and is able to apply in given situations. Skills often are divided into basic and complex skills. *Basic skills* are elementary, purposeful actions, such as learning to manipulate eating utensils, a pencil, or a simple tool. *Complex skills* are integrated sets of actions to follow rules and to sequence and coordinate movements, such as learning to play games like football or to use a building tool. Answering the following questions guides practitioners to the next step of the analysis:

- Occupational therapy practitioners often must assess a person's cognitive abilities before determining his or her capacity to learn or *apply knowledge*. Does the activity require the participant to focus intentionally on specific stimuli, such as by filtering out distracting noises? Prerequisite performance components to be examined are level of arousal, orientation, and attention span.

- Does the person have adequate *skills* to support the efficient completion of the activity? Prerequisite performance components to be examined are motor control, praxis, body scheme, fine motor coordination and dexterity, crossing the midline, right–left discrimination, laterality, bilateral integration, and visual–motor integration.

- When engaged in the activity, what *thinking* processes (formulating and manipulating ideas, concepts, and images, whether goal-oriented, either alone or with others, such as creating fiction, providing a theorem, playing with ideas, brainstorming, meditating, pondering, speculating, or reflecting) does the activity require the person to use? Prerequisite performance components to be examined are memory, categorization, spatial operations, generalization, and concept formation. *Note.* Occupational therapists often must assess a person's cognitive abilities before determining his or her capacity to learn or apply knowledge.

- *Solving problems* requires that a person find solutions to problems or challenges to complete the activity. Simple problems involve a single issue or question. Solving complex problems requires that the individuals doing the activity consider multiple and interrelated issues or several related problems. To solve problems related to activities, people must identify and analyze issues, develop solutions, evaluate potential effects of the solutions, and execute the chosen solution. Prerequisite performance components to be examined are learning and memory.

■ *Making decisions* requires choosing among options, implementing the choice, and evaluating the effects of the choice, such as selecting and purchasing a specific item or deciding to undertake and undertaking one task from among several tasks that need to be done. Prerequisite performance components to be examined are memory, concept formation, categorization, and generalization.

Level of Arousal

Demonstrating alertness and responsiveness to environmental stimuli.

■ Does the time of day influence the person's arousal level?

■ What arousal level is needed to provide an adequate length of time to complete the activity?

■ Do fatigue and pain factors affect arousal level and ability to attend to task?

Orientation

Identifying person, place, time, and situation.

Orientation to person:

■ Does the activity relate to lifestyle?

■ Is the task or activity associated with a role that is meaningful to the person?

■ Could the activity be influenced by the person's routines (e.g., clean the bathroom on Tuesday or clean the bathroom when it needs cleaning)?

Orientation to place:

■ Does the activity require the person to know where he or she is?

■ Is the activity associated with a place other than the present situation?

Orientation to time:

■ Does the person need to know the exact time and date to engage in the activity or task?

Orientation to situation:

■ What is the relationship between the activity and the person's environment and roles?

■ Does the person need to know where he or she is to engage?

Attention Span

Focusing on a task over time.

■ How long must the person attend?

- Is vigilance required (e.g., high demands, sustained)? For how long?

- Will the person be required to disregard other irrelevant stimuli?

- Does the activity require the person to shift attention (e.g., frying eggs, making toast, pouring coffee while cooking)?

Motor Control

Using functional and versatile movement patterns.

- Does the activity require repetition? If so, what kind (e.g., putting a puzzle together, catching a ball)?

- Do numerous joints need to be controlled during the activity (degrees of freedom)?

- Does the activity require the person to inhibit movements to be most efficient (e.g., children using scissors)?

- Does the activity require constant or variable changes in speed of movement (e.g., dealing cards, playing jacks)?

- Is the pace of the activity externally or internally controlled?

- Does the activity require manipulation of tools or utensils (e.g., must control the tool as well as the limb)?

Praxis

Conceiving and planning a new motor act in response to an environmental demand.

- Does the activity require the person to assume a novel position (postural praxis) (e.g., yoga, martial arts, dance routines for the novice)?

- Does the activity require the person to plan movements that are not habitual?

- Does the activity involve the use of new tools or utensils?

- Does engagement require the person to have a plan?

- Is the activity new and unusual for the person?

Body Scheme

Having an internal awareness of the body and the relationship of body parts to each other. This component is closely related to kinesthesia and proprioception because it requires integration of sensation from muscles and joints.

- Does the activity require that the person have an appreciation for his or her body and be able to sense how the different parts work together (e.g., playing basketball)?

■ Does the activity require the person to have an internal awareness of body actions that must happen in a specific sequence (e.g., ballroom dancing)?

Fine Motor Coordination and Dexterity

Using small muscle groups for controlled movements, particularly in object manipulation.

■ What degree of isolated finger use is required?

■ How many grasp patterns are used during different functions (hook, cylindrical, spherical, three-jaw tripod, lateral pinch, tip-to-tip pinch, tripod)?

■ Does the activity require in-hand manipulation skills?

Visual–Motor Integration

Coordinating the interaction of information from the eyes and body movement.

■ What degree of eye–hand or eye–foot coordination is required (e.g., tracing, copying, pencil tasks, balance beam)?

Crossing the Midline

Moving the limbs and eyes across the midline sagittal plane of the body.

■ Does the activity require the person to scan the environment to find tools and utensils? If so, how frequently?

■ Does the activity require that the person cross the midline of the body with his or her arms or legs (e.g., dressing)?

Right–Left Discrimination

Differentiating one side from the other.

■ What degree of bilateral coordination is required to do the activity?

■ Does the person need to be able to use or apply right–left concepts?

■ Does the activity require that the person be able to follow verbal or written directions that require actions to the left, right, or both sides of the body?

■ Does the activity involve tools that require bilateral coordination and use of one hand as an activator and the other as an assist?

■ Does the activity require that the person differentiate right and left on another person (e.g., demonstrated instruction as in Aikido, karate, dancing)?

Laterality

Using a preferred or dominant hand or foot.

■ Does the activity or a task require a high degree of skill in which the person needs to use a preferred hand or foot (e.g., cooking, sewing, writing)?

■ Does hand or foot preference influence how smoothly or effortlessly the person performs the activity?

Bilateral Integration

Coordinating both sides of the body. Bilateral integration is considered a prerequisite for gross and fine motor coordination and affects acquisition of skills.

■ How frequently do both sides of the body have to cooperate during the activity?

■ Does one side of the body need to stabilize while the other side acts?

■ Does each side of the body simultaneously have to perform a different function (asymmetrical performance) during the activity?

■ Does the activity require that the person use both sides of the body in the same manner (symmetrical performance) (e.g., pushing, pulling)?

■ Does the activity require reciprocal patterns (e.g., bike riding, swimming, running, martial arts)?

Learning

Acquiring new concepts and behaviors.

■ Does the activity provide a structured learning experience?

■ Does the activity provide feedback about performance?

■ Is the activity an unstructured experience requiring spontaneous exploration?

■ What type of learning is expected (e.g., motor, verbal, feelings, attitudinal)?

■ Is the activity compatible with the person's learning style?

Memory

Recoding information after a brief or long period.

■ What are the memory requirements of the activity (e.g., immediate [1 minute], short term [longer than 1 minute, less than 1 hour], long term [more than 1 hour])?

■ If the activity requires long-term memory, what elements of long-term memory?

– Information related to personal experience (episodic)?

– Factual knowledge of the world (semantic)?

     −   Knowledge of the world or how to do something (procedural)?

■   Is the long-term memory modality specific (visual, auditory, verbal)?

Concept Formation

Organizing a variety of information to form thoughts and ideas. This component is related to the ability to categorize.

■   Does the activity require synthesis of ideas (e.g., formulate a hypothesis about the how or why)?

■   Does the activity require abstract thought processes?

■   Does the activity require symbolic thinking?

■   Does the activity require the person to question him- or herself or evaluate performance?

Categorization

Identifying similarities and differences among pieces of environmental information.

■   Does the activity require the person to group objects or information according to characteristics (e.g., visual features, tactile features, similarities, differences)?

■   Does the activity require mental grouping (e.g., playing cards, different name brands to be purchased, price differences, nutritional contents)?

■   Does the activity require construction where the person must understand how parts relate to a whole or how to break the whole down into its parts?

Spatial Operations

Mentally manipulating the position of objects in various relationships.

■   Does the activity require the person to mentally visualize different perspectives (e.g., two-dimensional diagrams, three-dimensional objects)?

■   Does the activity involve mental visualization of performance (e.g., how close one is to preferred performances)?

■   Does the activity require that the person visualize how the object or activity should look on completion (e.g., clothing on a hanger or self, how a table will be set for a dinner party, how a cake will look after baking)?

Generalization

Applying previously learned concepts and behaviors to a variety of new situations.

■   Can the activity be performed in different contexts (e.g., bathing at bedside, sponge bathing at sink, tub bathing)?

■　Does the activity provide opportunities to apply learned skills to a new situation?

GENERAL TASK DEMANDS

Completing an activity requires that people carry out simple or complex and coordinated actions. These actions are related to the mental, physical, and social components. Some actions are single simple tasks that are clearly defined or time limited, such as initiating a task or terminating the activity. Single complex tasks need to be carried out in sequence or simultaneously, such as arranging the furniture in one's home or completing an assignment for school. Further, activities are influenced by the persons who participate in them. Consideration of the following guides practitioners to the next step of the analysis:

■　A person's mental and physical status influence how he or she carries out *simple* or *complex tasks*. Prerequisite performance components to be examined are initiation of activity, time management, termination of activity, coping skills, and self-control.

■　Some activities are composed of *multiple tasks* that need to be carried out in sequence or simultaneously, such as preparing a multicourse meal, with each course requiring initiation and management of time. Space to prepare a salad, main course, and side dishes must be organized, and several tasks may occur together or sequentially. The salad and vegetables are washed together, and a sequence of peeling and chopping vegetables and salad ingredients may occur sequentially to complete the activity. Prerequisite performance components to be examined are initiation of activity, time management, termination of activity, coping skills, and self-control.

■　Simple tasks, complex tasks, and multiple tasks may be carried out *independently* or within a *group* setting. When tasks occur independently, prerequisite performance components to be examined are initiation of activity, time management, termination of activity, coping skills, and self-control. When tasks occur in a group, prerequisite performance components to be examined are social conduct and interpersonal skills.

Initiation of Activity
Starting a physical or mental activity.

■　Does the activity require a "self-start?"

■　Does the person have to plan the start (e.g., alarm clock)?

■　How motivating is the activity (meaningfulness, relevance)?

■　How would the psychological components affect this component?

Time Management

Managing "parcels of time" as they relate to the performance of tasks or activities. In this case, it is a prerequisite to attaining an acceptable balance of performance.

■   Does the activity require the person to plan and arrange time in order to complete the activity?

■   Is the activity performed in one session or over a number of sessions?

■   Are there set time restraints for portions of the activity (e.g., bake at 350° for 30 minutes)?

■   Is the activity part of a personal routine that has imposed time restrictions (e.g., morning care consisting of 10 minutes for shower, 10 minutes for dressing, and 10 minutes for grooming)?

■   Does the activity offer the opportunity to make choices about the use of time (e.g., a craft project where the detailing could require additional time because of increased interest or skill level)?

■   What degree of organization and timing is required?

■   Does the activity require an internal sense of time?

Termination of Activity

Stopping an activity at an appropriate time.

■   How engaging is the activity?

■   Can the person disengage at an appropriate time?

■   Is the activity rote and repetitive?

■   Is the activity self-limited?

■   What is the person's control over engaging in and disengaging from the activity?

Coping Skills

Identifying and managing stress and related factors.

■   Is this activity new for the person, or is it part of a personal repertoire?

■   Does the activity environment influence the perceived stress?

■   Does the activity provide an appropriate level challenge without promoting undue stress?

■   Are there aspects of the activity that might contribute to failure or perceived failure?

- Does the activity require "perfection," or is there a range of acceptable performance?

- Are there aspects of the activity that are externally controlled, or is the activity entirely internally controlled?

Self-Control

Modifying one's own behavior in response to environmental needs, demands, constraints, personal aspirations, and feedback from others.

- Does the activity, activity environment, or both provide for unexpected "glitches" (e.g., spillage, dropping of utensils or equipment, nonfunctioning appliance)?

- Does the activity incorporate constraints?

- Does the outcome of the activity lead to attainment of personal aspirations (goals)?

- Will activity performance be criticized? By whom (an authority figure, peer, friend, family member)?

- Does the activity challenge physical, social, or cognitive abilities?

Social Conduct

Interacting by using manners, personal space, eye contact, gestures, active listening, and self-expression appropriate to one's environment.

- In what type of situation does the activity occur (one to one, unstructured, parallel, structured activity group, structured verbal group [e.g., classroom, club, discharge-planning meeting])?

- Does the activity require cooperative behavior?

- What are the accepted personal boundaries of the activity (e.g., sport, card table)?

- Does the activity require appropriate interaction with an authority figure?

- Does the activity require the person to initiate and sustain logical conversation?

- Does the activity require the person to assert him- or herself appropriately (e.g., ask questions, make comments)?

- Does the activity offer an opportunity for the person to receive a negative response from others?

Interpersonal Skills

Using verbal and nonverbal communication to interact in a variety of settings.

- Does the activity require independence, cooperation, or competition?

- What degree of verbal interaction is required?

- Does the person have to ask for assistance during performance of the activity?

- Does the activity require active verbal participation?

- Does the activity require expression of emotions?

- Does the activity require casual conversation?

- Does the activity require specific nonverbal behavior, appropriate sitting posture (open, relaxed, formal subtle signs of active listening, changes in facial expression)?

- Could engagement in the activity result in criticisms?

- Does the activity require the person to assume an unfamiliar interaction style?

MOBILITY

Mobility is *changing body positions* or location by *transferring* from one place to another; by carrying, moving, or manipulating objects; by walking, running, or climbing; and by using various forms of transportation. Changing and maintaining body position may occur during performance of the activity. Prerequisite performance components to be examined are postural alignment, muscle tone, postural control, depth perception, and body strength. Answering the following questions guides practitioners to the next step of the analysis:

- Does the activity require changes in body positions?

- When completing specific tasks, must one get into and out of a body position?

- Does the activity require moving from one location to another, such as getting up from a chair to lie down on a bed and getting into and out of positions of kneeling or squatting?

- Does the activity require the person to change body position or maintain lying down, sitting, squatting, standing, kneeling, or bending?

- Does the activity require the person to move him- or herself from one surface to another?

- When completing specific tasks, must the person transfer?

- What kind of control does the person need to move from one surface to another?

Postural Alignment
Maintaining the biomechanical integrity among body parts.

- What degree of axial alignment does the activity require?

- Does the pelvic position change during performance of the activity (e.g., taking off shoes)?

- Does the activity require frequent changes in alignment (e.g., seated and reading, playing racquetball)?

- Does the activity require any rapid postural adjustments?

- What postures are needed to optimally perform the activity?

Observations and descriptions of specific changes in body position or the need to maintain positions should be noted. Describe any movement from one surface to another (transfer).

Postural Control

Using righting and equilibrium reactions to maintain balance during functional movements.

- Must alignment of the trunk and limbs be maintained?

- Does the position of the head change frequently?

- Must the person stabilize against the forces of gravity when engaged in the activity (lean forward, lean back, lean to the side)?

- Do changes in the base of support occur while engaging in the activity (two feet to one foot, sit to stand)?

- Does the activity require that the person be familiar with the demands of the activity so that he or she can anticipate the postural requirements?

- Does the activity have the potential for a sudden displacement of the center of gravity?

Depth Perception

Determining the relative distance between objects, figures, or landmarks and the observer and changes in planes and surfaces.

- Does the activity require the person to step down or up?

- Does the person have to make precise movements of the arms and legs to complete the activity?

- Does the person have to reach distances to acquire objects or complete activity?

- Does the person need to place body parts (e.g., foot, arms) in relationship to changing elements of the environment?

- Do aspects of the activity occur in different planes?

Body Strength

Degree of gross muscle power when body movement is resisted or is against gravity.

■ Is there sufficient muscle strength to perform the activity?

■ Does gravity influence the performance of the activity?

■ Does the activity require concentric, eccentric, or isometric muscle activity?

■ Where is strength needed (upper extremities, lower extremities, trunk)?

CARRYING, MOVING, AND HANDLING OBJECTS

Completing many activities requires that a person be able to handle, move, and manipulate objects with his or her upper extremities and hands. These movements may be gross motor, fine motor, or a combination of both. Sometimes, the actions required are small, demanding, intricate, coordinated finger movements. Other actions require lower-extremity strength and control. Answering the following questions guides practitioners to the next step of the analysis:

■ Are any of the following *upper-extremity movements* done while performing the activity: pulling; pushing; reaching; coordinated, turning or twisting hands or arms; throwing; or catching? Prerequisite performance components to be examined are range of motion, strength, and endurance.

■ Must the person move and manipulate objects with his or her upper extremities? Prerequisite components for *upper-extremity control* to be examined are range of motion, strength, endurance, stereognosis, kinesthesia, and figure–ground perception.

■ Must the person *walk* or use his or her *lower extremities* to complete the activity? Prerequisite performance components to be examined are range of motion, strength, endurance, and topographical orientation (walking).

Range of Motion

Moving body parts through an arc. Most activities that involve a physical action require some degree of active range of motion.

■ Are there any soft-tissue conditions that would affect range of motion (hyper- or hypomobility)?

■ Which joints are positioned statically, and which joints are active during the activity?

■ What degree of movement is required during the activity (beginning range, middle range, end range)? This can become very detailed in worker rehabilitation or biomechanical approach.

■   What movements are required of the head, neck, trunk, and limbs during the activity?

■   Does the activity or any task require the person to control movements at multiple joints (e.g., swinging a bat [shoulder, elbow, wrist, and hand])?

Strength

Degree of gross muscle power when body movement is resisted or is against gravity.

■   Is there sufficient muscle strength to perform the activity?

■   Does gravity influence the performance of the activity?

■   Does the activity require concentric, eccentric, or isometric muscle activity?

Endurance

Sustained cardiac, pulmonary, and musculoskeletal exertion over time.

■   What is the duration of the activity (time)?

■   What degree of exertion is required to perform the activity under "normal" conditions?

■   How repetitive is the activity?

■   Are portions of the activity resistive?

■   What is the fatigue level on completion?

Stereognosis

Identifying objects through proprioception, cognition, and the sense of touch.

■   Does the activity require the hands or feet to identify or manipulate objects without reliance on the sense of vision (e.g., reaching into a bag to find specific objects related to a task, reaching into a pocket to find a coin, reaching into a drawer)?

■   Do aspects of the activity require visual vigilance that may require the person to find, manipulate, or reach for objects outside the visual field (e.g., sewing on a machine, use of machinery)?

Kinesthesia

Identifying the excursion and direction of movement.

■   Does the activity require movements to be coordinated over multiple joints (e.g., shoulder, elbow, wrist, fingers)?

■   Does the activity require visual vigilance so that the person must rely on this ability to execute a variety of movements without the aid of vision (e.g., swinging a bat at a baseball, playing tennis, playing basketball)?

■ Does the activity require the person to change directions of movements (quick, slow, precise) (e.g., fingers during typing)?

Figure–Ground Perception

Differentiating between foreground and background forms and objects.

■ Does the activity require that the person be able to select an object or image from a competing condition (e.g., word search games, finding hidden objects)?

■ Does the activity require that the person be able to discriminate two-dimensional or three-dimensional figures to complete tasks?

■ Does the activity require that the person be able to discriminate objects from a cluster of objects (e.g., food in refrigerator, clothes in a closet, an object in a junk drawer)?

■ Does the activity require discriminating a figure or word from a page with multiple images?

Topographical Orientation

Determining the location of objects and settings and the route to the location.

■ Does the activity require the person to use maps or other guides?

■ Must the person be familiar with the surroundings to complete the activity?

■ Does the activity require the person to use verbal maps or directions?

■ Does the activity rely on the person's ability to identify visual landmarks or routes?

■ Does the activity require the person to use mental representation of surroundings (e.g., cognitive mapping)?

OTHER CONSIDERATIONS

Self-Concept

How one evaluates oneself as a person. Perceived self-efficacy, self-esteem, and self-concept are used interchangeably and are interrelated. Self-concept is how a person describes him- or herself and includes his or her beliefs, ideas, and attitudes about the self. How might this activity relate to the person's perceived self-efficacy?

■ Does the activity enhance the person's ability to deal with life events?

■ Does the activity enhance the person's ability to cope with the change that illness or injury presents?

■ Does the activity enhance the person's assessment of his or her own ability to change his or her life?

■ Does the activity enhance the person's satisfaction with a life role?

Self-Expression
Using a variety of styles and skills to express thoughts, feelings, and needs.

■ Does the activity allow the person to use a variety of skills to express thoughts, feelings, and needs?

■ What types of self-expression (verbal, written, artistic or creative) occur during the activity?

■ Does the activity provide the opportunity for imaginative play?

■ Does the activity permit different styles of "doing" (e.g., fast or slow tempo, temporal sequence, organization)?

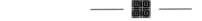

Exercise 4.1—Analysis of a Daily Life Activity

Consider the activity of frying an egg for breakfast or folding clothes. Think about the way that you normally do the activity. Follow the process outlined in this section. The purpose of this assignment is to appreciate that everything you do is potentially a therapeutic activity. Through the analysis you learn the component pieces outside the context of the real world of activities. In practice, occupational therapy practitioners perform activity analysis with consideration of the client's real activities, the context in which they are performed, and the meanings that the activities have for the client.

Activity Analysis Within the Context of a Frame of Reference

Activity analysis is a tool that occupational therapy practitioners use to determine the therapeutic potential of an activity and to analyze the activity for therapeutic purposes. As such, activity analyses provide the means for understanding the client and his or her ability to perform specific purposeful activities. Up to this point, activity analysis has been described as a process to examine or analyze specific activities. When activity analyses, however, are used within the framework of a frame of reference, a guideline for practice, or a conceptual framework, the framework provides the guidelines for the activity analysis. For example, if the occupational therapist is going to treat a client with left hemiparesis, the client will most likely have language skills intact. After screening the client, the therapist determines that the client's standing balance, postural control, and sitting balance are fair and that he has problems with upper-extremity motor control. On the basis of this information, the therapist determines that the neurodevelopmental treatment (NDT) approach is most appropriate to restore performance skills. Given that the client wants to dress himself, the therapist evaluates the client's performance of upper-body dressing, which is best done by having the client attempt to dress. The therapist then does an activity analysis of the way the client performs the activity, with special attention given to the client's neuromotor functioning.

Before observing the client attempting various activities, the therapist does an activity analysis of the typical performance of the various purposeful activities involved in upper-body dressing, which involves knowing the component demands of upper-body dressing. The demands of a shirt with buttons are different from the demands of a pullover shirt. In the case of the client with left hemiparesis where the NDT approach has been selected to guide intervention, the therapist attends to the motor and sensory demands of the trunk and upper extremities during dressing. The therapist uses the frame of reference to guide the focus needed as the client attempts to complete the activity.

Summary

The ability to analyze an activity competently is a critical piece in an occupational therapy practitioner's repertoire. Without the ability to analyze activities, the practitioner is left to use trial and error to plan and carry out interventions with clients. This chapter describes the development of activity analysis over the years, and no doubt there will be further development as the profession evolves. However, the ability to analyze the activity in the context of the person and his or her life will enable both the client and the practitioner to reach agreement on goals for the client. The chapter includes a comprehensive outline to approach activity analysis for the occupational therapy student and practitioner. Although the activity analysis may seem to be tedious and difficult to the beginning student, it is a process that gradually becomes integrated into a key aspect of clinical reasoning for practitioners as they use activities as therapeutic interventions. Additionally, although it may seem to a student or entry-level practitioner that activity analysis is not being done in reality the way that it is taught, occupational therapy practitioners integrate the process into their daily practices. ■

References

Allen, C. A. (1987). Activity: Occupational therapy's treatment method, 1987 Eleanor Clark Slagle Lecture. *American Journal of Occupational Therapy, 41,* 563–575.

American Occupational Therapy Association. (1994). Uniform terminology for occupational therapy—Third edition. *American Journal of Occupational Therapy, 48,* 1047–1054.

American Occupational Therapy Association. (2002). Occupational therapy practice framework: Domain and process. *American Journal of Occupational Therapy, 56*, 609–639.

Ayres, A. J. (1983). *Sensory integration and the child.* Los Angeles: Western Psychological Services.

Creighton, C. (1992). The origin and evolution of activity analysis. *American Journal of Occupational Therapy, 46*, 45–48.

Cynkin, S., & Robinson, A. M. (1990). *Occupational therapy and activities health: Toward health through activity.* Boston: Little, Brown.

Dunton, W. R., & Licht, S. (1957). *Occupational therapy principles and practice.* Springfield, IL: Charles C. Thomas.

Fidler, G. S. (1948). Psychological evaluation of occupational therapy activities. *American Journal of Occupational Therapy, 2*, 284–287.

Hinojosa, J. (1996). Practice makes perfect. *OT Practice, 1*(1), 34–38.

Hinojosa, J., & Kramer, P. (1998). Evaluation–Where do we go begin? In J. Hinojosa & P. Kramer (Eds.), *Occupational therapy evaluation: Obtaining and interpreting data* (pp. 1–15). Bethesda, MD: American Occupational Therapy Association.

Hopkins, H. L., & Smith, H. D. (1978). *Willard and Spackman's occupational therapy* (5th ed.). Philadelphia: Lippincott.

Kremer, A. R., Nelson, D., & Duncombe, L. W. (1984). Effects of selected activities on affective meaning in psychiatric patients. *American Journal of Occupational Therapy, 38*, 522–528.

Licht, S. (1947). Kinetic analysis of crafts and occupations. *Occupational Therapy and Rehabilitation, 26*, 75–78.

Llorens, L. (1973). Activity analysis for cognitive perceptual motor dysfunction. *American Journal of Occupational Therapy, 27*, 453–456.

Llorens, L. (1986). Activity analysis: Agreement among factors in a sensory processing model. *American Journal of Occupational Therapy, 40*, 103–110.

Llorens, L. (1993). Activity analysis: Agreement between participants and observers on perceived factors in occupation components. *Occupational Therapy Journal of Research, 13*, 198–211.

Mosey, A. C. (1986). *Psychosocial components of occupational therapy.* New York: Raven.

Neistadt, M., McAuley, D., Zecha, D., & Shannon, R. (1993). An analysis of a board game as a treatment activity. *American Journal of Occupational Therapy, 47*, 154–160.

Nelson, D. (1996). Therapeutic occupation: A definition. *American Journal of Occupational Therapy, 50*, 775–782.

Pedretti, L. W., & Wade, I. (1996). Therapeutic modalities. In L. W. Pedretti (Ed.), *Occupational therapy practice skills for physical dysfunction* (pp. 293–317). St. Louis, MO: Mosby.

Reed, K. L. (1986). Tools of practice: Heritage or baggage. *American Journal of Occupational Therapy, 40*, 597–605.

Trombly, C. A., & Scott, A. D. (1977). *Occupational therapy for physical dysfunction.* Baltimore: Williams & Wilkins.

War Department. (1944). *Occupational therapy.* Washington, DC: U.S. Government Printing Office.

World Health Organization. (2001). *ICF: International classification of functioning, disability, and health, Short version.* Geneva.

Appendix 4.A
Activity Analysis Form

Description of the Activity:

Tasks (Steps) Required to Perform the Activity:
1.
2.
3.
etc.

Materials, Tools, and Equipment (availability, cost, source):

Safety Precautions and Contraindications:

Time Needed to Complete: Hours: Minutes: Seconds:

The Person:
Roles:
- Present:
- Past:
- Future:

Relevance and Meaningfulness to the Person:
- Current:
- Past:
- Future:
- Values and Interests:
- Culture:
- Self-Expression:
- Self-Concept:

Context (interrelated conditions within and surrounding the client that influence performance):
- Physical (nonhuman environment):
- Social (significant people, social groups):
- Temporal (time):

Learning and Applying Knowledge

Activity Requires	Yes	No	Focus On
Watching			Visual reception, sensory processing
Listening			Auditory, sensory processing
Other purposeful sensing			Tactile, proprioceptive, vestibular, olfactory, gustatory, sensory processing

Sensory processing—using internal mechanism to process and respond to sensory input

Level of Influence	Observations:
☐ 0 ☐ 1 ☐ 2 ☐ 3 ☐ 4	

Visual reception—interpreting stimuli through the eyes, including peripheral vision, acuity, and awareness of color and pattern

Level of Influence	Observations:
☐ 0 ☐ 1 ☐ 2 ☐ 3 ☐ 4	

Auditory—interpreting and localizing sounds and discriminating background sounds

Level of Influence	Observations:
☐ 0 ☐ 1 ☐ 2 ☐ 3 ☐ 4	

Tactile—interpreting light touch, pressure, temperature, pain, and vibration through skin contact and receptors

Level of Influence	Observations:
☐ 0 ☐ 1 ☐ 2 ☐ 3 ☐ 4	

Proprioceptive—interpreting stimuli originating in muscles, joints, and other internal tissues that give information about the position of one body part in relation to another

Level of Influence	Observations:
☐ 0 ☐ 1 ☐ 2 ☐ 3 ☐ 4	

Vestibular input—interpreting stimuli from the inner-ear receptors regarding head position

Level of Influence	Observations:
☐ 0 ☐ 1 ☐ 2 ☐ 3 ☐ 4	

Olfactory—interpreting odors

Level of Influence	Observations:
☐ 0 ☐ 1 ☐ 2 ☐ 3 ☐ 4	

Gustatory—interpreting tastes	
Level of Influence ☐ 0 ☐ 1 ☐ 2 ☐ 3 ☐ 4	Observations:

Basic Learning

Activity Requires	Yes	No	Focus On
Copying			Recognition, form constancy, spatial relations, position in space
Rehearsing			Sequencing

Recognition—identifying familiar faces, objects, and other previously presented material	
Level of Influence ☐ 0 ☐ 1 ☐ 2 ☐ 3 ☐ 4	Observations:

Form constancy—recognizing forms and objects as the same in various environments, positions, and sizes	
Level of Influence ☐ 0 ☐ 1 ☐ 2 ☐ 3 ☐ 4	Observations:

Spatial relations—determining the position of objects relative to each other

Level of Influence	Observations:
□ 0	
□ 1	
□ 2	
□ 3	
□ 4	

Position in space—determining the spatial relationship of figures and objects to self and other forms and objects

Level of Influence	Observations:
□ 0	
□ 1	
□ 2	
□ 3	
□ 4	

Sequencing—placing information, concepts, and actions in order

Level of Influence	Observations:
□ 0	
□ 1	
□ 2	
□ 3	
□ 4	

Acquiring Skills

Activity Requires	Yes	No	Focus On
Applying knowledge			Level of arousal, orientation, attention span
Basic skills			Motor control, praxis, body scheme, fine motor coordination and dexterity, crossing midline, right–left discrimination, laterality, bilateral integration, visual–motor integration
Complex skills			
Thinking			Memory, categorization, spatial orientation, generalization, concept formation
Solving problems—simple			Learning, memory
Solving problems—complex			
Making decisions			Memory, concept formation, categorization, generalization

---

Level of arousal—demonstrating alertness and responsiveness to environmental stimuli

Level of Influence	Observations:
☐ 0 ☐ 1 ☐ 2 ☐ 3 ☐ 4	

Orientation—identifying person, place, time, and situation

Level of Influence	Observations:
☐ 0 ☐ 1 ☐ 2 ☐ 3 ☐ 4	

Attention span—focusing on a task over time

Level of Influence	Observations:
☐ 0 ☐ 1 ☐ 2 ☐ 3 ☐ 4	

Motor control—using functional and versatile movement patterns

Level of Influence	Observations:
☐ 0 ☐ 1 ☐ 2 ☐ 3 ☐ 4	

Praxis—conceiving and planning a new motor act in response to an environmental demand

Level of Influence	Observations:
☐ 0 ☐ 1 ☐ 2 ☐ 3 ☐ 4	

Body scheme—having an internal awareness of the body and the relationship of body parts to each other

Level of Influence	Observations:
☐ 0 ☐ 1 ☐ 2 ☐ 3 ☐ 4	

Fine motor coordination and dexterity—using small muscle groups for controlled movements, particularly in object manipulation

Level of Influence	Observations:
☐ 0 ☐ 1 ☐ 2 ☐ 3 ☐ 4	

Visual-motor integration—coordinating the interaction of information from the eyes and body movement

Level of Influence	Observations:
☐ 0 ☐ 1 ☐ 2 ☐ 3 ☐ 4	

Crossing the midline—moving the limbs and eyes across the midline sagittal plane of the body

Level of Influence	Observations:
☐ 0 ☐ 1 ☐ 2 ☐ 3 ☐ 4	

Right–left discrimination—differentiating one side from the other

Level of Influence	Observations:
☐ 0 ☐ 1 ☐ 2 ☐ 3 ☐ 4	

Laterality—using a preferred or dominant hand or foot

Level of Influence

□ 0
□ 1
□ 2
□ 3
□ 4

Observations:

Bilateral integration—coordinating both sides of the body

Level of Influence

□ 0
□ 1
□ 2
□ 3
□ 4

Observations:

Learning—acquiring new concepts and behaviors

Level of Influence

□ 0
□ 1
□ 2
□ 3
□ 4

Observations:

Memory—recoding information after a brief or long period

Level of Influence

□ 0
□ 1
□ 2
□ 3
□ 4

Observations:

Concept formation—organizing a variety of information to form thoughts and ideas

Level of Influence	Observations:
☐ 0 ☐ 1 ☐ 2 ☐ 3 ☐ 4	

Categorization—identifying similarities and differences among pieces of environmental information

Level of Influence	Observations:
☐ 0 ☐ 1 ☐ 2 ☐ 3 ☐ 4	

Spatial operations—mentally manipulating the position of objects in various relationships

Level of Influence	Observations:
☐ 0 ☐ 1 ☐ 2 ☐ 3 ☐ 4	

Generalization—applying previously learned concepts and behaviors to a variety of new situations

Level of Influence	Observations:
☐ 0 ☐ 1 ☐ 2 ☐ 3 ☐ 4	

General Task Demands

Activity Requires	Yes	No	Focus On
Simple task			Initiation of activity, time management, termination of activity, coping skills, self-control
Complex task			
Multiple tasks			
Independent performance			
Group performance			Social conduct, interpersonal skills

Initiation of activity—starting a physical or mental activity

Level of Influence	Observations:
☐ 0 ☐ 1 ☐ 2 ☐ 3 ☐ 4	

Time management—managing "parcels of time" as they relate to the performance of tasks or activities

Level of Influence	Observations:
☐ 0 ☐ 1 ☐ 2 ☐ 3 ☐ 4	

Termination of activity—stopping an activity at an appropriate time

Level of Influence	Observations:
☐ 0 ☐ 1 ☐ 2 ☐ 3 ☐ 4	

Coping skills—identifying and managing stress and related factors

Level of Influence	Observations:
☐ 0 ☐ 1 ☐ 2 ☐ 3 ☐ 4	

Self-control—modifying one's own behavior in response to environmental needs, demands, constraints, personal aspirations, and feedback from others

Level of Influence	Observations:
☐ 0 ☐ 1 ☐ 2 ☐ 3 ☐ 4	

Social conduct—interacting by using manners, personal space, eye contact, gestures, active listening, and self-expression appropriate to one's environment

Level of Influence	Observations:
☐ 0 ☐ 1 ☐ 2 ☐ 3 ☐ 4	

Interpersonal skills—using verbal and nonverbal communication to interact in a variety of settings

Level of Influence	Observations:
☐ 0 ☐ 1 ☐ 2 ☐ 3 ☐ 4	

Mobility

Activity Requires	Yes	No	Focus On
Changing and maintaining body position			Postural alignment, postural control, depth perception, body strength
Transferring oneself			
Observations and descriptions:			

Postural alignment—maintaining biomechanical integrity among body parts

Level of Influence	Observations:
☐ 0 ☐ 1 ☐ 2 ☐ 3 ☐ 4	

Postural control—using righting and equilibrium reactions to maintain balance during functional movements

Level of Influence	Observations:
☐ 0 ☐ 1 ☐ 2 ☐ 3 ☐ 4	

Depth perception—determining the relative distance between objects, figures, or landmarks and the observer and changes in planes and surfaces

Level of Influence	Observations:
☐ 0 ☐ 1 ☐ 2 ☐ 3 ☐ 4	

Body strength—degree of gross muscle power when body movement is resisted or is against gravity	
Level of Influence ☐ 0 ☐ 1 ☐ 2 ☐ 3 ☐ 4	Observations:

Carrying, Moving, and Handling Objects

Activity Requires	Yes	No	Focus On
Upper-extremity movement			
Lifting			Range of motion, strength, endurance
Carrying			
Upper-extremity control			
Fine hand use			Range of motion, strength, endurance, stereognosis, kinesthesia, figure–ground perception
Hand and arm use			
Moving objects with lower extremities			Range of motion, strength, endurance
Walking and moving			Range of motion, strength, endurance, topographical orientation

Range of motion—moving body parts through an arc	
Level of Influence ☐ 0 ☐ 1 ☐ 2 ☐ 3 ☐ 4	Observations:

Strength—degree of gross muscle power when body movement is resisted or is against gravity

Level of Influence	Observations:
☐ 0 ☐ 1 ☐ 2 ☐ 3 ☐ 4	

Endurance—sustained cardiac, pulmonary, and musculoskeletal exertion over time

Level of Influence	Observations:
☐ 0 ☐ 1 ☐ 2 ☐ 3 ☐ 4	

Stereognosis—identifying objects through proprioception, cognition, and the sense of touch

Level of Influence	Observations:
☐ 0 ☐ 1 ☐ 2 ☐ 3 ☐ 4	

Kinesthesia—identifying the excursion and direction of movement

Level of Influence	Observations:
☐ 0 ☐ 1 ☐ 2 ☐ 3 ☐ 4	

Figure–ground perception—differentiating between foreground and background forms and objects

Level of Influence	Observations:
☐ 0 ☐ 1 ☐ 2 ☐ 3 ☐ 4	

Topographical orientation—determining the location of objects and settings and the route to the location

Level of Influence	Observations:
☐ 0 ☐ 1 ☐ 2 ☐ 3 ☐ 4	

5

The Occupational Profile

Judy Urban Wilson, MA, OT

What we do and what we think about what we do make up who we are. We act, and we react. Sometimes, we choose a line of action. Other times, we act because we believe we can do nothing else. These daily actions are the occupations that define us, to ourselves and to others.

Health means access to and participation in these occupations. When we become disconnected from these occupations, our sense of who we are is at risk. Threats to our health as defined by our ability to engage in occupations include a sudden or gradual change in body structure, paucity in available occupations, or a change in context.

Occupational Profile Definition

The fundamental purpose of occupational therapy intervention is to ensure that a person can participate in meaningful life activities, or occupations (American Occupational Therapy Association [AOTA], 2002). Because the key features of occupations are their personal meaning, the specifics of the occupations vary from person to person. Occupational therapy intervenes to link a person to what defines him or her.

If the objective is to engage people in occupations, then the first responsibility of the occupational therapist is to identify what the client's occupations are. The occupational profile is the set of activities, routines, and roles that describe a person at one point in time. In practice, the occupational profile is the imperfect collection of data the therapist collects to try to capture the individual client's living occupational profile.

The occupational therapy literature has had an ongoing discussion on how to define *occupations, roles, activities,* and *lifestyles* (e.g., AOTA, 1997; Kielhofner, 1983, 1985, 1992; Kramer, Hinojosa, & Royeen, 2003; Nelson, 1996; Trombly, 1995). All

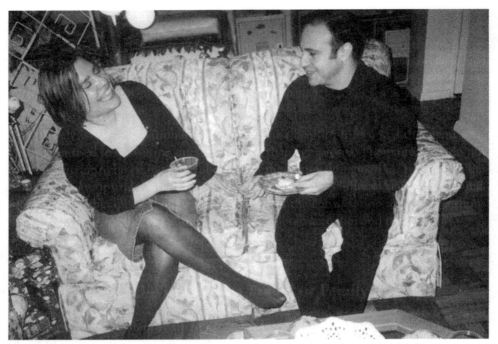

Figure 5.1. Some of the occupations we cherish most are those that we think of least as occupations. Deborah and Jeremy enjoy socializing with friends.

these terms express human action and try to capture their meaning to our lives. In practice, occupational therapists need to identify and analyze these terms in relation to each client. Recently, the AOTA defined the *occupational profile* in the official document, *Occupational Therapy Practice Framework: Domain and Process,* as "information that describes the client's occupational history and experiences, patterns of daily living, interests, values, and needs" (AOTA, 2002, p. 616). This is a lot of information. In fact, it is the person's whole life.

Biography, however, is not the occupational therapist's goal. The focus of the occupational profile is on the mundane rather than on the big events. The story of the person's accident itself or of his or her life accomplishments is relevant to the occupational profile for their effects on the person's roles and daily activities but not for the events themselves. During the evaluation, the therapist seeks specific features of the client's story. The therapist looks for descriptions of activities performed, patterns of behaviors, and where and with whom the client performs activities. Further, the occupational therapist examines data to determine what makes an activity meaningful or important to the client and, thus, identifies the client's occupations.

When a client seeks occupational therapy services, not all of his or her occupations are impaired, changed, or threatened. An occupational therapist delves more deeply into the areas that the client identifies as a problem or area of concern. The therapist uses the occupational profile process to obtain information that clarifies the

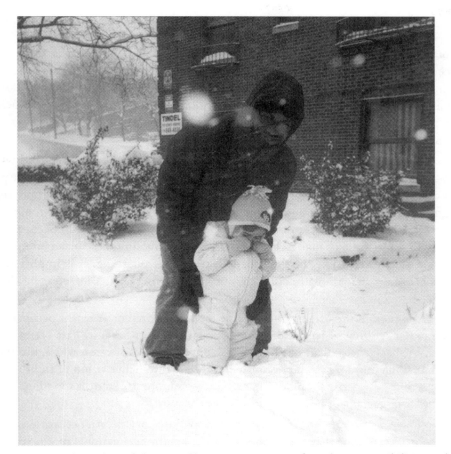

Figure 5.2. In his role as father, Mark's occupations stem from his responsibilities to keep Morgan warm and safe and to teach her new play skills in her first winter storm.

client's priorities, needs, and values. Data from the profile give the therapist a picture of the client as a real person in his or her own unique life, with his or her defining values, activities, and occupations.

Exercise 5.1—Personal Profile

What occupations make up your own profile? Which occupations are the most important to you? Why? Pick one occupation and list all the activities that it includes. Where do you perform these activities? With whom? What is unique about how you do these activities?

The Time Dimension

Obtaining an accurate occupational profile requires that the occupational therapist focus on present or recent occupations. These occupations are most relevant to the client's present sense of self and current circumstances. If illness or injury has caused an unfavorable change in activities or occupations, then the occupations just before the change make up the most critical profile. These occupations may reflect best the client's values, goals, ambitions, and aspirations.

Current occupations and activities are especially critical to understand when the client's present occupations form a negative sense of self, such as an abusive parent or a "helpless invalid." If the client is performing activities because of physical, cognitive, psychosocial, or environmental limitation, then the therapist must consider how these limitations influence the client's abilities to engage in occupations. If the client desires a change in these occupations, targeting these occupations may become a central goal of treatment. In all treatment planning, it is important to know current occupations because they are the starting points for creating therapeutic change.

Even though the occupational profile focuses on present or recent occupations, some understanding of past and future occupations is important. Past occupations helped to shape the present ones and are a source of experience on which the client can draw. In addition, it is important to appreciate the client's vision of future occupations. The past occupations and the future aspirations are sources for adjustments or renewals in occupations as the client moves forward.

Time is a defining dimension of any occupational profile. An occupational profile is not a job résumé that builds over time. Rather, the occupational profile is a continually morphing entity. Part of our challenge is to determine what spaces in the continuum provide the most relevant pictures of the person's occupations for planning interventions.

A person's roles and routines are shaped by past, present, and future. People's occupational profiles change as they mature and in response to life events. A child stops playing with toy trucks and becomes interested in baseball. A student graduate becomes a worker. A worker retires. A woman gives birth. An aunt becomes ill, and her niece takes her in. Each of these transitions would change the person's occupational profile. In some cases, the occupational therapist is working with a client who is transforming in response to some event that changed the client's occupational profile. The client was injured or got sick, which changes his or her pattern of daily life and daily activities. In other cases, the client comes to the therapist because of an unsatisfying or destructive condition that influences his or her occupational profile. Whether a client is changing because of a causal event or circumstances, a therapist must learn about the client's prior occupational profile, current occupational profile, and needs and wants to include in the profile for the future.

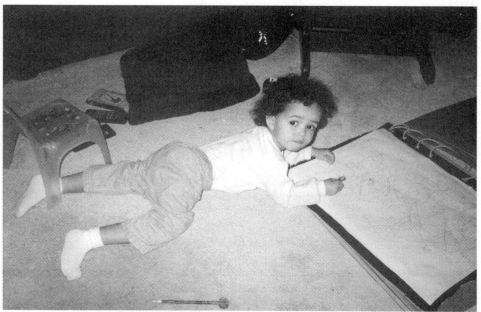

Figure 5.3. Two-year-old Morgan's consuming occupation of play is the means by which she gains new developmental skills.

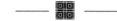

Exercise 5.2—Reflection on Personal Profile

Reflect again on your own occupational profile. When has it changed? What past occupations do you no longer have? What impact do these prior occupations have on your present occupations? What occupations do you aspire to in the future? Do these aspirations shape any of your present occupations?

_____

Case Scenario

For each of the following cases, which time period in the clients' occupational profiles should be the strongest focus for the therapist for treatment planning? Why?

Maria is an 11-year-old girl who broke her radius playing soccer in her town league. She is in sixth grade and has applied to a specialized science school for next year. She has several neighborhood friends with whom she plays on weekends. Maria lives with her mother and little brother. Her dad disappeared 2 years ago.

Maureen is an 87-year-old woman with depression who was referred to a day psychiatric treatment program. She has been a widow for 30 years and retired 2 years ago from her work as a secretary. After retirement, she moved away from where she had lived her whole life, leaving friends and sisters, to move in with her daughter and son-in-law in another state. Maureen now watches a little television, knits, and tries to help her daughter around the house. She reports that her relationship with her daughter has become very strained.

Alex is a 4-year-old boy with severe developmental delays. He lives with his two parents, a 1-year-old brother and 6-year-old sister. His siblings play with him on the mat in the playroom. He has an adapted highchair in which his mom and dad feed him. They transport him in an adapted stroller. Mom hopes to start Alex in the town's mainstreamed school system next year.

Data Collection

The process of gathering the information that forms the occupational profile is time consuming and lengthy. It begins at the moment of meeting the client and continues throughout the span of the occupational therapy intervention. An evaluation generally starts with an interview. Much of the most important data the therapist learns, however, the client does not share until rapport is established. So, the intervention plan changes as the intervention goes along.

INTERVIEW

The therapist continually refines interviewing as he or she interacts with clients and other professionals. As occupational therapy students, we learn the fundamentals of good interviewing. The key to good interviewing skills is not in the questions but in effective listening. From listening closely to what the client says, the therapist decides what questions to ask. Once the dialogue has begun, the therapist seeks clearer details and brings up topics to explore other areas. The therapist probes for clarification and understanding.

People are not used to being asked about exactly how they do every task in their day. Asked what they do in the morning, many answer that they get up and go to work. The occupational therapist however, wants and needs to know when clients get up, what kind of bed they sleep in, who is in the bed, where they go next, whether they wear slippers, and whether they brush their teeth first or drink their coffee first. The only way the therapist can learn this information is to ask clear, probing questions.

The therapist treating a client with a broken finger will ask more about how the client holds the toothbrush and squeezes the toothpaste and less about the bunny slippers. For the client with depression, however, the therapist would not care so much about the grip on the toothbrush but may focus on the time or the regularity of the tooth-brushing routine. The therapist uses clinical judgment and knowledge about the client's condition in shaping the interview.

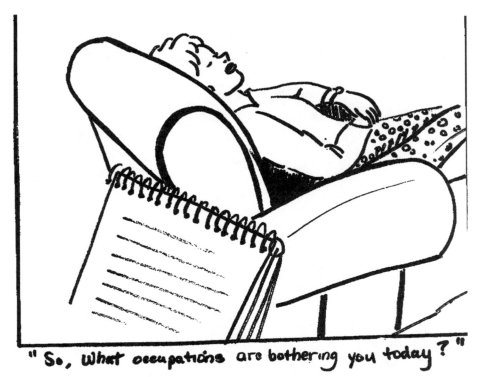

Figure 5.4. A cartoon that captures the complexity of activities included in human occupation.

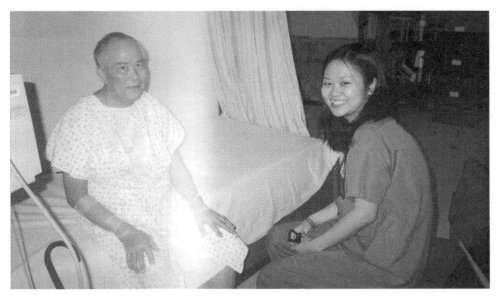

Figure 5.5. Occupational therapist Diana interviews Wing Ming as an essential tool in obtaining the occupational profile.

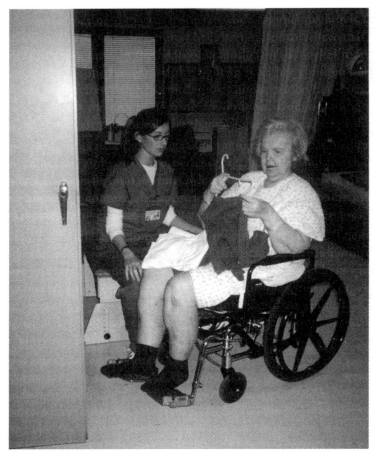

Figure 5.6. To prepare Margaret to go home, occupational therapist Danielle needs to find out the layout of her home, where she keeps her clothes, who puts them away, whether she stacks them or hangs them, and what she is open to changing.

Rarely is the occupational therapist the first health professional the client sees. Clients get used to answering questions about their symptoms. Therefore, they do not expect someone to be asking them about what they enjoy doing in their free time, what community groups they are involved in, and what responsibilities they have at home. Occupational therapists therefore need to refocus the conversation and ask questions in multiple ways to find out about the client's full life activities and occupations.

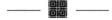

Exercise 5.3—Interview a Friend or Family Member

Interview a friend or family member about his or her present occupational profile. Do not interview an occupational therapy practitioner. Find out about the person's daily routines, his or her responsibilities, and what he or she does with regard to work and leisure activities.

––––––––––––––

Sometimes, simply asking the client is not effective. The client may be a young child, confused, or unable to communicate. In these cases, the therapist can usually turn to family members. Along with the therapist's own observation, the family has much more extensive experience with the client and can give a fuller description. In some cases, the family may be considered a client, and a therapist may work closely with the family to develop intervention priorities. A mother may want to be able to fit her daughter into a car seat to ease transportation to school. A son may worry about his elderly mother wandering into the kitchen and turning on the stove.

There are times, however, when a client cannot speak for him- or herself, nor can family or friends speak for the client. This scenario includes both clients who are unable to communicate and those who are resistive to treatment because of confusion or depression. In these cases, a standard interview will be unproductive. The occupational therapist becomes a puzzle solver who must piece together a hypothesized profile. This profile is constantly updated from the general social data available, from pieces of conversations with the client, and from the client's reaction to activities. Success, however, relies on the resistance waning as rapport builds during the treatment process.

––––––––––––––

Case Scenario

Ling Mei is an elderly Chinese woman who had suffered a severe stroke and who was found on the streets of Chinatown. In the inpatient rehabilitation unit, Ling Mei claimed that she was fine and asked that someone take her to the statue of Confucius where she could sit and panhandle "and I'll be fine." She had had significant frontal lobe damage impeding awareness and limited cognitive skills. Her resistance to formal testing impeded the accuracy of the neuropsychological evaluation. The occupational profile became especially critical when the occupational therapist needed to report to the team whether Ling Mei was ready to be discharged safely to the community.

Case Questions. Could Ling Mei resume her previous activities adequately without social support? What skills should the therapist consider as survival skills in the city? What occupations would you guess made up her profile recently? What activities would you try with Ling Mei to see how she responds?

––––––––––––––

PARTICIPANT OBSERVATION

When evaluating a client, a therapist often uses ethnographic techniques and skills. Whereas the goal of an ethnographer is to study an individual, the occupational therapist's goal is to use these techniques to obtain greater understanding of the individual as a person. The therapist begins to learn about the client and his or her life with a general interview to establish rapport and to get to know each other. After establishing rapport and becoming comfortable with the client, the therapist engages in participant observation. Participant observation is a research technique in which the researcher carefully watches people as they carry out activities or engage in activities with other people in order to learn about the people and their lives. Whereas the ethnographer values not influencing the research participants, a therapist enters into interactions with clients with the purpose of understanding the person so that he or she can develop appropriate interventions for change.

In the framework collaborative process model (see Figure 5.7), the occupational therapist, occupational therapy assistant, and client work together in the process of service delivery. The therapists and client jointly engage in the activities making up the intervention; therapists interact; and rapport builds. Even where rapport is difficult to develop, over time our interactions with each other, family members, and other professionals broaden the therapists' picture of the client and the client's abilities and areas of difficulty. As part of occupational therapy, therapists use activities pertinent to the client and to many in the client's personal context. This activity plan is the therapist's "fieldwork" from which observations are made.

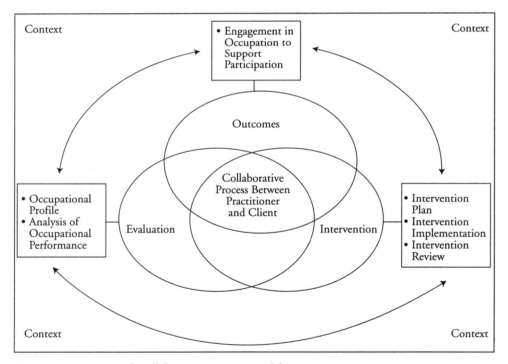

Figure 5.7. Framework collaborative process model.

Note. From "Occupational Therapy Practice Framework: Domain and Process," by the American Occupational Therapy Association, 2002, *American Journal of Occupational Therapy, 56,* p. 614. Copyright 2002 by the American Occupational Therapy Association. Reprinted with permission.

Participant observations provide the therapist with new details about the client's performance in context. They support or contrast with what the therapist learned during interviews and discussion with the client and his or her significant others. As the client chats with the therapist, he or she shares information that triggers new ideas and new questions from the therapist for a fuller occupational profile. A level of intimacy develops between client and therapist. As the relationship develops, the client may reach a point where he or she shares more personal and, therefore, vulnerable information.

While the therapist enters the world of the client, the client, through the shared experience of the intervention, is learning an occupational therapy perspective. As the client understands occupational therapy better, he or she becomes more self-directed in the process. A client may see him- or herself doing more activities and identify which activities he or she wants to work on next to pursue a valued occupation. The client may bring up an old hobby or a long-held aspiration as he or she perceives that occupational therapy may be able to help him or her do these occupations. Some clients take more of a partnership role during intervention. Some identify meaningful occupations and clearly understand the potential of the occupational therapy process. Others need more direction and may focus on specific activities without a clear understanding of how intervention relates to their occupations.

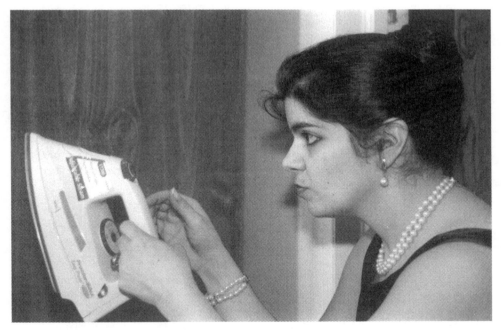

Figure 5.8. As a friend and bridesmaid, Alysia uses the occupation of ironing, even in pearls.

Case Scenario

Martha is a 40-year-old woman with major depression and a borderline personality who was referred to an outpatient psychiatric treatment program. On the initial interview with the occupational therapist (along with the chart review), she shared that since what she calls her "meltdown," she has been cutting herself and, as a result, is on leave from her job as a music teacher in the local school system. Her husband also is a local teacher. She has two daughters, one in college and one doing well in high school. She reported that when she was growing up, her mother had been domineering and emotionally abusive and forced her and her sisters to be performers all their lives. Martha had been sexually assaulted as a child and harbored a lot of anger toward her mother for never stopping or addressing the abuse. She describes herself as shy. Presently, Martha cannot tolerate crowds and is very uncomfortable around other people. The therapist observed that Martha's social interactions were stunted.

The initial treatment plan included relaxation techniques for social situations and to help manage anger in relation to her mother; building self-esteem, beginning with emphasizing her successes, such as her two daughters; coping strategies for interacting with her mother; and graded resumption of social activities, with the eventual goal of returning to work. Returning to work was especially difficult because in the small town everyone knew why Martha was on leave. She eventually did return to work. Another big success was attending a concert of her favorite singer.

After more than 1 year in treatment, small comments from Martha began to emerge while talking with the therapist, such as fear in her voice at the mention of bringing financial problems to her husband and complaining about cleaning mouse cages that her husband brings home from his classroom. At a program family event, the therapist noted that Martha was hyperattentive to her husband and that her husband seemed aloof. Additionally, others in the program complimented Martha on the town-wide children's concerts she once led, about which she seemed proud but reserved and reluctant.

Martha's confidence was growing, which allowed her to answer as the therapist began to question more about her marriage. Slowly, the therapist learned that Martha's husband was neglectful, emotionally abusive, and forced her into an introverted role in response to his high achievement. The treatment plan changed to focus on her developing occupations outside her marriage.

Over time, Martha began jogging daily; resumed playing the organ in church; made new friends; took on a caregiver role with her mother, who had suffered a stroke; played piano for the town Christmas show; and restarted the town-wide children's concerts.

Case Questions: Why could Martha discuss her marriage later in treatment and not in the beginning? How did this change the treatment plan? How did the revelation about her marriage change the meaning of her past occupation as performer? How might the revelation about her marriage affect her social relationships? What did the therapist observe about Martha's occupations through interaction in activities with Martha?

The occupational therapist often uses more advanced methods of data collection when constructing the client's developing occupational profile. During this process of advanced data collection, the therapist begins to use the information from the client's occupational therapy profile to influence intervention choices and approaches. As the therapist learns about the client's occupations and related activities, whether past or future, the therapist acknowledges occupations that are still attainable or are especially self-affirming. The therapist emphasizes activities that help the client to see his or her capabilities and encourages the client to actively choose what occupations he or she wants to set as goals. The discourse between the client and therapist is the first step in empowering the client to make changes for a healthier, fuller life.

As with all ethnographers, the occupational therapist brings to the process his or her own worldview. The therapist conscientiously considers what questions to ask. What is relevant? What does the therapist need to know for a fuller understanding of the client and his or her life situation? How does the client's culture influence his or her beliefs, values, and behaviors? Questions are derived from the therapist's interaction with the client, observation of the client, and interactions with the client's significant others. The therapist recognizes that his or her personality and interaction style influence interactions with the client and considers these data to further understand the client. The therapist knows that he or she is influenced by the theories and frames of reference used, by medical knowledge about the diagnosis and prognosis, by experiences with other clients, and by personal experiences and prejudices (Urban, 1998a, 1998b).

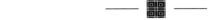

Exercise 5.4—Martha's Occupational Profile

In the case of Martha, how did the therapist use the occupational profile as a tool? Think about which occupations the therapist reinforced as part of the treatment plan. Which past occupations opened new occupations for her?

How Context Affects the Occupational Profile

An activity out of context loses its meaning. *Contexts* are the factors that are within the person or surround the person and influence his or her performance of activities and occupations. Contexts can be external or internal to the client. Internal contexts include the person's physical, social, and virtual realities. Internal contexts include the person's personal and spiritual beliefs. Context also can have time and space dimensions. Time dimensions are the time of day or the person's age. Space dimensions are the physical features, such as the size of the room (AOTA, 2002). The occupational profile identifies the contexts relevant to each activity. The contexts of an occupation are the primary elements that individualize them. The context shapes how the tasks are performed, where they take place, and how important they are.

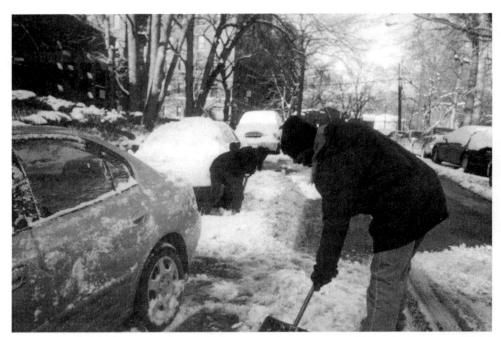

Figure 5.9. Mark does not enjoy shoveling snow, but it is part of his valued occupation of driving.

Self-care is an occupation in everyone's profile. Self-care, however, is different for everyone. A woman may need to wear nylons to work, another to church. One woman may wear sneakers every day; another may have been raised to believe that sneakers are unfeminine. One may dress in the bedroom, another in the locker room. One may believe that at her age she has earned the right to have her children help her dress. Another would go barefoot before admitting she cannot put on her shoes herself. The elements affecting just the task of dressing are limitless. Understanding the specifics relevant to the person are the critical data that give the occupational profile shape.

Context also influences the process of obtaining the occupational profile. Issues of class, social norms, and personal experiences of the client and the therapist shape the therapeutic relationship and, in turn, what information is shared. As the therapist learns more about the context, the approach may be adjusted. Sometimes, a clearer occupational profile will emerge as the therapeutic relationship develops.

Ultimately, the therapist must respect the gaps in the profile. The occupational profile obtained is never complete. What the therapist needs is identification of the occupations, with their contexts, that the person is willing to address with the therapist at that time. Less obvious is the occupational profile's impact on context. This perspective emphasizes that people are active forces in their contexts. Our occupations bring us places and link us to people. Through our occupations, we have the power to change our physical and social environments.

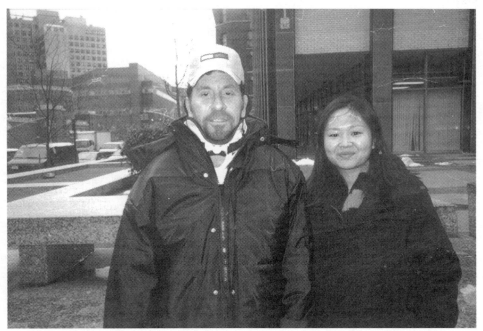

Figure 5.10. Therapy brings the occupational therapist Diana and her client Ronald outside because that is a physical context he will act in after discharge.

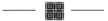

Exercise 5.5—Personal Occupations

Think about one of your occupations, for example, the occupations related to your role as a student. Reflect what contexts shape how you perform your occupations related to school. What are the personal meanings of these occupations to you? Include cultural, physical, social, personal, spiritual, temporal, and virtual contexts. How do the details of your occupation differ from someone else you know with the same occupation?

The Occupational Therapy Evaluation

The occupational therapy evaluation has two components: the occupational profile and the analysis of occupational performance. While the occupational profile is the starting point, these two aspects of the evaluation process are not sequential steps. The process of *evaluation* is a continuous interplay between the occupational profile and the analysis of occupational performance (AOTA, 2002).

The occupational profile identifies which occupations need to be evaluated for occupational performance. It pinpoints which occupations are priorities for intervention and what configuration of activities currently defines that occupation for the client. The therapist can then evaluate the client's performance on these activities. As the therapist analyzes the client's actual performance of the specified occupations, he or she observes the individual details of the client's task execution, which flesh out the profile. People have difficulty describing their habits and routines because these things are so ingrained that they do not think about them anymore. As the client does the task, or tries to do the task, the therapist sees what the client is able to do and what he or she needs to know about the activity.

With the new details observed about the client's occupational performance, the therapist now can ask more questions, which further clarify the occupational profile and, in turn, refocus the direction of the evaluation of occupational performance. Likewise, as the therapist identifies specific skill deficits through the evaluation's analysis, the therapist will be able to anticipate what areas of occupations may be problematic and concentrate the questions there. For example, for a client with limited elbow flexion of the nondominant arm, the therapist will delve more deeply into the areas of applying make-up rather than doing nails and golfing rather than reading.

Case Scenario

Enrique is a 22-year-old man with a traumatic brain injury who was recently discharged from an inpatient rehabilitation hospital and referred for outpatient services. In the occupational therapist's initial interview, Enrique says that he is having no problems. He lives with his mother. Every morning he gets up and gets his daughter ready for school. He spends his day helping around the house and taking care of his daughter. Enrique is eager to return to work but is concerned that he may not be able to return to construction work because his leg bothers him sometimes.

The therapist's formal testing showed severe disorganization, memory deficits with instructions, inefficiency, and multiple errors in task performance. The therapist decides to ask Enrique's mother about his daily routine. His mother reports that he sleeps late every day. He cannot pick out his own clothes, even though he has always been a meticulous dresser. She takes care of his daughter. She does not let him out alone because he gets lost. She worries when she goes to work because Enrique left the stove on one time, and she is afraid that he will wander off.

Case Questions: What information for the evaluation do the discrepancies in reports give us? What suspicions do you think the therapist had that made her ask the mother for the same information she had asked of the client? What occupations does the client value? Which occupations are problematic? How does the additional information change the occupational focus of treatment?

Observing a person's occupational performance, particularly in context, is an intimate act. As these activities are shared, the dialogue between the therapist and client begins to develop; this is when the therapist learns the most about the client's occupational profile.

With a new injury or illness affecting occupational performance, the occupational therapy evaluation may be the first time clients are attempting some of the tasks important to their occupations, which places them in a vulnerable moment. What they were or were not capable of changes as they confront familiar tasks with new difficulties. In response, their priorities and values in their occupational profile shift.

This shift is emotionally charged. Often, clients struggle down a tumultuous road toward new self-perceptions, which are tied directly to the occupational profile. They are struggling to gain a vision of themselves in the future, with which they set their goals and give meaning to their present (Morris, 1994). This metamorphosis spans the evaluation and the intervention stage.

Intervention and the Occupational Profile

The constant adjustment of the occupational profile is most extreme with an acute injury or illness. Occupational therapy *intervention,* however, signifies a point of change for all clients. Even with healthy populations, if they are seeking an occupational therapy consultation, they are looking for ways to improve how they are performing or to decrease risk factors in their occupations. As change occurs, the client's present occupational profile and the vision of the future, in terms of occupations, also changes.

The occupational profile influences intervention by identifying the client's needs and priorities for intervention. When asked, many clients' goals are too general to use as treatment goals: "I want to go home." "I want to be like I used to be." "I want to walk." "I want to get better." The occupational profile gives the therapist data with which to interpret these goals into treatment. In the client's array of occupations, where did the person walk, what activities are necessary to survive at home, which occupations are presently "worse" than before?

The occupational profile is important in choosing types of interventions. It identifies what activities are significant for the client and provides a rich source of ideas for the intervention plan's purposeful activities. The therapist seeks purposeful activities that draw on the client's interests in order to be engaging and motivating for the client. Participating in purposeful activities will build the foundation upon which the client's occupations can emerge.

The occupational profile also aids the therapist in choosing a method to approach a goal. Knowing how the client has adapted his or her occupations at previous stages of life can help with the selection of an approach to which the client will be receptive. Where will the client be open to making changes? Would the client rather scale back the performance of an occupation or completely redesign how to fulfill a role?

—— ▦ ——

Exercise 5.6—Lifestyle Redesign

Read the story of Penny in Florence Clark's "Occupation Embedded in a Real Life: Interweaving Occupational Science and Occupational Therapy" (Clark, 1993). Consider these questions: Which occupations from childhood helped Penny to reform her occupations after the "big A?" Which occupations does Penny value most? What occupations did she modify to fulfill her roles? What are new occupations that she has taken on to fulfill old roles?

The intervention process makes a continuous impact on the occupational profile, creating the "dynamic assessment" (AOTA, 2002, p. 631) that overarches evaluation and intervention. The client's awareness of what he or she can and cannot do increases. The therapist exposes the client to new experiences that may open possibilities in the client's eyes. The client travels through different emotional responses to the changes. Plus, as all this happens, the client–therapist relationship is forged, and new revelations or understandings emerge about the occupational profile.

Case Scenario

George is a 27-year-old who recently suffered a T-4 spinal cord injury and has a complete paraplegia. He has hope for walking and returning to rock climbing and camping. He feels despair at times, convinced that he cannot even shave or feed himself. Sometimes, he just wants to indulge in his role as son and let his mother baby him, bathing him and combing his hair. Other times, he feels empowered, such as his first time propelling himself in a wheelchair around the hospital unit.

George's occupational profile in relation to the present and the future responds to his occupational performance in the evaluation and in ongoing treatment. Sometimes his only goal is to go home as soon as possible, with his mother and sister caring for him. Sometimes, he can only address his occupations within the hospital stay, such as his self-care, his exercises, and his leadership role among other patients, but cannot discuss going home. Still other times, he has many questions for the occupational therapist about how accessible public transportation is and asks for information about wheelchair sports.

Case Questions: Which activities will the occupational therapist encourage? How can George's treatment plan capture his changing occupational profile and his changing focus? Which occupations are most urgent in treatment planning as his inpatient stay nears an end? How can his present activities help build up his ability to support longer-term occupations?

Outcomes and the Occupational Profile

Beginning in the evaluation process, the occupational profile is a tool to set specific outcome measures. With the *fundamental outcome* defined as "engagement in occupation to support participation" (AOTA, 2002, p. 614), the occupational profile provides information about which of the client's activities and occupations are desired, valued, and needed. Participation in life is specifically defined, and anticipated, through the client's occupational profile.

Most specific outcome measures derive from the occupational profile. Successful performance of those occupations that were client priorities is the most basic and clear outcome measure. The profile identifies the client's valued roles. Role competence may be achieved by successful implementation of changes in the occupations demanded by that role for a successful outcome.

The outcome measure of adaptation needs to specify from the occupational profile what life changes confront the client and how they will influence his or her participation in life activities. Life activities that have personal meaning form the

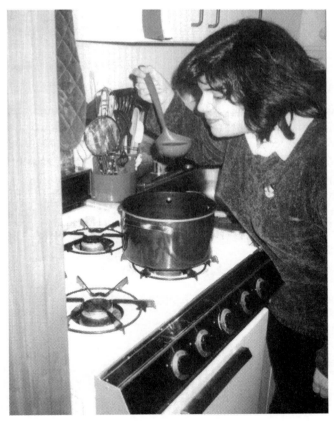

Figure 5.11. Alysia loves to throw a party, and to carry out that occupation, she is warming her wassail.

client's occupations. If in the past the client used actions that resulted in personal dissatisfaction, then changes in actions that give satisfying results are successful outcomes. For example, in one occupational profile, a client describes a series of job losses, each time because of fights with his coworkers. This occupational profile is not satisfactory to the client, who desires change. The outcome measure is the change in behavior that allows the client to maintain a job.

Setting outcomes is where the dimension of time in the occupational profile is critical. To set outcome measures, the therapist draws on the client's anticipated occupations and how soundly they are based on past occupations and behaviors. Interventions must be realistic and include the client's vision with regard to his or her desired future occupations. Therefore, outcome measures are reworked throughout the intervention process as the client and therapist reconfigure the occupational profile.

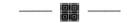

Exercise 5.7—Lifestyle Redesign Application

Review several of the cases presented in this chapter (Maria, Maureen, Alex, Martha, Ling Mei, Enrique, Penny, George). Identify appropriate outcome measures for each.

Summary

This chapter explains what it means for therapy to be occupational in practice. I try to keep it practical in showing that the long heritage of occupational therapy is present in our daily work. I could not cite references for each idea because my thoughts here are rooted in a wealth of occupational therapy literature that has brought me to where I am now. My ideas are not new but, rather, basic occupational therapy. What I hope I can offer readers are reflections on occupation from the clinic floor. Keeping my focus on the occupational profile reminds me who we are professionally and propels me to continue growing as an occupational therapist. ∎

Acknowledgment

Martha case study provided by Kathy Urban, MA, RN.

References

American Occupational Therapy Association. (1997). Statement—Fundamental concepts of occupational therapy: Occupation, purposeful activity, and function. *American Journal of Occupational Therapy, 51*, 864–866.

American Occupational Therapy Association. (2002). Occupational therapy practice framework: Domain and process. *American Journal of Occupational Therapy, 56*, 609–639.

Clark, F. (1993). Occupation embedded in a real life: Interweaving occupational science and occupational therapy, 1993 Eleanor Clarke Slagle Lecture. *American Journal of Occupational Therapy, 47*, 1067–1078.

Kielhofner, G. (1983). Occupation. In H. L. Hopkins & H. D. Smith (Eds.), *Willard and Spackman's occupational therapy* (6th ed., pp. 31–41). Philadelphia: Lippincott.

Kielhofner, G. (Ed.). (1985). *A model of human occupation: Theory and application.* Baltimore: Williams & Wilkins.

Kielhofner, G. (1992). *Conceptual foundations of occupational therapy.* Philadelphia: F. A. Davis.

Kramer, P., Hinojosa, J., & Royeen, C. B. (Eds.). (2003). *Perspectives in human occupation: Participation in life.* New York: Lippincott, Williams & Wilkins.

Morris, J. (1994). Spinal injury and psychotherapy in treatment philosophy. In G. M. Yarkony (Ed.), *Spinal cord injury: Medical management in rehabilitation* (pp. 223–229). Gaithersburg, MD: Aspen.

Nelson, D. L. (1996). Therapeutic occupation: A definition. *American Journal of Occupational Therapy, 50*, 775–782.

Trombly, C. A. (1995). Occupation: Purposefulness and meaningfulness as therapeutic mechanisms, 1995 Eleanor Clarke Slagle Lecture. *American Journal of Occupational Therapy, 49*, 960–972.

Urban, J. (1998a). *A critical analysis of "cultural sensitivity" in health care practice.* Unpublished master's thesis, Hunter College of the City University of New York, New York.

Urban, J. (1998b, June 3). *Cultural issues in occupational therapy.* Presented at the 12th International Congress of the World Federation of Occupational Therapists, Montreal, Canada.

6

Activity Synthesis as a Means to Occupation

Paula Kramer, PhD, OTR, FAOTA
Jim Hinojosa, PhD, OT, FAOTA

The magician's sleight of hand is smooth and sinuous, creating an illusion of reality that is not really there. The audience members watch in awe, trying to reconcile the reality that they know exists with what they think they are seeing. It seems so simple, yet creating the illusion is so complex. In many ways, this is much like the activity synthesis the occupational therapy practitioner creates. Make no mistake, the occupational therapy practitioner does not perform magic. Yet, the practitioner puts so much thought into developing and creating activities (something common to everyday life) for the client that the process becomes as complex as the magician's illusions.

Activity synthesis occurs in everyday life, yet people do not conceptualize the development of activities as synthesis. Occupational therapists, however, view activities and their synthesis in a complex and theoretical way, building on what people do on a daily basis. Despite the fact that activity synthesis is central to the art and practice of occupational therapy, very little has been written specifically about this aspect of intervention. Within this chapter, activity synthesis is viewed as a means toward the ability to participate in occupations.

Activity Synthesis in Everyday Life

> All thought, in its early stages, begins as action. The actions which you have been wading through have been ideas. . .but they had to be established as a foundation before we could begin to think in earnest. (White, 1977, p.11)

Activity synthesis is not unique to occupational therapy; it occurs in everyday life in a much more simplistic form. Synthesizing activities is something that people take for granted. When we present a task to a child and meet with resistance from him or her, we frequently will change or modify the task to engage the child and cut down on the resistance. For example, many young children do not like clothes put over their heads, occluding their eyes. When the parent turns this into a game, saying, "Where did Johnny go?" when putting the shirt over Johnny's head, the child often will laugh rather than be frightened. The parent has just adapted or synthesized the activity for engagement and success. People often modify, adapt, or synthesize activities without even thinking. If one is tired when doing a task standing up, he or she will try to find a way to do the same task sitting down. Sometimes, this way is as simple as pulling up a chair, and other times, it requires moving to another area with a different-height table or counter so that the task can be done sitting down. On the most simplistic level, synthesis is simply changing or creating an activity so that an individual may engage in it successfully.

Although people naturally modify activities so that they can complete them successfully, they do not adapt the activity in any organized way. No theoretical rationale exists for the adaptation of the activity; they rely on what appears to be "common sense," looking for a simple change in the activity that will bring about success rather than looking at the activity as a whole. Occupational therapy practitioners, however, use activity synthesis in an organized manner often determined by a specific theoretical perspective.

Activity analysis and synthesis have long been considered important tools for occupational therapy practitioners (Mosey, 1981). They have been discussed as sepa-

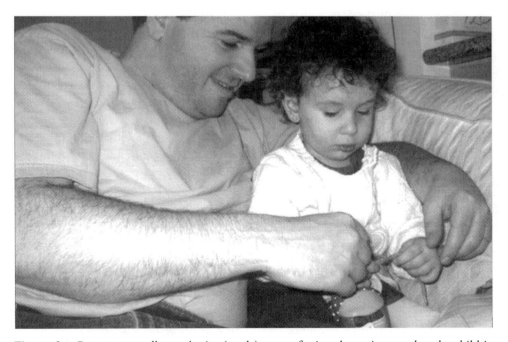

Figure 6.1. Parents naturally synthesize (grade) steps of tying shoestrings so that the child is successful.

rate processes that are integrally connected with providing the practitioner the means to understand and use purposeful activities. Two processes, activity analysis and activity synthesis, are used together for the benefit of the client. Nelson (1997) characterized *occupational analysis* as "what occupational therapists do" (p. 15), incorporating the importance of synthesis. *Occupational synthesis* is grounded in the occupational forms that determine the meaningfulness and purposefulness of an occupation to the individual. Synthesis is considered to be this intellectual process and part of the clinical reasoning and decision-making aspects of practice (Mosey, 1996; Nelson & Jepsen-Thomas, 2003).

From a therapeutic perspective, activity synthesis begins with the practitioner's conception of how to adapt an activity that the client wants or needs to do. It is up to the client and the practitioner to determine the importance of these actions, to think them through, and to use this combined thought and action process as the foundation for activity synthesis. The way occupational therapy practitioners understand, analyze, and use activity synthesis, however, is unique.

Perspectives on Activity Synthesis, Occupation, and Participation

In occupational therapy professional education, much time is spent on activity analysis, with very little time spent on activity synthesis. Hence, students and clinicians get the impression that activity analysis is more important and significant to the intervention process than synthesis. The assumption is that once the clinician understands the step or stage of the task that is problematic to the client, intervention can take place, and the client can complete the task. This assumption may or may not be accurate. In fact, a constant interplay exists between analysis and synthesis.

Let us take a step backward. Before analysis or synthesis can take place, the clinician needs to understand the client and his or her life situation. This involves understanding the client's personal goals and desires, capacities, and limitations. These personal goals and desires may depend on context, and in some cases, goals and desires may be those of the family or society and may depend on life situations. Then goals and desires need to be explored within the context of capacities and limitations. Although there is a desire to achieve something, there may not be the capacity for that achievement. The client comes to this process with a very personal understanding of him- or herself and where he or she wants to be in the future. Activities can be synthesized only once the practitioner has a clear understanding of the client.

Identifying and defining potential goals for the intervention requires negotiation and collaboration between the client and practitioner. This process goes two ways, with each way involving specific aptitudes. The practitioner brings a clinical understanding of the client's condition from a medical and psychosocial perspective and understands the potential sequela of the disease process. The client has his or her unique sense of self and a strong understanding of his or her own drive and aspirations to achieve the goal. Together, the practitioner and client develop goals that define the course of treatment and the outcomes of intervention. Ideally, the goals should relate to the occupations in which the person will engage in the future and how he or she will be able to participate in life and society.

The next step is to complete an activity analysis, thus giving the occupational therapist or occupational therapy assistant a rudimentary understanding of the tasks that may be adapted or changed. With this understanding, the therapist can now take this knowledge and begin to design or create activities that meet the client's needs.

Before actually moving to the synthesis of an activity, the therapist needs to consider theory. The therapist chooses a theoretical perspective, model, or frame of reference that will suit the client's needs and goals. Putting together his or her professional knowledge, the expected outcomes of the therapeutic process, and the client's (or family's) mutually agreed-on goals, the synthesis begins. This process begins with defining the key elements of the activity. One can adapt an activity only so much until it becomes something else. For example, is it still baking if there is no oven or heat involved? Is it still baseball without a ball and bat? When these key elements are no longer present, the activity is no longer the same.

With the activity analysis and the theoretical perspective, the therapist can now take this knowledge and begin to design or create activities that meet the client's needs. Once the activities are created and presented to the client, the therapist observes client performance and continually reanalyzes what is occurring for the client in order to adapt and resynthesize the activity to meet the client's goals. This process is ongoing and dynamic. Sometimes, the activity needs to be reconstructed or synthesized in a different way to allow the client to be successful. Analyzing the activity is not enough, understanding how one can synthesize an activity is equally important. Both are important tools for occupational therapy practitioners.

Activity Synthesis in Occupational Therapy

Occupational therapists and occupational therapy assistants have an organized conceptual approach to activity synthesis. The activity is viewed as a whole, and an activity analysis is done to break it down into component parts. The final step in the process is to synthesize or re-create the activity with change, modification, or adaptation to allow the client to achieve success in the task. Synthesis involves more than just the activity; it involves the personal meaning of the activity, the interaction involved, and the context of the activity. It involves layering all parts of an activity to create a whole. For occupational therapy practitioners, synthesis is complex. It is adapting and grading activities, modifying activities, and creating new activities. It can be used as part of an evaluative tool or the intervention process. Activity synthesis can be used to evaluate performance within a context, teach a new skill, refine a skill, or maintain one's functional status or performance ability. The creative process of synthesis requires a thorough understanding of the activity, a visualization of the goal, and the end-product one wishes to achieve.

Occupational therapy practitioners view synthesis in the context of the person as an occupational being. The following questions are asked: Who is the person involved in the intervention process? What occupations are important to this person? How do specific purposeful activities relate to these occupations? Does the accomplishment of a purposeful activity build on or allow this person to engage in meaningful occupations at his or her current stage of life?

The Synthesis Process

Traditional activity synthesis is based on activity analysis when we have taken the activity apart to explore and understand its component tasks. Synthesis requires that we reconstruct the activity, incorporating the client's therapeutic goals, areas of strength and limitations, and the therapeutic relationship. The activity is reconfigured in ways that allow the client to approach it with minimal fear of failure and with greater potential for success. This section discusses the process of adapting and grading activities, modifying activities, and creating new activities. These processes overlap and may not be mutually exclusive. Although each process is addressed individually as though it is distinct, in practice one or more processes may be used in combination. As with learning any process, it is important that each component (process) be appreciated and understood in relationship to the others. Through understanding components, a distinct knowledge of the whole synthesis process is attained.

Adapting and Grading

Guided by a theoretical perspective, *adaptation* involves a change to the environment or the activity and not a change to the person. Adaptation of activities, therefore, involves changing the environment in which the activity occurs or changing the activity itself rather than working to bring about change in the person doing the activity. When a client has difficulty with a task or activity, the activity is adapted for the client. This process begins with an activity analysis that considers the activity, the context in which it will be done, and the capabilities of the client. After analyzing the activity or completing the activity analysis, the therapist uses the theoretical perspective to decide how the activity should be adapted or changed to meet the client's abilities so that the client can do the activity in a specific context. For example, with a rehabilitation frame of reference, the therapist can simply provide the client a spoon with an adapted handle, have the client change his or her position when engaging in the task, or have the client sit down during the activity for energy conservation. If a therapist selected a different theoretical perspective, the adaptation also can involve a more complicated process where the activity itself is changed.

——— ⊞ ———

Exercise 6.1—Adaptation

Think about an activity that you adapted to make your life easier. Reflect on the adaptation. How did you figure out the appropriate adaptations? Because you knew your capabilities and had a goal in mind, how did that influence the way you approached the adaptation?

——— ⊞ ———

Exercise 6.2—Adapting an Activity From a Developmental Perspective

Observe children playing in a playground or a schoolyard. Select one activity that they are playing. Using a developmental perspective, how would you adapt the activity so that a child in a wheelchair could participate?

——— ⊞ ———

Exercise 6.3—Adapting an Activity Using a Sensory Integration Frame of Reference

Adapt a playground activity for a child with tactile defensiveness using a sensory integration frame of reference.

———————

Grading an activity is a common way of adapting an activity. Although a basic principle from learning theory, grading is almost universally used by occupational therapy practitioners. For this reason, it is critical to think about grading and how it is used in the context of specific theories that guide intervention. Grading can involve simplifying the activity, making the activity more complex, modifying the sequence or physical nature of the activity, or modifying the amount of time it takes to do the task. Simplifying the activity, or grading the activity down, entails making the activity easier in some way for the person. For a child who is learning how to undress himself (an acquisitional frame of reference), grading might involve pulling off his socks after the sock is rolled down off his heel or removing his pants after the fastenings have been opened. In this case, the practitioner may do a part of the task for the child and have the child do the remainder. Once the child has accomplished this segment of the task, the task can be made slightly more difficult, grading the activity "up" rather than "down." Grading a task down allows the client to feel successful and gain confidence so that he or she is willing to try more difficult types of tasks, to develop skills, or to build on a previously acquired level of skill.

——— ⊞ ———

Exercise 6.4—Grading an Activity

Select an activity that you are very competent at doing but that one of your class-mates cannot do. If you are good at playing chess, the piano, or baking, then select a student who does not know how to play or bake. Develop and carry out one teaching session with your classmate. How did you grade the activity so that the other person would have a positive learning experience? How would you have graded the activity for a different person?

_____

Whether adapting or grading, theoretical perspectives often require that the physical nature of an activity be changed by modifying the materials used in a task. From a developmental perspective, if a child has difficulty building with wooden blocks because they are hard for him or her to grasp and lift, then cardboard or foam blocks could be provided that are lighter and easier to grasp. This adaptation allows the child to play with blocks without having adequate grasp for lifting. The adaptation here is grading the activity down so that the child can use his or her strength and skills to participate in the block-building.

Modifying Activities

Activity modification does not involve changing the activity itself. The purpose and goal of the activity are the same when modifying an activity, but the sequence or time requirements of the tasks that make up the activity are altered. Modifying the sequence of tasks involves changing the order in which tasks are done so that the person can engage in the task more successfully. This approach is used frequently in energy conservation, for example, having the client change the order in which he or she performs activities of daily living (ADL) tasks to avoid walking up and down stairs or back and forth across a room. The client accomplishes the ultimate goal of dressing him- or herself more efficiently.

——— ⊞ ———

Exercise 6.5—Altering the Sequence of Tasks

Think about the way that you accomplish the self-care occupation of getting ready for work in the morning. List the tasks that you do to accomplish each activity (e.g., personal hygiene, selecting clothes, dressing). Select one activity. Consider how you would change the sequence of the task if you had to get ready in a shorter period of time one morning.

_____

Performances (the actual doing) of the tasks involve a time factor. They have to be done either within a specified amount of time or at a specific time of the day or year; otherwise, they are not functional. In the therapeutic environment, the timing of a task can be modified, or the time requirements of a task or the activity can be changed. The client can take a longer time to complete the task without repercussion, or dressing can be done in the middle of the day rather than in the morning. Once a client has mastered an activity within an extended time frame, the tasks' time requirements can be decreased. For example, when first working with a child learning to put on a pullover shirt, the child might be allowed to take as much time as he or she needs. Slowly, a time requirement would be added. After the child has mastered putting on the pullover shirt in a reasonable amount of time, the child might be asked to put on a button-down shirt in the same amount of time, even though this shirt is more difficult to put on. The task of putting on and fastening the shirt is layered to make each task more complex than the previous one while using a time requirement as an important component. Many activities are not functional if they cannot be done within a specified time; that is, for a child to spend a half hour putting on a shirt would not be considered functional.

———— ⊞ ————

Exercise 6.6—Altering the Timing of Tasks

Select an activity at which you are really good. Determine how much time it takes you to do the activity from beginning to end. Divide the time in half and do the activity. How does it affect your performance? Now, double the time that it takes to do the activity. How does this affect your performance?

_____

Creating New Activities

The most complex type of activity synthesis is creating new activities. This synthesis occurs after evaluating a client and determining the areas that require intervention, and in response, the practitioner creates an activity specifically for the client. There are two different ways in which the therapist engages in creating new activities. This "creating" may arise from the practitioner's responsibility to present a specific level of challenge to the client and thus promote growth. The other type of "creating" may be based on the occupational needs and desires of the client to move to a certain level. It is important to note that creating an activity is at a different level than grading and adapting because an entirely new activity will emerge from this process rather than a modification to the previous activity.

Some theoretical perspectives and frames of reference, such as neurodevelopmental treatment and sensory integration, almost define the role of the therapist as the creator of activities. This responsibility is defined as the role of the therapist based on the client's therapeutic needs and the goal of the frame of reference to promote future growth and skills. The client collaboration is secondary and derived from engagement in the task. If the client does not engage, the therapist must create new activities to entice the client.

In other theoretical perspectives and frames of reference, such as occupational adaptation and occupational performance, the creation of activities comes from the client and is based on perceived occupational needs. This synthesis requires skill, creativity, and an in-depth understanding of the client. The resultant activity is based on an understanding of the client, his or her interests, and his or her problem areas and goals and has a "just-right fit" for the client. It is not based on activity analysis but is client centered. Within this type of synthesis, the nonhuman environment plays a very important role. The practitioner, therefore, also gains an understanding of both the human and nonhuman environment and creates activities that will engage the client based on his or her occupations. For example, if a pet is important to the client and the practitioner can involve the care of that pet in an aspect of the intervention, then the client will be more likely to engage in that intervention.

Case Scenario

Janet, a woman with multiple sclerosis, is confined to a wheelchair and resides in a nursing home. Before she came to the nursing home, she raised several dogs who were very important to her. The nursing home has a pet therapy dog, and the occupational therapist found that Janet was much more likely to come to groups when the therapy dog was present. The therapist's understanding of Janet's interest in pets allows him or her to design activities that will fit with Janet's interest.

Exercise 6.7—Creating a New Activity

Determine a goal that you have for a skill that you would like to develop. After selecting the skill, look around your home and develop an original activity that you could engage in that would develop the skill.

Exercise 6.8—Creating New Activities With Defined Developmental Goals

You have been hired to work in a new occupational therapy practice with limited space and materials. All that you have in the treatment environment are two chairs and one small table. You also have in the supply closet masking tape, a box of colored 1-inch blocks, and two boxes with 12 pencils (unsharpened) each. You have two children scheduled for the day: Steven, a 19-month-old boy with developmental delays functioning at about a 9-month developmental level, and Shana, a 3-year-old with cerebral palsy spastic diplegia. Develop goals for a treatment session for Steven and Shana and develop an activity using only the materials, supplies, and environment described.

— ▦ —

Exercise 6.9—Creating New Activities Based on Occupational Needs of the Client

Diego is a 12-year-old child with attention deficit disorder with hyperactivity. He wants to join the local Little League team but needs to develop basic skills in baseball and self-control. Create an activity that will move Diego toward his goal of playing on the team.

Connecting Synthesis With Occupation

All these examples of synthesis require skill on the part of the occupational therapy practitioner. First, the practitioner needs to understand the activity and its importance to the client as well as its relationship to the client's occupations. Why is this activity important to the client? How does this activity relate to the client's occupations? What role will it play in his or her life? How will it help the client to engage in meaningful occupations? To accomplish this successfully entails engaging the client, developing rapport, and developing an understanding of who the client is as a person. Then, using the creative process within a theoretical framework, the practitioner devises or synthesizes activities that will meet the client's needs. If the client has no interest in the activity or does not see it as meaningful to his or her life, then he or she will only go through the actions without a personal investment. Further, the client may not be self-motivated to participate in the activity, and the therapeutic value will be minimized. To be successful, the synthesis of activities has to take the client into account. Some theoretical perspectives explicitly address personal motivation; others address meaningfulness to the client. When motivation is not a major concept in the theoretical framework chosen, other theoretical perspectives may need to be introduced to explore personal motivation. Occupational therapy practitioners should not make assumptions about a client's motivation.

Context also should be considered when the synthesis of activities is related to intervention. The ultimate goal is for the client to be able to perform the activity in the real world, not just in the simulated environment of the occupational therapy practice setting.

Importance of Activity Synthesis to Intervention

When people have done a particular task for many years, frequently it is difficult for them to change or modify the way that they do that task, even if they are having difficulty completing the activity in their traditional manner. For example, if one is accustomed to preparing a meal standing at the kitchen counter and has limited standing tolerance, then the person can move that meal preparation to the kitchen table to complete the task sitting down. Yet, it is sometimes difficult for people to make such adjustments. When people have always done tasks that are important to them and find that they can no longer do those tasks in the same manner, making modifications to those tasks often is very difficult for them. For example, when cleaning one's home becomes too strenuous or difficult, some obvious options include getting assistance from others, cleaning one room each day until all are done, or doing minimal cleaning. Some of these options may be more acceptable to some people than other options. For some people, getting assistance with cleaning is not an acceptable option because cleaning house has been one of their life's occupations; for others, doing minimal cleaning may not be an acceptable option because people have different beliefs and practices when it comes to cleanliness.

Case Scenario

Betty chose to adapt the task of house cleaning in a way that was meaningful to her. She knew that objects she had collected over the years needed to be washed periodically but did not like the thought of having other people handle them. These objects were on high shelves, out of reach without climbing on a ladder. She did her own analysis of the task. As a senior citizen, she was aware that climbing on a ladder was not an acceptable option because she would risk falling, which could result in an injury. Betty hired someone to help her but was very clear in defining the role this person would take. This person was to do the climbing to get the objects down from the shelf, and Betty would wash them and direct where they were to be put back in place. This modification allowed Betty to have control over the task, handle the things that were precious to her, and avoid the parts of the activity that could be potentially dangerous to her.

How do occupational therapy practitioners use activity synthesis as part of their intervention? Where does activity synthesis fit into the overall intervention process? As presented in this chapter, activity synthesis is the reasoning process that guides us on how activities are used. When activity synthesis is used in an intervention, it is used within a frame of reference or a theoretical context.

Occupational therapy intervention is based on a theoretical perspective, frequently referred to by a variety of names, including models of practice, theoretical orientations, guidelines for intervention, or frames of reference. In the rest of this chapter, we use the term *frames of reference* to include all interventions that are theoretically based. Synthesis is based on the practitioner's skills and abilities, his or her understanding of the client and the client's needs, the context in which the activity will occur, and the frame of reference that the therapist has determined to be the most appropriate for the client. Use of the frame of reference forces the synthesis to take place in the context of theoretical information. The theoretical information that underlies the frame of reference will guide what is actually done. Thus, the actual synthesis occurs within the parameters of the frame of reference and how the frame of reference directs practitioners to use, adapt, modify, or create the activity.

Case Scenario

Juan, an 8-year-old boy, was referred to occupational therapy for a handwriting problem. After a comprehensive evaluation, the occupational therapist assigns Juan to an occupational therapy assistant to implement a program to develop hand coordination for writing based on muscle strengthening using the biomechanical frame of reference. The therapist selected the frame of reference because she had determined that Juan has poor muscle strength and has limited experience with fine motor activities. The intervention must be done within the context of Juan's class. After meeting Juan and reviewing the recommendations and discussing the frame for reference with the therapists, the occupational therapy assistant, using activity analysis and synthesis, determines that Juan should use an adapted pencil while writing and paper with raised lines that will give him more sensory feedback. Additionally, the assistant observed what computer-time activities were done in the classroom. After careful analysis of what Juan does on the computer, the assistant decides to change the keyboard to one that provides more resistance and to raise the keyboard so that Juan has to use more shoulder motion.

Case Scenario
(Continuing With the Case of Juan)

If the occupational therapist has decided to use a frame of reference based on play and theories of psychosocial development outside of the classroom environment, the occupational therapy assistant would begin by focusing on Juan's personal interests, analyzing those purposeful activities, and synthesizing them as guided by the frame of reference. An understanding of theories of psychosocial developmental suggests that an 8-year-old boy would be expected to relate to others in a competitive manner. Juan enjoys the game Connect Four®. The objective of this game is to pick up small checkers and put them into a vertical form in order to line up four in a row. The occupational therapy assistant involves Juan in creating a new competitive game. Guided by this perspective, the assistant competes with Juan using the new rules that they develop together. To make the game address some of Juan's motor needs, they decide to place the checkers under various heavy objects around the room. Before putting the checker in the board, Juan and the assistant must balance themselves in prone over a small ball, using the nondominant hand to balance and support weight. Additionally, a 2-pound weight is placed on Juan's dominant hand.

All occupational therapy practice should be based on theoretical information or rationales. Activity synthesis is used by the practitioner within the context of that theoretical information. It is not separate or outside of the theoretical framework but is guided by the theoretical framework. The frame of reference, theoretical perspective, or framework guides the practitioner in his or her activity synthesis.

Activity Synthesis as a Medium for Intervention

Typically, occupational therapy practitioners think about activity synthesis as a medium to use when treating a client. It is generally something that is used to improve function once a deficit has been identified. Activity synthesis, however, can be used in many more ways that are creative. It can be used to evaluate client performance, teach new skills, refine a skill, and maintain functional status or performance abilities. This section presents the use of activity synthesis for all of these purposes.

In the synthesis of activities, the practitioner needs to be artful in developing or choosing an activity that suits the client's needs from a functional perspective and the client's interests from a personal perspective. If both needs and interests are not met, then the activity will not be successful in achieving its goal. The occupational therapy practitioner first takes the time to learn about the client, focusing on who he or she is as a person and his or her strengths and limitations. Then the practitioner identifies goals for the intervention and the client, with his or her input. This may involve analyzing the client's performance in particular activities and identifying performance components that are interfering with successful completion of the task. It also may involve some aspect of client education to increase the client's awareness of how performance can be improved or how performance in a particular area is affecting overall functioning. Activities then are synthesized with the client so that they are meaningful and beneficial to the client.

Case Scenario

Janay has a weakness in her hands. She enjoys baking and has an interest in baking bread. When first synthesizing activities for Janay, the therapist considered using modeling clay as a therapeutic intervention, but Janay showed no interest in working with clay. Baking bread, however, requires kneading the dough, which also will strengthen the hands, and it provided Janay with an activity that is meaningful and pleasurable to her. Baking bread proved to meet Janay's personal and therapeutic needs, leading potentially to a more successful intervention.

Synthesis is not concrete. It does not follow a step-by-step process; there are many different ways to go about it with no one way being right or wrong. But several elements should be present for synthesis to be successful. These elements are developing an understanding of the client, including what is important to this person; analyzing activities to determine how deficits are interfering with performance; and selecting a frame of reference that will help the client to overcome his or her deficits. Additionally, together with the client, the practitioner identifies or devises activities that will help the client to overcome his or her deficits or develop the skills necessary for successful task performance.

Exercise 6.10—Synthesizing Activities Using a Frame of Reference

You have just been assigned to a new client, Malcolm. He has a right hemiplegia secondary to a cerebral vascular hemorrhage. Before this trauma, Malcolm was an engineer working for the U.S. Navy. He had a very high-level position designing equipment for ships. His hobbies included building things for his family and home, using multimedia (e.g., woodwork, electricity, mechanical devices). Choose a frame of reference or a theoretical perspective and synthesize several activities for this client using that perspective and incorporating Malcolm's personal interests. Describe the activities and how they reflect both his interests and the theoretical perspective you have chosen.

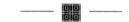

Exercise 6.11—Activity Synthesis in a Clinical Environment

Observe an intervention with a client. Identify the activities that have been synthesized for the client. Try to identify the type of theoretical perspective that provides the foundation for this intervention. Have the activities been synthesized specifically for this particular client? Can you determine the client's investment in the intervention? Are you observing artful practice?

Teaching New Skills

Using learning theories, a practitioner can use synthesis to teach new skills. This type of intervention is what an occupational therapy practitioner typically thinks of as activity synthesis. How does one devise a meaningful activity that will assist the client to develop new skills? Expanding on an example given previously, when teaching a child to do clothes fastening, one may first work on the skill in isolation on a doll and then make it more complex by translating the same skill into fastening one's own clothing. In this situation, the practitioner is identifying the skills that need to be developed and creating activities that will promote the development of that new skill.

Case Scenario

Ayisha has difficulties with the skills of money management. She does not watch how much money she gives to the store clerk and does not count her change. The therapist uses an acquisitional frame of reference and sets up a simulated store. Ayisha must pay for everything that she wants from the store, and the therapist works with her on management within this context. Periodically, the therapist takes on the role of consumer and has Ayisha take the role of cashier. Through this activity, the therapist can begin to teach Ayisha basic skills necessary for developing the ability to manage her money.

Refining a Skill

Similarly, a practitioner can use activity synthesis to refine a skill, again using learning theories. Once a basic skill level has been attained, the practitioner can enhance and embellish the activity to make the required skill level more complex. When working on developing communication skills with a client with psychosocial dysfunction, the practitioner might first work on having the client say "Good morning" to others in a protected environment, such as a therapy group, and then work on conducting an entire conversation. Although the activity synthesis might begin in a protected environment, eventually the skills would need to be tested in the real world to determine their viability.

Case Scenario

Sam is developing social skills in a group doing role-playing. He then tries out the skills he has acquired in a real situation. The therapist works with Sam on refining his behavior in the "real-world" environment. Is he dressed appropriately to go out shopping? Does he make eye contact with store personnel? Can he ask questions appropriately if he needs to find an item he wants to purchase? Can he handle money responsibly?

Activity Synthesis for Evaluation and Support of Functional Performance

Up to this point, activity synthesis has been discussed as an intervention process used to bring about change in the client. The use of theory in this process has been stressed. At the beginning of this chapter, however, it was postulated that activity synthesis occurs in everyday life. In some cases, the emphasis may not be on the theoretical base of the synthesis but on the use of activities and activity synthesis as a tool. Occupational therapists often use this tool to evaluate client performance and to support functional performance.

Activity synthesis can assist the therapist in evaluating a client's performance within a context. The therapist may first see whether a child can close a zipper on a doll or on an ADL board. The therapist may then observe the child's ability to close a zipper on his or her own clothing. It may be easy for a child to close a zipper on an ADL board or on a doll, but it is critical for the child to be able to close a zipper on his or her own coat. The therapist uses the synthesized activity to evaluate the child's performance within two different contexts and by doing so can determine whether intervention is necessary and how then to intervene.

Case Scenario

A therapist works with Bob on developing social skills. In a group, Bob role-plays purchasing an item in a store. During the role-playing, the therapist observes how Bob handles himself, whether his verbalizations are appropriate, and his ability to count out money to pay for the item. Based on Bob's ability to perform in the role-playing situation, the therapist can take Bob into an actual store and observe his abilities in a real context rather than in a simulated situation. The therapist uses these observations to give feedback to Bob and to develop a plan for intervention.

Maintaining Functional Status or Performance Abilities

A fundamental assumption of occupational therapy is that people are more likely to engage in activities that are meaningful to them; in other words, these activities are purposeful. Purposeful activities are both meaningful and goal directed. Occupations encompass purposeful activities. As occupational therapy practitioners, we believe that engagement in occupations keeps people healthy. Therefore, a primary goal of the occupational therapy process is to assist people in finding meaningful occupations, to help restore function so that they can engage in personally chosen occupations, and to help explore various options that will allow them to engage in occupations.

Synthesis can be used to maintain a person's functional status or performance ability. If a client has been working on strengthening her hands and has achieved an acceptable level of strength, then it would be incumbent on the practitioner to work with the client to synthesize activities that would maintain that level of strength after completion of intervention. Such activities would have to be of sufficient interest to the client so that she would want to continue doing them to maintain her hand strength, thus creating meaningful occupations for the client. If the activities devised held no interest for the client, there would be little incentive to continue with them. Therefore, the synthesized activities would have to incorporate purposeful and meaningful occupations for the client. Squeezing theraputty may not be a meaningful occupation, but molding clay into animals that could be given as gifts might be more important to this individual. In this case, activity synthesis is based on the fundamental assumption of the profession rather than on a theoretical perspective.

Case Scenario

Olivia has had difficulty with range of motion of the shoulder. She has received intervention and has been responsive to therapy. She can now raise her arms to 180° of shoulder flexion. The therapist initially suggested that Olivia do exercises to maintain this ability, but Olivia did not follow through on the exercise program. The therapist then did a home visit and suggested that Olivia place the dishes that she used most on the second shelf in her cabinets so that she would have to reach for them. Olivia was willing to do this, and the maintenance of her shoulder range became a part of her everyday life.

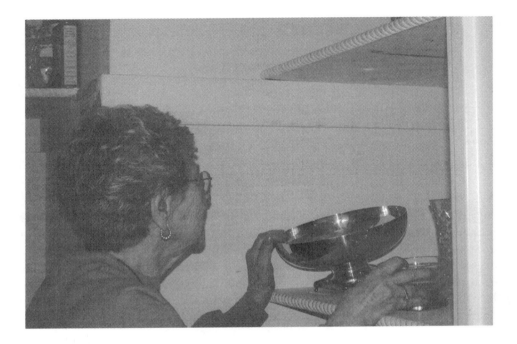

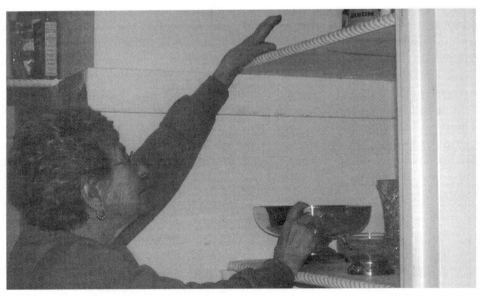

Figure 6.2 and Figure 6.3. Dishes are placed on the second shelf so that the woman can maintain shoulder range of motion.

Artful Practice and Occupational Synthesis

Activity synthesis requires artful practice on the part of the occupational therapy practitioner. It is not something that can be taught easily. It is, in part, the product of experience. One does not start out as an artist. First, one learns how to use and play with materials; learns techniques; develops skill with the materials; and, finally, develops a personal style. These are the prerequisites to becoming an artist. Once a person has the basic skills, he or she may be able to develop into an artist, but it takes time, practice, and experience. The same is true of the occupational therapy practitioner. Initially, the practitioner starts out as a novice, with a technical or procedural understanding of what is going on with the client. With time and experience, the practitioner develops into an expert. Once one has more expert-level skills, he or she can develop synthesis as an effective tool and become an artful practitioner. This level of skill requires considering not only the client's disability and functional level, but also the client as a person.

The clinical reasoning process is part of the art of practice. The practitioner develops reasoning skills in different areas and during different stages of professional development. Some aspects of clinical reasoning include scientific reasoning, narrative reasoning, pragmatic reasoning, and ethical reasoning (Schell, 2003). These different types of reasoning are discussed in depth in Chapter 7, "Activity Reasoning." Clinical reasoning skills develop as the practitioner matures and gains experience. Engaging in synthesis in practice, however, involves more than just reasoning; it involves understanding the client, his or her life, and oneself as an occupational therapy practitioner. Experience contributes to the ability to be an artful practitioner and allows the practitioner to try various approaches, develop a range of techniques and responses, and develop higher-level interaction skills. Having a multitude of experiences with clients with various disabilities and in various settings expands one's repertoire. All of these experiences provide the practitioner with options for intervention as well as with options for interaction. Knowledge gained from experience is not necessarily an expansion of theoretical knowledge but an expansion of practical knowledge and a greater understanding of the self and the human condition, all of which are essential for occupational synthesis. The practitioner has a clearer understanding of the role of activity and occupation in the client's life and is able to creatively match intervention with the client's needs. Artful practice requires an understanding of the individual and incorporates the individual as an active participant in the process. The art comes from within the practitioner and not from a greater understanding of theory (Schell, 2003). It is a personal and professional development, not exclusively an intellectual development.

Although the art of practice does not come from an understanding of theory, it does occur within a theoretical context. The practitioner should choose a theoretical framework or frame of reference that will fit the setting, the needs of the client, and his or her own knowledge base. The choice of a theoretical approach and, therefore, the choice or synthesis of activities should consider all of these things and not be based on one area alone. Understanding personal, organizational, and client contexts is complex but critical to effective practice.

If one practices artfully, then it can be assumed that occupational synthesis will take place. But what exactly is occupational synthesis? Our view of occupational synthesis is that this process takes place within the client. Whereas activity synthesis is done by the practitioner, occupational synthesis is done internally and sometimes unconsciously by the client. Once the client has received occupational therapy and has engaged in tasks and activities that have improved functional performance, the client develops a sense of which of those activities are meaningful occupations for him- or herself. Those occupations become a part of that person, occupations that he or she is willing to continue to do to maintain functional performance. For example, in the case of Olivia, placing the dishes she uses frequently on a higher shelf helped her to maintain the range of motion in her shoulder. If reaching up has become part of her occupational synthesis, then she would keep her dishes on the higher shelf and incorporate this activity into her daily life. If engaging in stretching activities daily reduces stiffness in a client, then the ongoing use of these activities have become part of this individual's routine and, thus, have been synthesized into his or her daily life. In this view, the occupational therapy practitioner provides activities and options for the client as a means of intervention; the client then incorporates some of these activities into personally meaningful occupations. The occupational synthesis then takes place within the client, as the client chooses those occupations to continue as part of everyday life.

Occupational synthesis takes place within the client; the artful occupational therapy practitioner creates the circumstances in which this process can take place. The practitioner uses his or her knowledge of human occupation integrated into theoretically based guidelines for intervention to provide activities and opportunities that the client uses for occupational synthesis. The definitive goal of occupational therapy is to provide interventions that will produce the desired changes so that the recipients of service can participate in occupations that are personally significant for them (Hinojosa, Kramer, Royeen, & Luebben, 2003). How do occupational therapy practitioners facilitate the occupational synthesis? They facilitate opportunities for occupational synthesis to occur by providing interventions that are relevant and creative.

It should be noted that the perspective we propose is not consistent with that proposed by Nelson and Jepson-Thomas (2003). They defined *occupational synthesis* as what the practitioner does. They do not use the term *activity* at all. We believe that what the practitioner does is "activity synthesis," whereas "occupational synthesis" occurs within the client.

Artful practice requires that the practitioner experience the treatment with the client. The practitioner uses him- or herself and his or her life experience as an active agent of change to design and implement treatments (Weinstein, 1998). The practitioner reflects on what is happening to continually modify, adapt, or change the intervention process or activity. As proposed by Schön (1983), the art of professional practice is built on a professional's reflection-in-action. An artful occupational therapy practitioner thinks about and examines what is happening during treatment. Beyond the theoretical perspective, the practitioner experiences what is happening

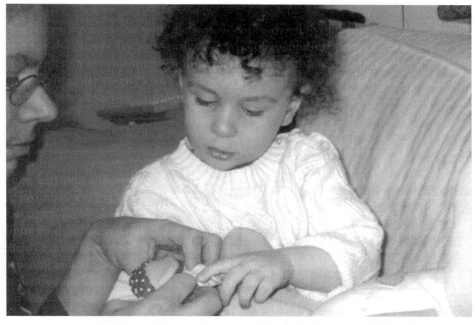

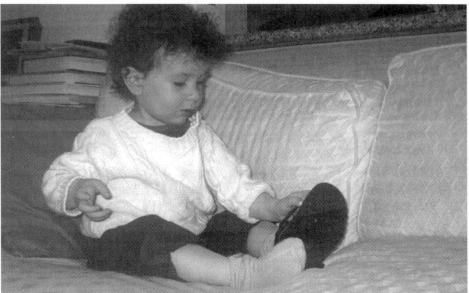

Figure 6.4 and Figure 6.5. The child who is learning to dress himself practices on a doll; this activity naturally transfers to the occupation of self-dressing.

and is prepared to change strategies spontaneously. In some cases, modifying the activity, the environment, or the interaction will help to make the treatment more effective for the client. In other situations, when the predicted changes are not happening, the practitioner decides to change the intervention. In these cases, the artful practitioner proposes new hypotheses and implements the revised intervention. These modifications ensure that occupational synthesis takes place and that treatments are related to the client's future occupations.

When interventions are relevant, the client is able to transpose the tasks or activities easily into his or her real-life occupations. Relevant interventions are judged by two criteria. First, are they appropriate for addressing the client's deficits? Second, are they pertinent to the client's life situation (e.g., goals, values, culture, lifestyle) as defined by the client? Occupational synthesis is more likely to take place when the occupational therapy program is relevant to the client. The practitioner begins this process by considering the following four questions to ensure that the client's life situation is being addressed:

1. Do I understand the client's occupations?

2. Do I respect the client's occupations and personal choices?

3. Do I understand the client's activity patterns, particularly in relation to his or her cultural significance, and do I respond to them appropriately?

4. How do my client's occupations influence others in his or her daily life?

Following reflection on this first set of questions, five additional questions have been identified (Hinojosa, 2003) that an occupational therapy practitioner might ask to assess the relevance of his or her interventions with regard to the concept of occupation:

5. Are my interventions reflecting an understanding of the client's life situations and his or her culture?

6. Have I developed an understanding of my client's occupations through discussions with him or her?

7. Have I considered clear ethical reasoning when developing my interventions within the context of the client's goals, priorities, and capacities?

8. Are my interventions based on an understanding of how the client defines his or her occupations?

9. Do my interventions result in enabling the client to engage in occupations and increase his or her life satisfaction?

Developing meaningful intervention using synthesis is a complex process. The practitioner usually starts by developing an understanding of activity synthesis. At the same time, he or she is developing sound clinical reasoning skills and, over time, gains experience to develop the art of practice. With experience, the practitioner comes to understand the critical role of the client and his or her unique situation. This process is not necessarily linear, but it is one that takes time and experience to develop. Once this development has occurred, occupational synthesis can be facilitated, and intervention becomes truly meaningful. The ultimate demonstration and most valuable outcome of occupational synthesis can be observed when the client engages in his or her chosen occupations in real life rather than in an artificial clinical situation.

Summary

Activity synthesis is something that occurs in everyday life. People constantly develop occupations and activities that are meaningful to them. They modify and change activities so that they can perform them successfully. Activity synthesis appears simple because it is so common. But most people do not synthesize activities in an organized and systematic manner. True activity synthesis is a complex skill, yet very little has been written specifically about the topic. Occupational therapy practitioners approach activity synthesis from an organized theoretical perspective requiring an understanding of activity analysis; underlying components; the context; and, of course, the client. Further, activity synthesis is influenced strongly by the frame of reference chosen for intervention and the artfulness of the practitioner. Activity synthesis is a critical function of the occupational therapy practitioner, used frequently in day-to-day interventions. If used successfully in the intervention process, activity synthesis should result in occupational synthesis within the client.

Both activity synthesis and occupational synthesis are complex processes. The practitioner needs to understand what synthesis is and the difference between activity synthesis and occupational synthesis. Then, through ongoing development, reflection, and experience, the practitioner becomes both skillful and artful in developing interventions that are meaningful for the client. ∎

References

Hinojosa, J. (2003). Occupation and continuing competence: Part II. *OT Practice, 8*(14), 11–12.

Hinojosa, J., Kramer, P., Royeen, C. B., & Luebben, A. (2003). The core concept of occupation. In P. Kramer, J. Hinojosa, & C. B. Royeen (Eds.), *Perspectives in human occupation: Participation in life* (pp. 1–17). Philadelphia: Lippincott, Williams & Wilkins.

Mosey, A. C. (1981). *Occupational therapy: Configuration of a profession.* New York: Raven.

Mosey, A. C. (1996). *Applied scientific inquiry in the health professions: An epistemological orientation* (2nd ed.). Bethesda, MD: American Occupational Therapy Association.

Nelson, D. L. (1997). Why the profession of occupational therapy will flourish in the 21st century, 1996 Eleanor Clarke Slagle Lecture. *American Journal of Occupational Therapy, 51*, 11–24.

Nelson, D. L., & Jepson-Thomas, J. (2003). Occupational form, occupational performance, and a conceptual framework for therapeutic occupation. In P. Kramer, J. Hinojosa, &

C. B. Royeen (Eds.), *Perspectives in human occupation: Participation in life* (pp. 87–155). Baltimore: Lippincott, Williams & Wilkins.

Schell, B. A. B. (2003). Clinical reasoning: The basis of practice. In. E. B. Crepeau, E. S. Cohn, & B. A. B. Schell (Eds.), *Willard and Spackman's occupational therapy* (10th ed., pp. 131–139). Philadelphia: Lippincott, Williams & Wilkins.

Schön, D. A. (1983). *The reflective practitioner: How professionals think in action.* Basic (Basic Books, Inc., Publishers): New York.

White, T. H. (1977). *The book of Merlin.* Austin: University of Texas Press.

Weinstein, E. (1998). *The nature of artful practice in psychosocial occupational therapy.* Unpublished doctoral dissertation, New York University, New York.

7

Activity Reasoning

Fran Babiss, PhD, OTR/L

Professionals whose work requires collaboration with the people they treat have an enormous responsibility. An inevitable moment comes during an occupational therapy student's fieldwork when this enormity becomes very tangible. This reality is expressed often in the form of fears about saying or doing the wrong thing with a client. That "what if" is the starting point of clinical reasoning. It is an awareness of the power that each of us has to effect destiny through the choices we make. Never is there a guarantee that what we say or do will have the outcome for which we strive, but we are responsible for taking action, and the job of the practitioner is to develop the skill to make such choices.

I have had students ask me, "How did you know what to say to that client?" The attempt to operationalize the decision-making process is complex. Reasoning about activities and occupation is how we make decisions about what intervention course to pursue with a client. Can we make the best decision? How do we know we have taken the right course, and essentially, how do we go about the process of deciding what purposeful activities to choose in working with others?

This chapter assists readers both in the process of becoming more aware of the concept of reasoning about activity and in engaging in clinical reasoning. It is filled with examples and exercises designed to give you the opportunity to think about your thinking.

—— ▦ ——

Exercise 7.1—Making a Decision

Take a few minutes now to reflect on the way in which you decided to become an occupational therapist or an occupational therapy assistant. Think about your age at the time of the decision. What was going on in your life? Did you have other career choices from which you fixed on occupational therapy? Can you tease out the cognitive and emotional mechanisms you used to settle on your chosen course? More importantly, can you remember what happened immediately following the point at which you made the decision?

———————————

Most often, individuals do not function in a metacognitive mode. By this, I mean that it is a rare occurrence to think about our own thinking in an overarching manner. Therefore, it is a difficult task. Whether it is something you are aware of or something you develop over time, decision-making and reasoning about activity and occupation are skills you will need to hone as a professional. You may not be able to make the right decision, but you can learn to make the best decision.

Definitions

Many years ago, when I was beginning my study of occupational therapy, I was told repeatedly that practitioners worked *holistically*. What this meant was that I paid attention not only to the physical or mental health concerns of a person, but also to the interaction among body, mind, and spirit. I still believe this holistic view to be true, and it contributes to the intricacy of reasoning about activities and occupations. It makes definition of the concept very difficult. As Hinojosa and Blount stated in Chapter 1, "having a definition does not necessarily simplify one's understanding of a phenomenon or the issues that it raises." It is, however, a starting point, and the inherent difficulty supports the argument for looking at the concept of clinical reasoning from a pluralistic standpoint.

Clinical reasoning is complex (Mattingly & Fleming, 1994), and many definitions exist. Consistent with my views of clinical reasoning, Schell (2003b) defined it as a process that is both complex and multifaceted. She went on to define *clinical reasoning* as "the process used by practitioners to plan, direct, perform, and reflect on client care (p. 131).

Building on Exercise 7.1, think about what happened to you once you decided to become an occupational therapy practitioner. A decision is nothing more than what I think, until I begin to take action based on the decision. This is the planning stage of clinical reasoning. At first, deciding to become an occupational therapy practitioner looks no different from deciding to become a black belt in karate. The way in which you or anyone else knows that a decision has been made is by the behavior in which you engage after having made the decision. This is the performance stage of clinical reasoning. Imagine deciding to become an occupational therapist or an occupational therapy assistant and finding a *sensei* based on that decision.

A decision that Mr. Ames will need 120° of forward shoulder flexion to permit him to return to his job stocking shelves in a warehouse makes clear a course of action designed to assist him in a return of range of motion. Complexity enters in the form of deciding just what to do to implement that increase in movement. In addition, how do we know that Mr. Ames really wants to return to work, and can we provide an environment for him that approximates closely the conditions of his workplace? A dozen more questions can and should be asked before action can take place.

Clinical Reasoning—A Very Brief History

A close examination of the process of clinical reasoning was a natural development in the maturation of occupational therapy as a profession. Cohn (1991) traced the origin of the inquiry to Joan Rogers's 1983 Eleanor Clarke Slagle Lecture devoted to explicating clinical reasoning (Rogers, 1983). In the closing, Rogers spoke of the need to examine thinking more systematically for the purpose of making it accessible to the profession. She connected correctly an improvement in one's art of practice with a greater awareness of the ways in which we think about that practice.

Based on this beginning, Mattingly and Fleming (1994) worked with the American Occupational Therapy Association (AOTA) and American Occupational Therapy Foundation (AOTF) to conduct an ethnographic study to begin to explain the thinking that takes place when occupational therapists solve treatment problems. Today, clinical reasoning has been incorporated into occupational therapy curricula to address the expanding knowledge required of practitioners. This addition is based on the following premises: With the ability to perform reasoning about activities and occupation, occupational therapy practitioners should be able to solve treatment problems that exist outside of their experience or training, and learning how to think about a profession improves the ability to engage meaningfully in that profession. Throughout their professional careers, practitioners continue to develop their clinical reasoning skills.

The Underlying Framework

The catalyst for much of the thinking about thinking in occupational therapy is based on the work of Schön (1983). In addition, Dreyfus and Dreyfus (1986) contributed to our understanding of the movement of the practitioner from novice to expert. This section summarizes the work of Schön and that of Dreyfus and Dreyfus so that readers can have a better understanding of the development of the categories of clinical reasoning in occupational therapy.

The Reflective Practitioner

Schön's (1983) work is credited as the starting point for the exploration of the workings of clinical reasoning in the occupational therapy profession. His area of exploration was the development of professions, more specifically how professions acquire their particular knowledge. He created this epistemology of practice based on the premise that most practicing professionals know more in practice than they can verbalize. This situation is what I wrote about in the beginning of this chapter and represents the strongest argument for participating in the training of occupational therapy students as they keep thinking about choices made in practice. When asked how decisions are made during practice, the occupational therapy practitioner is sometimes at a loss to explain the process. This not being able to say what we know (p. 49) is what Schön explored.

The task for professionals is to develop an art of practice in spite of the multiplicity of frames of reference that exist. Schön (1983) believed that the conflicts and difficulties that exist in solving professional problems are what allows a person to grow in his or her ability to solve these problems artfully, and I agree. Pluralism is healthy for a profession (Mosey, 1985), and the art of practice can be developed regardless of the techniques chosen:

> It is true that there is an irreducible element of art in professional practice, it is also true that gifted engineers, teachers, scientists, architects, and managers sometimes display artistry in their day-to-day practice. If the art is not invariant, known, and teachable, it appears nonetheless, at least for some individuals to be learnable. (Schön, 1983, p. 18)

Schön (1983) labeled the simple application of learned techniques of practice as *technical rationality*. The movement to full professional status of an artful practitioner involves moving from what he termed *knowing-in-action* to *reflection-in-action*. Knowing-in-action involves the concept of *tacit knowledge*, a term credited to Polanyi (1962, 1974) that describes a form of knowing without knowing how we know. For example, you may have no difficulty knowing that you like or dislike a certain work of art, but you might not be able to say what it is that makes you like or dislike the artwork. In the same way, we use language often without the slightest understanding of its grammatical underpinnings. A sentence may be dissonant to our ears, but we would be challenged to provide the grammatical rule that is the cause of our discomfort. Similarly, a practitioner may interact with or choose a purposeful activity with an individual without any ability to explain why a statement was made or an intervention chosen.

Much knowing-in-action is a function of experience as a practitioner. As the practitioner experiences situation after situation, a database is built. After time and repetition, the connection between experience and action becomes separated, much in the same way that a person can daydream driving home from work, yet find him- or herself at the front door without any difficulty. While writing this chapter, I asked many therapists to pay attention to their thinking about what they did as they practiced, and some likened the experience to "waking up." This is not to say that many occupational therapy practitioners sleep in practice but that certain practices become so automatic that they melt from our awareness. These experiences become tacit knowledge. Hence, the question from a student, "How did you know how to do that?" is an opportunity to explore knowing-in-action and make the tacit explicit. Then, a piece of the art of practice becomes learnable.

Danger lurks, though, in the habituation to tacit ways of applying clinical knowledge, which is addressed by the cliché, "When all I have is a hammer, the whole world looks like a nail." In my practice, I have come to specialize in working with people with borderline personality disorder. As a result, I often see the patterns associated with this disorder in many of the clients with whom I work. This perspective creates a tunnel vision that negates the possibility of entertaining other possible explanations for the way in which a client functions, which was made explicit by an occupational therapy student who had worked in the school system for many years before pursuing a career in occupational therapy. During an occupational therapy activity, a client got up from the table and took a lap blanket from a chair, reseating herself wrapped in the blanket. After the group, the student and I were reflecting upon the group, and I described the client's behavior as a need to direct the group's attention to her because the group was focused on another client. The student opined that perhaps the client's behavior had been an indication of a need for tactile pressure because she was starved for sensory input. I will return to this example in the discussion of reflection-in-action.

Reflection-in-action is a characteristic of a professional who is practicing at the highest level of expertise. It is the ability to reason about what is going on as it is in process. Schön (1983) saw reflection-in-action as the positive outcome when the professional is confronted by a situation that falls outside the applied science of technical rationality, the experience of knowing-in-action, and catapults into a world of problem solving in which he or she must entertain new thinking and actions:

> Many practitioners, locked into a view of themselves as technical experts, find nothing in the world of practice to occasion reflection. They have become too skillful at techniques of selective inattention, junk categories, and situational control, techniques which they use to preserve the constancy of their knowledge-in-practice. For them, uncertainty is a threat; its admission is a sign of weakness. Others, more inclined toward and adept at reflection-in-action, nevertheless feel profoundly uneasy because they cannot say what they know how to do, cannot justify its quality or rigor. (p. 69)

At this point, it is helpful to return to the previous anecdote in which the practitioner and the student had such different explanations for the behavior of the client who wrapped herself in a blanket. In terms of reasoning about the incident, each person saw it through the lens she had been using, either sensory or psychological. Either conclusion could lead to such differences in intervention, even interventions that could be counterproductive for the client. Schön (1983) spoke of a virtual world (p. 157) in which the student and supervisor can imagine a situation without being in the situation. Although this strategy works for the architect planning on paper or the psychotherapist analyzing the transference, it is not helpful in this situation because not enough information is available about the client. The answer to the problem of the need for attention versus the need for tactile pressure can be solved by reflection-in-practice, which involves continued observation of and interaction with the client. As it turned out, by asking questions and providing different input, the client seemed to be in need of both tactile input and the attention of others and provided a learning experience in creating interventions that worked along both axes. Schön likened reflection-in-action to a form of research designed for learning new and different ways of thinking about phenomena. It challenges the practitioner to stretch the limits of his or her knowledge.

Schön (1983) acknowledged the value of experience in passing on the skill of being a reflective practitioner. The movement of a practitioner from novice to professional is another area of professional development that has a strong impact on reasoning about activity.

Activity Reasoning and Experience

Suppose you were told that in order to become an expert practitioner you would have to rely on intuition? In other words, what you could learn by rules, regulations, and experience was not enough. If learning the rules and exceptions were enough, the problem of computer artificial intelligence would have been solved by now. Dreyfus and Dreyfus (1986), brothers who are professors of philosophy and industrial engineering, have explored the progression of individuals from novice to expert in different careers and skill acquisitions. Their investigations provide a framework for understanding growth in the ability to reason about activities as a function of time and experience. The five stages that an individual may pass through are:

1.   Novice

2.   Advanced beginner

3.   Competence

4.   Proficient

5.   Expert.

STAGE 1—NOVICE

The beginner who is learning a new skill is taught to recognize certain features and rules that are based on features of the task at hand. For example, when a novice dancer is learning to dance a waltz, the order of the steps is the focus of the activity. The rules about the order of steps in the dance are what Dreyfus and Dreyfus (1986) referred to as "context-free" elements because they can be recognized without a need to be aware of anything else that is happening (p. 21). In fact, the novice dancer might not be able to learn the steps of the dance if she had to focus on anything other than the rules for the steps. The novice could not account for the crowd on a dance floor or the dance style of a partner. It would not be possible for the novice to carry on a conversation while dancing a waltz.

Novice occupational therapy practitioners beginning school 25 years ago were given rules for mental health practice in their introductory classes. At that time in the history of the profession, students often were taught exact prescriptions of activities to be used with clients, with much of it based on psychodynamic theories of the meaning of symbols. They were taught that male clients would prefer leather- and wood-working and female clients would be motivated by needlework crafts. When they wrote papers for school, these students followed these rules assiduously.

STAGE 2—ADVANCED BEGINNER

At this stage, the learner of a new skill or profession is continuing to gather more context-free facts. The context they perceive is becoming larger because of the experience gained through practicing in concrete situations in the world. The learner is beginning to gather a database of situations with which past experiences can be compared. Thus, the advanced beginner begins to use situational cues for reasoning and practice. The dancer begins to be able to look around the dance floor and negotiate and adjust steps so as not to collide with others. Knowing the steps was not enough. To survive on the dance floor, one must learn to avoid others in the same space.

In the mental health clinic it did not take long to gather a collection of situations in which the "gender" of a craft was often a useless rule. From these experiences, practitioners learned that, although preference for activities might still relate to generalizations about gender, asking a client what he or she enjoyed doing had more value and helped the practitioner to establish a rapport with the client. The rules these practitioners had learned as novices did not serve them well in each real-world situation.

STAGE 3—COMPETENCE

At this point in learning a skill or profession, the learner has amassed so many context-free rules and situational experiences that a feeling of being overwhelmed can ensue. So much is known that extracting the significant from the irrelevant is difficult. The competent professional adopts or is taught a hierarchy of decision-making to assist him or her in making a way through the confusion of too much information. At this level, the learner begins to have a sense of responsibility for the outcome of a decision, and this emotional involvement is critical to the move to the level of competence. Our dancer now is able to decide that dancing close to the judge of a dancing contest is the most important task and feels confident in moving close to the judge while dancing. Other components of the dance do not require intense focus anymore. The steps of the waltz are second nature, the synchronization with a usual dance partner is established, and the dancer rarely bumps into other couples on the dance floor. Thus, she is able to begin to plan and establish goal-directed behavior in the larger environment.

At this level, practitioners working in a mental health setting have had experience with hundreds of clients and several dozen activities. Access to all of this information allows them to begin to construct a form of triage in activity selection. A competent practitioner can interact with a client in a way that allows him or her to understand that the client's self-esteem is so damaged that an activity in which a successful outcome is ensured is of primary importance. After that decision, an exploration of the type of activity in which the client might be motivated to engage might follow. In other words, it is a search for an activity that is meaningful to the client. It is then the task of the competent practitioner to adapt and grade the client's choice to ensure a positive outcome. The practitioner has an emotional stake related both to empathy for the client and a desire to make the right choice in activity with the client. Dreyfus and Dreyfus (1986) stated that many individuals do not develop beyond this level of skill because to do so would entail moving into intuitive levels of thought and action.

STAGE 4—PROFICIENCY

The proficient practitioner functions without a conscious reach for rules, situations, or hierarchies. *Intuition,* as described by Dreyfus and Dreyfus (1986), consists of a "holistic understanding" (p. 109) in which response to patterns occurs without having them deconstructed into component parts. It is knowing the right thing to do without thinking about why it is the right thing to do. It is akin to the concept of *flow* as described by Csikszentmihalyi (1990) as a seamless flow of activity. The proficient practitioner functions effortlessly. The proficient dancer is at one with her body, partner, the dance floor, and the entire experience in which they exist.

A proficient mental health practitioner senses when a client is ready to tackle a more challenging task, tolerate an intervention about his or her behavior, or take an interpersonal risk. The practitioner does not break down the client's interactions or behavior into units but looks at the entire client moving through the environment. It is this level that is difficult to explain to the novice student because it goes beyond the simple acquisition of thousands of hours of experience. It is a leap into the intuitive realm that many practitioners never make.

STAGE 5—EXPERT

Dreyfus and Dreyfus (1986) said, "When things are proceeding normally, experts don't solve problems and don't make decisions; they do what normally works" (p. 31). Being one with what a person does is the essence of expertise. The move from proficiency to expertise mirrors that of the move from advanced beginner to competence. As the advanced beginner accrues more and more situations and rules, he or she groups them together to improve his or her decision-making skills. In the same manner, the proficient learner groups intuitive experiences into larger chunks so that thinking recedes and acting and living become one. As long as things unfold as usual, the expert will not make mistakes. The dancer on the floor will waltz in a way that all can recognize as expert, but to say why would be to break the experience into parts that would render it incomprehensible as a whole. If asked what makes her an expert, the waltzer may not be able to say, because at this level, such a question is akin to asking her what makes her who she is.

An expert practitioner in mental health practice might be able to sense that a client is in acute distress, even if the client is not manifesting symptoms. Many of my peers relate experiences of becoming disquieted by the behavior of a client during a group. They could not tell me why, but they knew somehow that increased intervention or even intervention of a more restrictive nature might be necessary. They could not tell the client's psychiatrist why they requested an immediate consult, but in most instances, they were correct in their belief. They did not think but acted according to instincts they could not identify.

The five stages from novice to expert along with the concept of reflective practice provide a structure around which a discussion of the different types of reasoning occupational therapy practitioners use can proceed.

Types of Reasoning About Activity

This section describes ways of looking at the complexities of clinical reasoning as they relate to occupational therapy. This subject is abstract, and readers are advised to compare the perspectives presented with his or her own thinking, reasoning, and decision-making processes.

The Therapist With the Three-Track Mind

The concept of the occupational therapy practitioner operating in three spheres of reasoning emerged from the clinical reasoning studies conducted by Mattingly and Fleming, which were supported by the AOTA and AOTF (Mattingly & Gillette, 1991; Mattingly & Fleming, 1994). This small qualitative study examined the reasoning of a small group of therapists with a specialization in physical disabilities as they provided treatment.

PROCEDURAL REASONING

When you engaged in thinking about the process of deciding to become an occupational therapist or occupational therapy assistant in Exercise 7.1, you were engaging in procedural reasoning. The practitioner who thinks about the activities he or she might use with a client to improve on the client's functional limitations is engaging in procedural reasoning. The evaluation process, focusing on the relationship between performance in daily life and the barriers to engagement and participation in daily activities, requires the ability to reason in a procedural way. The connection between this evaluation and the creation of an intervention plan is procedural as well.

Mattingly and Fleming (1994) distinguished between the procedural reasoning of an occupational therapist and that of a physician engaging in medical reasoning. The goal of medical reasoning is to postulate a diagnosis. Occupational therapists do not engage in diagnosis, but they work with the functional sequelae of diagnoses (A. C. Mosey, personal communication, 1986).

An experienced practitioner has a great deal of past information from which to refer in order to identify patterns and offer hypotheses about what might work with a client. Through a form of what I call "cognitive figure–ground," practitioners sort and sift through the information gathered while speaking with and observing a client. The practitioner pushes aside what he or she reasons to be irrelevant and extraneous in the hope of finding what is meaningful and worthy of attention. As Mattingly and Fleming (1994) stated, this type of thinking does not take place without the other two tracks operating in concert.

INTERACTIONAL REASONING

Relationships form the context within which practitioners function. During evaluation, the dialogue in which we engage is part of the intervention. The way in which we interact with a client can determine the efficacy of the entire course of treatment. Interactional reasoning is all of the ways in which we determine to communicate with and listen to a client. Experienced practitioners develop what they would call an instinct for knowing how to speak with clients.

The most powerful and meaningful intervention is that which allows the client to determine what goals are important to him or her. Collaboration with a client is essential to this process. Beginning practitioners have to juggle so many new ideas, thoughts, frames of reference, and facts that the simple act of listening to the story of a client becomes lost. Yet, it is this very act that can lead the practitioner to the point where the direction to take with a client becomes clear.

In addition, knowing how to speak with a client allows us to provide encouragement and motivation in a positive manner. This is not to say that reasoning about the interaction is to create a positive relationship. Often, the hardest concept for an occupational therapy student to grasp is that our job is rarely about being liked. We need to be honest and say the things that will move a client to pursue his or her goals. Using interactional reasoning skills, we can judge the point at which we can push a client to move beyond the safety of the movements he or she has been trying around the house or the interactions he or she has been risking with his or her spouse.

Interactional reasoning requires that practitioners know themselves well. The things that we say have to be a match for our personalities and styles, or they will not be taken as genuine. The question becomes, What do I need to communicate with this client, and how shall I express it so that it is coming from me? If you have a sense of humor, it can be used to connect with a client, as can a very serious nature. A practitioner has to have the ability to observe the effect of his or her interaction on others and adapt or alter it when needed.

CONDITIONAL REASONING

The joy of working with clients comes from the moment when the narrative they are sharing rings with meaning for them and allows you a glimpse into the world of the other. For example, Martha, a young woman with borderline personality disorder who refused to sit during her interview, became engrossed in her telling of what it is like to be in her head: "It's like in the movies, when those whirling disks are chasing the star, and she just escapes one, when, just like that there's another and another, and she can't keep up. I feel like I'm being chased and captured." Thanks to her eloquent metaphor, I was able to ask her whether she wanted help learning how to control the whirling disks. For the first time during the occupational profile process, she sat down, made eye contact, and seemed to be listening to me. All at the same time, I watched her movements in space, I watched the room in which she sat, and I listened to her words. For a brief moment, I entered her world, and she was ready to begin to do the things she needed to do to decrease the disorganization and emotional pain. This type of reasoning will be addressed further in the section on narrative reasoning.

The holistic roots of the profession of occupational therapy suggest the need for conditional reasoning in that it provides the connection from meaning to action. Conditional reasoning is the ability to place thinking in an environmental context at the same time that thinking takes place in a context that is beyond the bonds of strict linear cognition. It is phenomenological, creative, and imaginative. It is the synthesis of all of the other forms of reasoning, some of them beyond what is known explicitly.

The phenomenology of the client is of paramount importance in conditional reasoning. The practitioner's task is to understand how the client makes meaning out of his or her life and the activities it comprises. As with clinical reasoning, conditional reasoning is difficult to conceptualize.

Mattingly and Fleming (1994) said, "We think that conditional reasoning revolves around the ways that therapists think about which of the actions that the patient takes have potential for meaning-making" (p. 198). They believed that meaning-making connects with activity in three ways, which they label as *intentionality, habits,* and *symbolic meaning.* This connection is an integral one for occupational therapy practitioners. It is the framework for the jump from meaning to action.

Intentionality implies choice. Consider the thinking involved in collaborating with a client about the choices he or she will make about purposeful activities and occupations. Our goal is to see to it that the client is choosing activities that will allow him or her to move back into his or her life, but the ideas we have may not match those of the client. A weak grasp may preclude tooth brushing, but the client may want to be able to pick up a fork first. In a clinic, devoid of forks and toothbrushes, we may be working with pencils and pick-up sticks. The idea of doing an activity with many useful applications and outcomes is one of the caveats Mattingly and Fleming (1994) identified. Most people's conception of occupational therapy practice is based on a linear observation of activity provision. They are not aware of the clinical reasoning in the form of conditional reasoning that is the impetus for the choice of purposeful activities. What looks like playing pick-up sticks to an observer may mean independence in feeding to the practitioner and the client. The richness of the many layers of meaning for the client and the practitioner often is misperceived. When we explain to clients what we are doing and why, we let them into our phenomenology and provide them with the opportunity for greater understanding of the power of occupational therapy.

Habit is a word that has its origins in the very beginning of occupational therapy. Habit training harkens back to the earliest days of the profession. Life is made up of a series of routines and rituals that simplify and secure meaning. Practitioners understand the importance of habits to people whose daily routines have been interrupted by disability. The meaning of a morning cup of coffee is far grander than the mechanics of the praxis that brings the coffee to the lips. Although importance of praxis may not have been apparent when one did not have to think about how his or her body moved in space, it is of the utmost importance when it prevents the event from happening.

On an even more ephemeral level, the symbolic meaning of activity is critical to the clinical reasoning skills of the practitioner.

Exercise 7.2—The Macramé Lesson

Read the following case and identify when the therapist uses instances of procedural, interactive, and conditional reasoning.

Case Scenario

Thinking about thinking is not always an exercise that results in the outcome that is expected. The most glaring example of this that I have experienced came in working with a young woman, Roxanne, who came to day treatment after a long inpatient stay for depression, several suicide attempts, and severe self-mutilatory behavior. Although she was a respiratory therapist and social worker, school had always been difficult because of what she called her learning disabilities, which made it hard to process information and directions. Roxanne had not been able to maintain her employment in respiratory therapy because she could not arrange the equipment correctly when she was under pressure. When stressed, she became unable to tell left from right, a disability that could result in the death of a patient. At the time of this interview, Roxanne had no plans to return to work.

During my interview with Roxanne, she helped me to see how important it was to her to be able to spend some time with her children. She had great difficulty engaging in arts and crafts secondary to her perceptual difficulties, a symptom of her learning difficulties. She asked me whether I could teach her a craft that she could do with her children. She challenged me by letting me know that it would be a difficult undertaking. She suggested that she be taught to do macramé so that she could make the knotted friendship bracelets popular at the time. I agreed and made plans to carry out this activity. As she left for the day, Roxanne turned to me and said, "Get a good night's sleep before we meet again. I want you to have the stamina to make it through." I knew Roxanne well enough at this point that I understood her statement as a way of feeling close to me. Roxanne was extremely bright and liked when those around her spoke in an intellectual way; sarcastic language was very acceptable. In an instant I had a riposte that may have sounded inappropriate had a student been watching, but it was the right thing to say to Roxanne: "Oh, but I shall endeavor to have you in knots *tout à fait*." The word "endeavor," the use of French, and the sarcasm and play on words were all chosen to establish a bond and to compliment Roxanne on her brightness.

My reasoning after the interview followed this path. First, I believed that macramé was a purposeful activity that the client had identified as meaningful. The chances of Roxanne being motivated to engage would be high. Second, in this case, macramé would be a purposeful activity that made up a piece of the occupations of child care, leisure, and social interaction, adding to the repertoire of the client. Third, I was familiar enough with the activity to know that I could break it down into component parts that could be taught by rote over and over until the client could perform it in spite of perceptual difficulties. I believed that I had thought about the most important aspects of the task, had strategies for the intervention, and was confident that the experience would be a positive one.

In fact, the experience was a very positive one. Although it took a long time for Roxanne to master the basic square knots of macramé, she was able, eventually, to repeat the "mantra" I used to help her remember the steps involved in making the knot. At one point, Roxanne told me that using the phrase, "crossover in front," was confusing. Eventually, we figured out by trial and error that saying, "lay the cord on top of the macramé," allowed her to visually process the act. By the end of the session, Roxanne had begun to make an interlocking strand of knots and said that she would teach her son and daughter how to make the knots using the way in which she had been taught. I knew that written instructions would be unintelligible to her without a reader, but I gave her sheets with instructions and macramé cord to take home anyway.

After Roxanne left, I basked in the self-satisfied glow that is the prize of every therapist who knows the joy of a session that goes well. Roxanne was grateful, and I was fulfilled by having planned a useful intervention. I felt I had provided Roxanne with something that would improve her ability to engage in life in a meaningful way.

The next week I asked Roxanne how her arts-and-crafts session with her children had fared, and she told me that it had gone well. Now that she could master the basic knots she wanted to go on to do the finer work of making the friendship bracelets. But first, she wanted to tell me why she had adored the activity most of all. I was all set to hear how wonderful it had been to be provided with a means of interacting with her children in a meaningful and "mommy-like" way. Roxanne whispered to me, "I can't tell you what it meant to me that you let me take string home. You know I tried to kill myself three times when I was in the hospital." I was stunned. I believed that I had thought about what the ideal activity would be, why it was ideal, how to present it to Roxanne, and even how the outcome of the activity might be. Yet Roxanne focused on the interaction and relationship between us. I adjusted my response based on this surprise and told Roxanne that I trusted her and would be glad to spend a few more hours teaching her how to make the friendship bracelets. In the end, Roxanne did master the macramé, and went on to trying to learn to knit, but could not master this activity successfully.

PRAGMATIC REASONING

Health care has undergone major changes since the inception of managed care, and it is these changes that are taken into account by pragmatic reasoning (Schell & Cervero, 1993). Pragmatism was identified by Schell and Cervero after they completed a literature review on the topic of clinical reasoning. Pragmatic reasoning is similar to conditional reasoning in its recognition of the integration of environmental and personal factors but goes farther to embrace the phenomenology of the therapist, the input of the treatment team, and the political–economic factors of present-day health care. The difference between the 10-page treatment plans done for school assignments and the one-goal plans created for a 2-day length of stay for a patient in a hand surgery clinic are enormous.

ETHICAL REASONING

Within the context of pragmatic reasoning is the thinking that is done with regard to ethics. The mechanics of managed care and caps on reimbursement are often in conflict with both the needs of the client and the desire of the practitioner. How is reasoning affected when a therapist determines that a client requires 6 months of rehabilitation and the reimbursement is for 10 visits? How does one construct a context of improvement under these constraints? The opposite is just as common an occurrence. In my practice, the criteria for treatment at a partial hospital level of care are quite specific. Often, a client no longer meets these criteria but has been certified for additional days of treatment. The right thing to do is to discharge the client to a less-structured level of care, but this is not what happens in every case. When I deem that the continued care of the client for 1 or 2 days will prevent or forestall a relapse or rehospitalization, I may make this choice. In the same way, I would advocate for a client who was being discharged before receiving maximum benefit from the intervention, if I believed that he or she could benefit from additional treatment.

The concept of ethics lies outside of the scope of this chapter, but it is mentioned as another aspect of the complexity involved in clinical reasoning. The decisions we make about what we do need to be reasoned about in terms of whether it is the right thing to do. Ethical reasoning is a part of this process.

NARRATIVE REASONING

"Whether I shall turn out to be the hero of my own life, or whether that station will be held by anybody else, these pages must show." (Dickens, 1849/2000)

We are all the heroes of our own lives, and the way in which the story comes out has a lot to do with health and illness. Mattingly, Fleming, Schell, and others stressed the importance of the client's meaning-making in clinical reasoning. Each client's story is unique and carries the seed of intervention. Narrative is the story we tell of illness and wellness. Narrative is how the practitioner fashions a view of the future world of the client. Often, there can be disparity between this vision and the reality of the ensuing course of treatment (Mattingly & Fleming, 1994; Schell, 2003b). In the story of Roxanne, I envisioned her bonding with her children and teaching them an activity. What occurred was on the surface as I had envisioned, but the meaning for Roxanne was worlds apart from my view.

Listening for the meaning in the narrative requires the skills of an experienced clinician. Narrative reasoning exists on two levels. First is the life story of the client as it unfolds during evaluation and continues in treatment. Second is the narrative constructed by the practitioner as intervention is designed and implemented.

The key task for the practitioner who wishes to reason in narrative form is to listen, listen, listen. The story emerges through the storytelling. A beginning student is juggling so many impressions and ideas in his or her mind that the art of active listening can be lost. As experience begins to make it easier to focus attention, the student can relax in the story of the client. In my own work (Babiss, 2003), the story became the method for making decisions about ways of improving outcomes. I let the client tell me how the next chapter of her story should proceed. This can be invaluable in those instances when you are troubled by some aspect related to treatment with a client. It is always worth the time and effort to sit with a client in order to allow meaning to emerge. Often, the experience is quite intense when a client can see that you "get it," and his or her world opens to you.

Case Scenario

Chris is a handsome young man who was a brilliant student with a few good friends, a loving mother, and an obsession with flying. In his first year of aviation school he began to hear voices, which continued until he was forced to leave school and enter a psychiatric hospital. After the inpatient stay, the story he had written for himself—college graduate, pilot, husband, and father—was dashed. "I was going along fine, and then I was *plucked* out of life," he said with tears in his eyes. Chris's story highlights the temporal quality of narrative. He believed that his life was traveling a path and that its trajectory was assured.

On hearing this narrative of an interrupted history, the practitioner reasoned that there was some validity to Chris's assertion of being "plucked" from life but believed that he had been removed only from the life he had envisioned. Together with Chris, the practitioner determined that the task ahead was to write a new story and allow the narrative to unfold in a new and different way.

In a description of a book of his short stories, the author William Trevor said, "It's not as rose-tinted a world, as most people would like it to be. But the people in my stories and novels are not ragingly desperate; they have…come to terms, and coming to terms in itself is quite an achievement" (as cited by Allen, 1998, p. 7). It seemed that Chris's main task would be to write a new story of coming to terms with what he could do now, and the job of the practitioner would be to work with Chris on editing his life.

The narrative of the practitioner was grandiose and spectacular but acknowledged the reality that Chris could not hope to fly again because of his psychiatric history. The practitioner's plan involved exploring with Chris the support activities involved in aviation. Chris's loss of narrative rendered cooperation difficult initially, but eventually he determined that he wanted to become involved in the construction of airplanes. This goal set the path that permitted the practitioner to work with Chris on constructing a daily life built around purposeful activities that would ensure that Chris's story would not face a major disruption. Chris worked out a daily schedule, independently figuring out that setting the alarm on his aviator's watch would remind him to take his medications, with which compliance was critical to maintaining his stability and function. Chris had a very supportive mother who was instrumental in providing a home environment in which he could remain independent, but supported.

Together, Chris and the practitioner researched schools, and he chose one far from the hospital. He applied to the school, visited it with his mother, and was accepted. It was determined that he would remain at home until the next school semester 3 months away. During that time, Chris came to the hospital and worked on work and study skills. He wanted his story to be one of someone who could concentrate in school despite the voices, which still plagued him from time to time. He worked on the computer in the clinic and showed slight improvement with time.

In addition, Chris made friends with several other clients in treatment. His story of the roles that had been disrupted made it difficult for him to see himself as a peer to them. As time passed, however, he realized that he had more in common with them than he had thought at first. The practitioner's story of Chris's life in the clinic before returning to school contained chapters on his connecting with other people, so she constructed group experiences and even the placement of chairs in the computer room to encourage spontaneous conversations.

The story ended for the practitioner when Chris and his mother moved to another state so that he could attend school. The last letter from Chris told of his moderate success in school and that he had a few friends. He was still sad about the change of his circumstances, but it seemed that he had come to terms with his new story.

Narrative reasoning for this practitioner helped her to enter into the world of the client in order to collaborate on the plot for future chapters. It is crucial to know what the client's story is so that effective interventions can be made.

Again, the most crucial element in narrative reasoning is listening. Without hearing what the client is saying, a practitioner is unable to place his or her reasoning skills into the world of the person with a disability. Peloquin (1993) addressed some of the beliefs that interfere with the ability to establish a full understanding of the client in his or her narrative. When we think of a client as, for example, "the right hemi," we are engaging in the reductionistic, monistic thinking that leads to applying techniques and rote exercises to a problem that may have more to do with a person's desire to pet her cat. Thus, to engage in meaningful narrative reasoning, one has to take the time to hear the story.

Exercise 7.3—Clinical Reasoning and Activity Choice

The following case scenario represents a unique instance of an individual with both mental health and physiological concerns. Read through the case and begin to think about the planning, performance, and reflection involved in working with this client.

Case Scenario

Gerard is a 55-year-old single man referred to the day program after an inpatient stay on the psychiatric floor of a major hospital. This is his first mental health hospitalization.

The information collected during the occupational profile revealed a man of many facets. Gerard is of medium height, slender, and graceful in his movements, all of which makes his story more remarkable. Gerard was a veteran of the Vietnam War, with the rank of captain. He watched as several of his men died in a helicopter that took off while he remained behind on orders from a superior. He commented that he has always felt guilty about this. After a 4-year tour, he returned home to find that his peers had gone to school, gotten married, and "moved on." He joined the city fire department where he worked for 20 years in some of the most dangerous neighborhoods in the city. On retirement, he sold the condominium in which he lived alone and moved into an apartment in the house of his sister and brother-in-law.

Gerard never married and attributed this to his use of alcohol throughout most of his life. At the time of his admission to the day program, he had not had a drink for several months. "Alcohol is the thing that destroyed anything good in my life." Gerard identified as an asset his desire to spend time with his family and as a weakness a fear of close relationships with people other than his family.

In retirement, Gerard taught himself to use a computer and started to work in construction with his brother-in-law. This vocation contributed to his current difficulties. While working on his sister's house, he fell from the roof, fracturing his spine, and crushing his right radius. Gerard's back healed, but he required surgery for his forearm, which has several internal stabilization devices in it. Gerard laughed ruefully as he said, "I set off the alarms at the airport now." Although Gerard went to therapy after the surgery, he remained unable to use his hand for carpentry and the computer keyboard. Besides computers, he identified golf and carpentry as avocational pursuits, all of which have been greatly hampered by the lack of range of motion. Frustrated with the difficulties with his hand, Gerard contemplated suicide, which necessitated the inpatient hospitalization.

As he began to realize that he would not regain full use of his right hand, Gerard began to experience what he described as anxiety attacks. He then remembered that in his last few years at the fire department he had become panicked and gone to speak with the fire department psychiatrist a few times. However, this was Gerard's first inpatient and subsequent day hospital encounter.

It was clear that more information was needed about the prognosis for Gerard's hand. A phone consultation was conducted with the occupational therapist who had treated Gerard. She reported that Gerard's internal fixation status would limit his wrist extension to 40° forever, but she believed that he could adequately accommodate for this with respect to the computer. Carpentry work, however, would be limited, unless he was able to change handedness for the use of tools.

Case Questions: What is the priority need for intervention with Gerard? Why did you make this choice? Suspend pragmatic and ethical concerns and make activity choices to provide intervention in the priority area. Reason about the importance of social components for Gerard in planning choice of activities.

The pragmatic realities of Gerard's case hampered greatly the realization of interventions that the treatment team reasoned to be meaningful. Gerard was discharged after 2 weeks, secondary to constraints of both his insurance company and the decrease in his acute psychiatric symptom of anxiety and suicidal ideation. The treatment team, working in a mental health environment, reasoned that the most important task for Gerard was to arrive at an acceptance of the restrictions in range of motion in his hand so that he could begin to move ahead with plans for avocational pursuits that took his limitation in hand function into account. Without acceptance, Gerard would have no motivation to act in a goal-directed manner oriented toward the future. Second, a review of Gerard's history seemed to suggest that he was not deeply concerned with the lack of intimate social relationships in his life and that the suggestion of 12-step attendance (Alcoholics Anonymous) would not be a good choice for him. Gerard seemed motivated to interact with family members and did not seem to value relationships outside of the family. Unfortunately, the treatment team did not get to enact many interventions with Gerard, beyond leaving him with the information about coming to terms with his hand injury.

New Directions in Clinical Reasoning

In my opinion, recent work in the area of clinical reasoning in occupational therapy has taken a step toward a more reductionistic view of the phenomenon. Schell (2003a) has begun to look at clinical reasoning as a cognitive activity, which it is, and to suggest the use of mental models as a means of making practice more efficient. Mental models were suggested first by the philosopher Craik (1967, p. 59), who posited that people used a "small-scale model" of reality in order to be able to predict events and explain phenomena. Although Schell did acknowledge a drawback to fitting people into scripts and schemata, she was supportive of mental models. I acknowledge that there is almost nothing a thinking practitioner can do to avoid categorizing and pattern recognition, but grave danger exists in adopting this habit as a means of making work more efficient. Johnson-Laird, Girotto, and Legrenzi (1998) warned against the dangers of reasoning using mental models. Individuals who create mental models make explicit very little as they focus on the implicit information in their models. This use of mental models creates an environment in which the possibility of considering alternatives that lie outside the mental model is diminished. The authors provided an example of a grievous error of this nature, which occurred during the nuclear crisis at Three Mile Island. The rise in temperature in the plant was ascribed to a leak. The staff did not entertain other explorations, which would have revealed that the valve was stuck in an open position. Their actions were guided by a faulty mental model, and the result was a disaster. Practitioners with less experience may welcome the ease of mental models, but the difficulty of changing one's models can be too strong to reject.

The art of practice is born of treating each client as if he or she were a completely new experience because he or she is a new experience. If I start out working on pattern recognition and mental models, I may remain within this framework and never grow into the seasoned professional who has the ability to look outside of the cubbyholes I have created. A "typical hemi" is never just that.

Knowing More Than We Can Say

Thinking about our thinking, the act of metacognition, is a laborious task. When asked to think about the way in which you decided to pursue a career in occupational therapy, you could probably discern a linear path that you followed in making the decision. Identifying the intangible factors that affected your decision is not a straightforward activity. Time spent examining the way in which your mind handles information and experiences can result in a significant improvement in your ability to reason about activities.

A structured portal into your thinking about thinking is the examination of your style of learning new information. Learning style models abound, and a student or practitioner who is interested in exploring how he or she learns what he or she knows is advised to choose a taxonomy that feels suitable to his or her needs. Gardner (1983) and Kolb (1984) offered learning style models based on, respectively, looking at seven types of intelligence and at experiential learning. Gardner asserted that intelligence is not one discrete measurement but that there are seven dimensions. For example, over time I have come to know that my strongest areas of intelligence are linguistic and spatial. Therefore, when learning new material or working with new clients, I read and observe as much as I can. It is the reason I am drawn to qualitative, narrative information gathering. The seven types of intelligence are (a) logical–mathematical, (b) linguistic, (c) musical, (d) spatial, (e) bodily–kinesthetic, (f) interpersonal, and (g) intrapersonal.

Kolb's (1984) work on experiential learning is similar to Schön (1983) in that it is based on doing and reflection. He reasons that individuals learn through doing and thinking about what they have done. For further information on learning styles, the reader is referred to the references for this chapter.

A practitioner who wishes to expand the ability to know without knowing and improve his or her prowess in the intuitive leaps that characterize a seasoned clinician is advised to practice some form of self-awareness technique. Meditation, yoga, and journal writing are all satisfactory means of expanding one's inner life. The more awareness you have of the way in which you make sense of the world, the better your ability to understand how this view affects your reasoning.

Case Studies—Activity Reasoning in Action

This chapter concludes with two examples of treatment interactions contributed by two occupational therapists. I asked each to think and reason about the choices they had made. The narratives provide a glimpse into the activity reasoning of a novice and an experienced practitioner. As you read, think about how you might have reasoned about each situation.

Case Scenario: Jane

The following description of an assessment, treatment plan, and intervention was conducted by Ann Winter, an occupational therapy student who had worked many years as a certified occupational therapy assistant but was beginning to negotiate the transition to the role of occupational therapist. Much of what she wrote included her reasoning, and she was asked to also think and write about the decisions made in collaborating with this client. What follows is both a wonderful account of a creative novice practitioner and a metacognitive exploration of clinical reasoning. Winter's musings about her choice, made after the treatment, are presented in italics.

Jane is a 17-year-2-month-old girl adopted from Korea. She was diagnosed with left hemiplegic cerebral palsy at 8 months of age and acquired Prader-Willi syndrome when she was 3 years old in addition to an inoperable tumor on her hypothalamus. She has many of the symptoms and signs of congenital Prader-Willi, including low muscle tone, short stature, cognitive disabilities, problem behaviors, and a flaw in the function of the hypothalamus, resulting in chronic feelings of hunger.

Jane's brother, also adopted by the same American parents, displays no cognitive or physical disabilities. The ethnic disparity in the family is reported to have had no effect on Jane's social or school experiences. Jane's father has a drug and alcohol dependency and has emotionally abused Jane's mother for the past 15 years. Consequently, Jane's mother has assumed the majority of the responsibilities associated with Jane's care since infancy and, currently, has an order of protection against her husband. He has been out of the house for the past 6 months. There is no history of physical abuse to either child.

Jane's room is on the ground floor of a home that has been environmentally adapted to suit her needs in terms of bathroom requirements and front door accessibility. She requires moderate assistance to rise from a sitting position, ambulate, and perform bed transfers, oral hygiene, dressing, showering, and toileting. She is able to navigate independently in a motorized wheelchair when outside her home. Her bedroom is adjacent to the den, which houses a television, computer, and stereo system, all of which Jane is able to operate.

Jane attends a Board of Cooperative Education Services (BOCES) high school and participates in the 6-week summer session. She has been taking part in a prevocational program at her school where she assembles parts for test tubes a full day once a week and receives a weekly paycheck. She spends the other days working on academics. Jane reads at a third-grade level, and she can perform single-digit addition and subtraction problems. Jane is unable to speak and must use an augmentative communication device to converse. She acknowledged that she enjoys communicating over the Internet and stated that she loves "looking things up." Jane's IQ was measured on a standardized intelligence test as 77. She continues to receive physical therapy at school, but much to her mother's opposition, occupational therapy services were discontinued 3 years ago because her therapist believed that Jane had reached a plateau in terms of skill acquisition. Jane displays enthusiasm for school, and as long as her routine is not interrupted, she moves willingly through her day. Any change in the routine, such as a different bus driver, however, brings on an "emotional meltdown" in the form of a temper tantrum, according to the mother. In fact, a change in the bus driver has resulted on a few occasions in Jane's mother having to miss a day of work.

Jane has two close female friends she has known since kindergarten, and whenever possible, their mothers take them to the mall. According to her mother, Jane has not demonstrated an interest or curiosity about boys. The mother's extended family lives in New Jersey, and they visit whenever possible. Jane receives home health care 3 hours a day, 4 days a week, and 8 hours on Saturday to help alleviate the strain placed on her mother. Jane's father does not visit, nor does he contribute financially to the family.

Jane presents as a grossly overweight adolescent girl of short stature. At the onset of the evaluations she did not appear timid or fearful in the presence of the evaluating therapist and did, in fact, seem to be excited by the attention. Although Jane is nonverbal, she demonstrated exuberance by displaying a broad smile and waving her arms up and down. Jane's left arm is significantly weaker than her left leg and only moves slightly in momentum with her body during her excitement. She is able to use her left arm as an assisting extremity for stabilization of objects in various tasks, such as eating or writing.

During the interview, Jane was cooperative for approximately 15 minutes, oriented to the reason for the interview, and adept in the use of her communication device. She used her right index finger to operate her communication device and computer. Jane's cooperation lasted for a brief period, and her mother had to complete various portions of the interview process with Jane's approval. Jane made frequent nonverbal sounds, which her mother understood to mean that she wanted food. According to her mother, Jane requests food all day long, and as soon as she comes home from school, she listens to music, logs on to the Internet, or watches television, while repeatedly making requests for food. Jane's mother spoke with the therapist to point out that Jane has an ongoing obsession with the stories she had watched on the Lifetime Network. She speaks incessantly to her teachers about the melodramas, claiming that specific actors were actually involved in her life.

Evaluation. Jane was observed eating a lunch of scrambled eggs, using a gross grasp of her fork. Although she continually requests food and is morbidly obese, she is reportedly an extremely finicky eater and will eat particular food items, such as eggs and pizza, without demonstrating satiety. Following the evaluation, Jane was seated on the floor in front of the television set in the den with moderate physical assistance from her mother. She was clad in a T-shirt and underpants, which her mother stated is her usual attire for home. Jane is unable to toilet herself independently, and this state of undress is a convenience strategy. Jane ambulates in a waddling, unsteady gait and exhibits traits of classic Prader-Willi of obesity, hypotonia, and dried saliva at the corners of her mouth. She wears bilateral ankle-foot orthotics to enhance ambulation stability while at school and outside. Jane requires contact guarding only when wearing the orthotics. At home, she requires minimal to moderate assistance for all transfers and ambulation, and does not wear the orthotics.

Evaluation was performed in the home because Jane had finished the school year and had not yet begun the summer program. The two assessments used in this evaluation were the Canadian Occupational Performance Measure (COPM; Law et al., 1998) and the Comprehensive Occupational Therapy Evaluation (COTE; Brayman, Kirby, Misenheimer, & Short, 1976). *I chose the COPM for this client because this tool is a client-centered interview, one in which the therapist elicits information that the client identifies as pertinent. This particular adolescent has not had many opportunities in her life to be heard through her own "voice." She has had few opportunities to make her own choices because of her physical, communicative, and mental limitations that she rarely gets a chance to express her desired occupations, dreams, and desires as an adolescent girl. Many girls at her age have already started to choose elective classes in school, get a driver's license, research potential colleges, and think what to do on a Friday or Saturday night. This tool enabled Jane to "call the shots" in terms of desired roles as well as satisfaction with the roles that she currently engages in within the home, school, and community. Although her mother was available to add information on issues that Jane was not interested in answering, such as household management, Jane clearly had much to say about her desired occupations. I did not want to oblige Jane to answer structured questions that limited her thought process or imagination.*

The COTE scale was selected for Jane because, given the time allotment, it allowed me to observe Jane and look for specific behaviors that would be pertinent to her occupational performance in interaction with people and objects in the environ-

ment as well as in daily life tasks. The COTE is relatively easy to administer, and Jane's behaviors were observed throughout the entire process of interview, lunchtime, watching television, ambulating from kitchen to den, and operating her communication device. Therefore, the COTE seemed to be an appropriate complement to the COPM, as it required no additional effort on Jane's behalf with regard to the overall assessment, and it still afforded me very pertinent data regarding Jane's behaviors, such as appearance, activity level, interpersonal behaviors, and task behaviors.

The COPM comprises three sections consisting of self-care, productivity, and leisure. The client or caregiver prioritizes the occupations that the client needs or wants to perform within the client's typical daily routine. The respondent then rates the importance of each activity on a scale of 1 to 10. Jane was able to participate in the interview by means of her communication device, and her mother continued when Jane decided that she was finished. *The COPM was chosen because Jane has had limited opportunity to express her wishes for direction of treatment and self-selected priorities. Jane initially appeared to enjoy the fact that the interview was directed toward her, and she had the power to answer without judgment or censure.*

The problems identified as Jane's priorities offer valuable insight. Jane would like to spend more time on prevocational skills; improve her ability to cope with changes in routines; expand her range of socialization; participate in more school activities, such as cheerleading, chorus, and acting; and increase her scope of hobbies beyond that of television and computer. Jane indicated that she would like to be an actress and that, although she is in chorus and cheerleading at school, she doesn't get as many chances to participate in these activities as she would like. In addition, she only has prevocational training 1 day a week in which she assembles test tubes. As indicated on the scoring section of the COPM, Jane believes that she does a good job at her prevocational activity but is not satisfied with the work. *I postulated that an increase in activities that Jane finds interesting, satisfying, and meaningful will lead to enhanced socialization opportunities, coping strategies, and variation of recreational hobbies because motivation is a key element in the treatment of people with Prader-Willi syndrome. Thus, in pursuing activities that Jane finds interesting, valuable, and enjoyable and melding them into the repertoire of Jane's desired occupations (as outlined in the COPM), I hypothesized that she would be more likely to participate actively in those occupations and with a greater degree of satisfaction.*

The COTE scale is a behavioral rating scale used as an observation tool to identify behaviors relevant to a client's occupational performance in the interaction with objects in the environment and daily life tasks. The COTE consists of a single-sided sheet of paper, which incorporates 26 behaviors divided into three areas: general behavior, interpersonal behavior, and task behavior. The occupational therapy practitioner applies a rating scale of 0 to 5 to the client's level of functioning for each component of behavior (Kunz & Brayman, 1999). The COTE was used throughout the entire process of the interview, during which time Jane ate lunch, watched television, operated her communication device, and ambulated from the kitchen to the den. *This tool was extremely helpful in Jane's evaluation because it documented valuable information about Jane's behaviors while imposing no further demands on her attention. In evaluating observed strengths and weaknesses, treatment planning will be made easier.*

Jane's major identified areas of difficulty are independence, attention-getting behaviors, concentration, cooperation, decision making, coordination, and frustration tolerance. These behaviors correspond to the deficits indicated on the COPM and, in particular, the problems that Jane experiences in coping with changes. Challenges presented to Jane in the form of a new task, alteration in task, or unfamiliar peers and personnel may elicit an extremely negative response. It is therefore easier for those around her to "play it safe" rather than risk invoking a tantrum reaction from Jane.

Jane might benefit from treatment using interventions based on the model of human occupation (MOHO; Kielhofner, 1995). According to the MOHO, the person is perceived as an open and dynamic system in which the organization of cognitive processes, musculoskeletal integrity, and nervous system influence the individual's ability to successfully explore the environment. The MOHO suggests a human system that not only is in a constant state of organized process, but also comprises three subsystems: The volition subsystem refers to a person's ability to anticipate, choose, experience, and interpret his or her own occupational behavior; the habituation subsystem occurs when the human system acquires automatic and familiar performances as a result of recurrent patterns of occupational behavior; and the mind–brain–body performance subsystem incorporates the biomechanical components of the physical and mental features of the human. *This is also the reason why MOHO was chosen as a frame of reference for Jane's treatment. For example, interests, attraction, and preference for certain occupations and aspects of performance are vital components of MOHO. The primary method for arousing motivation in adolescents with Prader-Willi is to focus on their interests. Another component of MOHO, that of values, generally will follow suit after interest has been established within the adolescent's personal convictions and sense of obligation toward an occupation that he or she finds pleasant or interesting. The MOHO also incorporates occupational choice, and one of the key aspects of choosing the COPM was to allow Jane to give her "voice" to what she finds meaningful and valuable in her life. Knowing the personality traits of Jane as well as other people with Prader-Willi, I believed that motivation for occupation (Kielhofner, 1995) was the only way to elicit Jane's incentive to engage in desired occupations.*

Activity reasoning and use of evidence-based support. In performing the COPM, Jane was given an opportunity to prioritize her interpretation of the volitional structure of her life's routines. Providing a rationale for motivation is a key element in the treatment of people with Prader-Willi syndrome. Weber (1993) found that "based on past experiences, a combination of social reinforcement and token economy incentives work well to control and change behaviors" (p. 6). In exploring occupations that she may find valuable, enjoyable, and interesting, it is projected that Jane's sense of self-efficacy will improve. Furthermore, the adolescent with Prader-Willi syndrome is most comfortable with routine and repetitiveness in daily occupations. To meld the performances that Jane chooses into a habituation process, the collaborative team involved in her progress will "provide opportunity for increasing emotional adaptability by systematically and slowly changing structure" (Weber, 1993, p. 5). Jane has many physical issues that must be considered when planning treatment, and performance is greatly affected by the impairments associated with her dually diagnosed conditions. "Occupation requires us to use our bodies to traverse the geography and act upon the objects of a physical world" (Kielhofner, 1995, p. 116). Jane's mind–brain–body subsystem has been affecting her actions in an inefficient manner as a result of low tone, neurological deficits, and decreased cardiopulmonary energy. With the introduction of activity choices that address her volitional needs, it is anticipated that she will move along the continuum from the current state of parent-asserted helplessness, observed incompetence, and inefficacy toward occupational exploration. It is likely that she will gain a sense of competence and eventual mastery over chosen occupations.

Jane demonstrates a zeal for occupations that she enjoys as well as for independent thought processes pertaining to attractions and interests that trigger personal convictions. According to the COPM, Jane has the ability to attribute significance to certain occupations in which she would like to be engaged. The COTE scale revealed an adolescent girl who has a generally appropriate orientation to her situation and surroundings and the desire for increased socialization along with a highly animated and appealing affect.

After examination of the results of the COPM and COTE, Jane's primary areas where she exhibits deficits are socialization, play or leisure exploration, and vocational exploration. These skill areas are clearly prioritized within the initial assessment of the COPM, and the deficits observed within interpersonal behaviors and task behaviors of the COTE further support the concentration of intervention on these areas. Jane exhibited a lack of independent actions, self-assertion, and a plethora of attention-getting behaviors (noisemaking and waving her arms) during the meal and interview process. Her task behavior demonstrated poor concentration, poor coordination, and inadequate decision-making abilities. She lost interest in the interview and had no coping mechanisms to implement when frustration emerged. Jane could benefit from activities that provide an opportunity to develop a sense of efficacy and control in achieving desired behavior outcomes (Kielhofner, 1995).

Socialization is deemed a priority to be addressed within the treatment plan, and vocational exploration is the next concern. The most likely scenario for Jane's future is to reside in a group home and work in a sheltered workshop. Jane presently is dissatisfied with the work that has been chosen for her. Thus, the sheltered workshop activity in which she engages does not facilitate a sense of personal causation, values, and interest. A disconnection exists between the reality of her current and projected life management. Play and leisure exploration are Jane's concern as well as her mother's. It will benefit Jane both physically and socially to broaden her range of hobbies to include less-sedentary interests. Adolescents with Prader-Willi syndrome can benefit from activities involving muscular strength, endurance, cardiovascular endurance, and coordination (Weber, 1993). Her current lack of incentive to actively explore her environment reflects a dysphoric attitude toward physical activity.

Treatment planning. To facilitate improved socialization skills, performance components that must be focused on include increased problem-solving skills, attention span, interests in activities that she enjoys and that may be shared with others, social conduct, interpersonal skills, self-expression, coping skills and self-control for improved frustration tolerance, and assumption of roles for societal demands. Jane's strength, endurance, and gross motor coordination need to be addressed to enhance participation in many social activities.

When planning treatment for vocational performance, the occupational therapist must take into account many areas of concern. Some of them are deficits in fine and gross motor coordination, endurance, strength, attention span, problem solving, initiation of activity, role assumption of worker, interest in task, social conduct, interpersonal skills, self-expression, coping skills for transitioning to new tasks, time management, and the self-control to modulate behavior in response to new demands. Jane's present play and leisure activities require very little physical exertion. She identified interests in acting and cheerleading. She will have to work on improving strength and endurance, gross motor coordination, postural control, attention span, initiation of activity, and problem solving. She also needs to assume the role of an active participant; assess her values in determining that an activity is worth her effort; share her interest in the chosen activity; and improve social conduct, interpersonal skills, self-expression, coping skills, and self-control.

Short-term goal 1. With moderate verbal assistance, Jane will identify two alternative strategies that she may implement when presented with a group task that she either is not interested in or does not want to complete within 2 weeks in order to enhance her problem-solving skills within a social context.

Short-term goal 2. With moderate assistance, Jane will compile a list of at least five activities that she is interested in attempting and that require more than one person to perform within 1 week in order to increase self-expression pertaining to a social setting.

Long-term goal. Jane will demonstrate an improved ability to interact with peers in an appropriate contextual and cultural manner by participating in a group task consisting of at least three other group members, with close supervision for 20 minutes and requiring less than three verbal prompts to stay on task, within 4 months in order to promote her role as social participant.

Activity: Guess What I Am Doing? This activity is a form of charades, but it takes the game a few steps further into occupational reality. A minimum of two participants are needed.

1. The occupational therapy practitioner prints out different tasks and activities that occur in everyday life on index cards. For example, a card could specify brushing one's teeth, washing dishes, or making a bed.

2. Each participant gets a card when it is his or her turn, and he or she must act out the task on the card.

3. The other participant(s) writes down what he or she thinks the actor is doing.

4. The actor then tells the group what he or she has performed.

5. The participants will be encouraged to applaud the actor at this juncture.

6. Following the performance, with the occupational therapy practitioner's assistance, the group discusses whether any components of the task have been omitted in the performance. For example, if the task is brushing teeth, perhaps the actor has forgotten to replace the toothpaste cap or rinse off the toothbrush.

7. It is then the next person's turn to give a performance.

This activity has been selected for Jane because, as indicated on the COPM, she desires to participate as an actress in plays and make more friends. This activity gives Jane an opportunity to act and exhibit self-expression while integrating socialization skills into the group process. The game also gives Jane a chance to be part of the audience; therefore, she may practice waiting her turn, attending to task, and implementing problem-solving strategies if necessary during the course of the activity.

Guess What I Am Doing has a great deal of significance relating to Jane's projected future within a group home. Although it is anticipated that she will enjoy the experience of role-playing within the socialization of a small group, the tasks that are to be enacted mimic activities that are a part of Jane's daily routines. In fact, many of the tasks on the index cards can be modified to correspond to the self-care and productivity sections of the COPM. To become a successful member of a group home, it is in Jane's best interest to practice situations and tasks that may be expected of her. In this manner, she will help to establish a sociocultural fit that will apply to current and future relationships and environments.

Intervention. The second visit with Jane took place in the late afternoon on a day that she did not attend the summer program. Jane's mother invited Jane's two close girlfriends over, who know ahead of time that they would be trying out a game. The activity encouraged participation and engagement because the girls appeared motivated to act out the situations and were eager to respond with their deduction. They giggled at each other's portrayals and were able to identify the tasks. The tasks were purposely very simple, such as brushing hair or washing face, to reduce possible frustration. The game addressed the priorities and goals, as Jane was observed to wait her turn, interact appropriately, express herself, and clearly maintain attention for a full 10 minutes before she required redirection to the activity. She began to ask for food, and her mother told her that she'd have to wait.

I would have preferred to field test the activity within the setting of Jane's summer program where there would have been more adolescent participants. The benefit to testing the game within Jane's home was that there was a high comfort level. Nonetheless, if the test occurred at BOCES, there would have been a better environment to observe the efficacy of the components of the game and how they relate to

Jane's goals. The discussion component of the game (Step 6) is one that would be reserved for a group that has a relatively high attention span and frustration tolerance. It was apparent that each participant wanted to take her turn as soon as the previous actor's task was identified. They did not have the tolerance or interest in discussing whether any aspects of the represented task were omitted in the performance.

Case Scenario: Mr. Lamb

The following vignette was provided by Donald Auriemma, MSEd, OTR/L, BCN, who is an assistant professor of Occupational Therapy at York College of the City University of New York. He was pleased to write this case scenario because of his belief that the skill of reasoning about activities connects directly to the elegance of practice.

Mr. Lamb, at 78 years of age, was referred for occupational therapy services through a certified home health agency. I began this journey with a review of the documentation package. A broadly written referral requested both the evaluation and treatment of challenges to activities of daily living. Frequency of treatment was set at two to three times per week for 9 weeks. Mr. Lamb had arrived home after an inpatient stay for an exacerbation of congestive heart failure (CHF). His hospital stay was just one of several in the past few years for heart failure. An exacerbation of CHF was his primary condition, with severe osteoarthritis being the secondary condition. Cardiac precautions were clearly indicated. The medication list for Mr. Lamb was extensive. A preliminary picture was drawn of a person facing the challenges that the later stages of his diseases posed. I made an appointment for an initial evaluation.

As I approached his front door, I made my way up his four-step stoop, and the absence of handrails stood out. He called out for me to "just walk in" in response to my knock. A frail-appearing, well-spoken gentleman welcomed me. The sight of this unkempt person sitting on a stained and tattered couch struck me. A musty smell and strong body odor permeated the room. Signs of years of neglect marked the first floor of his home. Mr. Lamb immediately offered an apology for not being able to walk over to open the door. A combination of limited range of motion and multiple sclerosis in both lower extremities along with compromised cardiovascular endurance had left him unable to ambulate.

Who was this man sitting in front of me, and how did his life situation lead to this unsettling picture? Mr. Lamb, an effective historian, provided a vivid history. As a child, he emigrated to the United Stated from South America. Raised by his grandmother, he lived a childhood marked by extreme poverty and a strong religious tradition. As a young adult with limited education, he learned a trade and worked as a machinist. This occupation he loved. It afforded him the ability to live out a dream of purchasing a home and raising a family. His two grown children live out of state. Proudly, he explained how in his middle years he converted his oversized garage into a machine shop. There, for more than 20 years, he was able to support his family. Advancing CHF and osteoarthritis slowly robbed him of the ability to continue his business, maintain his home, move about, and ultimately perform much of his self-care. He had been married for more than 40 years. His wife needed to work long hours in a hair salon she was trying to sell. Somberly, he described how he spent both day and night on his living room couch. For approximately the past 3 years, his wife would provide him with breakfast, lunch, a clean urinal, and bed pan. He would stay alone until she returned from work. Recreation was watching television and an occasional visit from a friend or neighbor. His elderly wife usually returned home visibly exhausted. Because he was reluctant to further burden his wife with the assistance he needed, several days would go by before he had a bath or changed his clothes. A dust-covered standard walker stood in the corner of his room. It was the only piece of therapeutic equipment Mr. Lamb had.

Evaluation. During this visit, I completed the initial evaluation. Information obtained helped me to better understand Mr. Lamb's challenges and assets. His roles as a husband, provider, friend, and neighbor were no longer satisfying. His ability to spend time in his machine shop as a leisure pursuit was gone. Participation in the home maintenance, cleaning, and shopping was no longer possible. Rolling and sitting up in bed was possible, but ambulating was not. Physical assistance to transfer was required. If food was brought to him he could feed himself. Managing the clothes of his upper body was possible, but he required assistance with his pants, shoes, and socks. Bathing was limited to sponging with assistance. He would toilet himself with the use of a bedpan and urinal. Deterioration in key performance components appeared to have significantly contributed to these performance area declines. Significant limitations in range of motion were present in all extremities and trunk, more so in his lower extremities. General strength was fair-plus to good-minus. His endurance was significantly limited, with an estimated muscle endurance test level of 2.0 to 2.5. The high value he placed on self-reliance, ability to cope with demanding situations, interest in learning, strong interpersonal skills, and liberal health insurance were some of the outstanding assets.

Reasoning and treatment planning. I believed that a client-centered approach and early successes would lay down the foundation for allowing Mr. Lamb to believe change was possible. This approach could motivate optimal participation and create an effective therapeutic relationship, thus maximizing his functional potential. Collaboration with Mr. Lamb revealed that functional mobility was his number one priority. My thoughts focused on adaptations, equipment, and instructed skills. Mobility options needed to match his physical capabilities and not place a dangerous demand on his compromised cardiac function. Sliding transfers and manual wheelchair use were chosen. Both could use the greater strength and range in his upper extremities and allow for a rest period at any point when the physiological demand became too challenging.

Intervention. Mr. Lamb's couch no longer confined him. Independence was achieved by providing a hospital bed, drop-arm commode, and a manual wheelchair. He now slept on an electric hospital bed set up in his living room. Sleeping became more restful, and Mr. Lamb found it easier to breathe in a semireclined position. Using all four extremities, he could move about in a manual wheelchair, in a slow and effort-filled manner. Access to his living room, dining room, and kitchen was regained. Within 2 weeks, his world had expanded from his couch to the entire first floor of his home.

Mr. Lamb's next priority was to reduce the burden on his wife by gaining a greater capacity to perform his own self-care. A focus was placed partially on what compensatory treatments would best help meet his desires. Through training with the use of a dressing stick, sock aid, reacher, long-handled shoehorn, and buttonhook, he regained the ability to dress himself. Long-handled devices provided access to the distal parts of his body that limited joint range prevented him from reaching. Commode use replaced the need to use a urinal and bedpan. Wheelchair access to the kitchen sink afforded Mr. Lamb a consistent opportunity to sponge bathe and groom regularly. Now able to reach his refrigerator, Mr. Lamb could choose from a variety of prepared or simple-to-prepare foods. A reacher provided access to lightweight objects placed in closets.

During this same period he engaged in an exercise program designed to remediate endurance, range of motion, and muscle strength. Because of his frail health, frequent, brief, and mild bouts of exercise were thought to be the most beneficial and least risky. Therefore, the remediation program was split between being provided as a portion of the three-times-a-week visits and a home exercise program that was performed on nontreatment days. I believed that even small gains in these components of performance would positively contribute to regaining both the quantity and quality of Mr. Lamb's functional abilities, and they did. Gains contributed to achieving independence in more physically demanding, modified stand-pivot transfers. Manual wheelchair propulsion was performed with greater ease. Self-care activities were performed with a reduction in the number of rest periods required. Once again, Mr. Lamb was strong enough to open and close his heavy front door. Successes gained in these 6 weeks of the program continued to motivate Mr. Lamb.

Mr. Lamb was encouraged to broaden his thinking. A 3-week window for occupational therapy was left. Cognizant of the limited remaining time and projected discharge date, his interest shifted to regaining access to his community. I judged his limited endurance and the four steps to enter his home to be his greatest challenges. The acquisition of a power wheelchair and a ramp constructed by a neighbor met these challenges. Power wheelchair use afforded Mr. Lamb access to his beloved machine shop. Traveling four blocks to the local shopping area became possible. Moving through his community allowed him to engage again with friends and neighbors with whom he had lost touch. His power wheelchair served him well for neighborhood travel. A solution for traveling longer distances was desired. Returning to driving seemed impossible. Car-related costs and the physical demands of placing a wheelchair into a car were beyond his economic and physical capabilities. Cab service costs could not fit within his limited budget. A referral to a city-based transportation service was pursued. This low-cost service broadened access beyond Mr. Lamb's immediate community. For the price of public transportation, he was able to travel throughout the city.

Termination of occupational therapy services occurred, as planned, in the 9th week of sessions. Contact with Mr. Lamb was maintained informally after his discharge through an occasional visit or crossing paths while I traveled through his neighborhood providing services to others. Despite the continuation of the destructive course of the CHF and osteoarthritis and several more hospitalizations, greater participation filled his remaining years. For years, it made my day brighter seeing him talking to neighbors in front of his home or traveling about his neighborhood.

These two cases were very different. What they shared in common was a desire to enter the world of the client so that these therapists could collaborate in the creation of a meaningful environment for the client. Each therapist used different forms of clinical reasoning to achieve his or her objectives.

Summary

In this chapter we explore the many facets of reasoning about activity. The goal is to increase awareness of the nature and importance of how you reason about what you do with clients. The enormity of the responsibility for decisions made in collaboration is mitigated by a conscious attention to the task of clinical reasoning. One day, a student or client may ask why you did or said something as you go through your day as a practitioner. If you can answer the question, you will be on the way to becoming an expert practitioner who can balance self-awareness with an awareness of the needs of the client within the realities of the environment. It seems a worthwhile goal to strive for the ability to reason with awareness. ∎

Acknowledgments

I wish to acknowledge the invaluable contribution of Ann Winter and Donald Auriemma, occupational therapists who willingly examined their practice and gave of their words and time.

References

Allen, B. (1998, September 6). Fatal attraction [Review of the book *Death in Summer*]. *The New York Times Book Review, 7.*

Babiss, F. (2003). *An ethnographic study of mental health treatment and outcomes: Doing what works.* New York: Haworth.

Brayman, S. J., Kirby, T. F., Misenheimer, A. M., & Short, M. J. (1976). Comprehensive occupational therapy evaluation scale. *American Journal of Occupational Therapy, 30,* 94–100.

Cohn, E. S. (1991). Nationally speaking—Clinical reasoning: Explicating complexity. *American Journal of Occupational Therapy, 45,* 969–971.

Craik, K. (1967). *The nature of explanation.* Cambridge, England: Cambridge University Press.

Csikszentmihalyi, M. (1990). *Flow: The psychology of optimal experience.* New York: HarperCollins.

Dickens, C. (2000). *David Copperfield.* New York: Modern Library Classics. (Original work published 1849.)

Dreyfus, H., & Dreyfus, S. (1986). *Mind over machine: The power of human intuition and expertise in the era of the computer.* New York: Free Press.

Gardner, H. (1983). *Frames of mind: The theory of multiple intelligences.* Basic (Basic Books, Inc., Publishers): New York.

Johnson-Laird, P. N., Girotto, V., & Legrenzi, P. (1998). *Mental models: A gentle guide for outsiders.* Retrieved September 24, 2003, from http://www.si.umich.edu/ICOS/gentleintro.html.

Kielhofner, G. (1995). *A model of human occupation* (2nd ed.). Baltimore: Williams & Wilkins.

Kolb, D. A. (1984). *Experiential learning.* Englewood Cliffs, NJ: Prentice-Hall.

Kunz, K., & Brayman, S. (1999). The Comprehensive Occupational Therapy Evaluation. In B. Hemphill-Pearson (Ed.), *Assessments in occupational therapy mental health* (pp. 259–274). Thorofare, NJ: Slack.

Law, M., Baptiste, S., Carswell, A., McColl, M. A., Polatajko, H., & Pollock, N. (1998). *Canadian Occupational Performance Measure* (3rd ed.). Ottawa, Ontario, Canada: CAOT Publications.

Mattingly, C., & Fleming, M. H. (1994). *Clinical reasoning: Forms of inquiry in a therapeutic practice.* Philadelphia: F. A. Davis.

Mattingly, C., & Gillette, N. (1991). Anthropology, occupational therapy, and action research. *American Journal of Occupational Therapy, 45,* 972–978.

Mosey, A. C. (1985). A monistic or a pluralistic approach to professional identity? 1985 Eleanor Clarke Slagle Lecture. *American Journal of Occupational Therapy, 39,* 504–509.

Peloquin, S. M. (1993). The patient–therapist relationship: Beliefs that shape care. *American Journal of Occupational Therapy, 47,* 935–942.

Polanyi, M. (1962, 1974). *Personal knowledge: Towards a post-critical inquiry.* Chicago: University of Chicago Press.

Rogers, J. C. (1983). Clinical reasoning: The ethics, science, and art. *American Journal of Occupational Therapy, 37,* 601–616.

Schell, B. A. B. (2003a, October 6). Clinical reasoning and occupation-based practice: Changing habits. *OT Practice, 8,* CE-1–CE-8.

Schell, B. A. B. (2003b). Clinical reasoning: The basis of practice. In E. B. Crepeau, E. Cohn, & B. Schell (Eds.), *Willard and Spackman's occupational therapy* (10th ed., pp. 131–139). Philadelphia: Lippincott, Williams & Wilkins.

Schell, B. A., & Cervero, R. M. (1993). Clinical reasoning in occupational therapy: An integrative review. *American Journal of Occupational Therapy, 47,* 605–610.

Schön, D. (1983). *The reflective practitioner: How professionals think in action.* Basic (Basic Books, Inc., Publishers): New York.

Weber, R. C. (1993). Physical education for children with Prader-Willi syndrome. *Palaestra , 9*(3). Retrieved May 14, 2002, from Infotrac database, Article No. 115.

8

The Application of Activities to Practice

Ann Burkhardt, OTD, OTR/L, BCN, FAOTA

O n Ellis Island is a sign posted of a statement made by a young woman who immigrated:

> The whole experience was very frightening....They brought me up to a room....They put a pegboard before me with little sticks of different shapes and little holes....I had to put them in place, the round ones and the square ones...and I did it perfectly, "Oh, we must have made a mistake. This little girl...naturally she doesn't know English, but she's very bright, intelligent." So they took the cross (chalk mark) off me so we were cleared. (Victoria Scarfatti Fernandez, a Macedonian Jewish immigrant in 1916, interviewed in 1985)

Clearly, the puzzle she was given had neither context nor meaning to her. It was an ineffective tool to measure her intellect, but it was the best tool available to the examiners at the time. Time changes, people change and grow, but the underlying concept that activities have meaning when they are in context and perspective for the person endures.

Value and Use of Activities

Occupational therapy practice and beliefs support the value of activity as an effective tool in the process of change. The practice of occupational therapy values the use of activities in context to the concept of occupation. "Occupations are generally viewed as activities having unique meaning and purpose in a person's life. Occupations are central to a person's identity and competence, and they influence how one spends time and makes decisions" (Pierce, 2001). How each of us occupies our time relates to a number of variables and values. Current thinking in the field supports the belief that spirituality is one key to the meaning and value of activities. Two key concepts of spirituality are existentialism and metaphysics.

Existentialism is the symbolic meaning experienced through the performance or engagement in daily life tasks. For example, whenever I put my earrings in my ears, I remember what my grandmother said to me when I was 15 years old, "Earrings make you look so girlish. They give us each that little something extra, don't you see?" Existentially, putting on my earrings is a very spiritual activity for me. I valued my grandmother's opinion and words. There is personal, spiritual meaning for me when I engage in this activity because I remember my grandmother as I do it, and I loved her deeply.

Metaphysics is the perception that participation in activities in the earthly plane somehow correlates to our relationship to a higher power, such as God, a Great Spirit, or angels, or that a higher purpose in life exists. Metaphysical activities can include religious activities, but they may also include nonreligious activities that have deeper spiritual meaning. For example, doing activities to support one's church or spiritual community, such as stewardship activities, could have metaphysical meaning. Engaging in rituals, for example the symbolism of exchanging vows and rings in a wedding ceremony, has a metaphysical basis. The ceremony is spiritually symbolic to those who become married to each other. It represents a commitment to each other in the

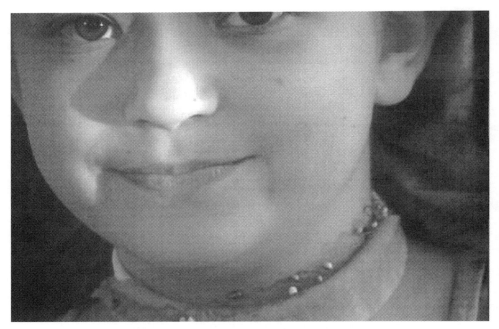

Figure 8.1. Occupations generally have more than one associated activity and numerous tasks that support engagement. This preteen girl has occupations of jewelry creator, collector, and jewelry "fashion bug." She creates her own designs; makes her own necklaces, bracelets, and earrings; and models her own creations. The tasks include imagining a design, stringing the piece, trying on the pieces, and modeling the pieces.

eyes of God and mankind. Additionally, the act of praying can be metaphysical. One could also argue that seeing the glories of nature in person could make people feel connected to the universe. Many people who see the Grand Canyon can support this notion. Being among a large number of people for an event, such as being in Central Park when John Lennon died, can be a metaphysical experience. Pilgrims who go to Mecca each year, Christians and Jews who travel to Jerusalem, all experience a heightened sense of connectedness to the universe in metaphysical terms when they partake in these journeys.

Occupational therapy practitioners use activities in proper context as related to the person being treated in order to effect change and restore meaning in life. Practitioners are agents of change. They promote change through the use of purposeful activities, in the context of real life and spiritual meaning, as a catalyst to the process of change. Purpose in doing the activity must be inherent for activity participation to be effectively used as a treatment modality. Using activities out of context or tasks that have no personal meaning to a client is futile and purposeless because such tasks are rote and repetitive and do not translate well to everyday existence or improve the quality of life.

"Context is an overarching, underlying, embedded influence on the process of service delivery" (American Occupational Therapy Association [AOTA], 2002). Contexts influence the client's performance and the process of service delivery. There are external contexts, such as the physical setting and its requisite social and virtual contexts, and there are internal contexts, such as what the process of "doing" means to the person while he or she is attempting to practice or engage in the process of the activity itself. Occupational therapy practitioners may be interacting with individuals on a personal basis, within a group, or as part of population-related work (e.g., data gathering during research, advocating for social change, sharing information in an educational context).

Several of our colleagues (e.g., Neistadt, 1994; Trombly, 1995) have studied the outcomes of activity use. Separately, they have found that people perform tasks with greater ability when a task is in context for them. Reaching for an object one wishes to use, for instance, results in better reaching ability than reaching for an object in a simulated circumstance. Clearly, there is more to using activities than the physical subcomponents of the task. People perform better under normal, contextually relevant circumstances.

This concept may seem revolutionary to some occupational therapy practitioners. In the 1970s and 1980s, many practitioners used activities that were meant to transfer subcomponents of activities into a later, greater functional purpose. At that time, it became popular to use cones, blocks, puzzles, and other therapeutic activities to try to develop subcomponent skills. This concept is viewed as part of a bottom-up approach to treatment. Subcomponents of activities (specific tasks) rather than the functional activities themselves were used to promote change. Some motor learning frames of reference still promote this approach to a certain degree. They propose that using subcomponents of activities can promote the acquisition of the skill needed to engage in occupational performance. Other occupational therapy practitioners who use a motor learning frame of reference focus treatment on those tasks that promote the actual acquisition of the desired skill in context (e.g., forming a fist with one's hand on the handgrip of a walker rather than gripping a cone). The act of gripping, in context, should promote a better functional outcome.

In the 1990s, a movement began to use actual participation in daily living tasks therapeutically rather than to focus on subcomponents as a first line of action in treatment. This top-down approach to treatment relies on having people in treatment do their daily life tasks as the evaluation and treatment focus. The tasks observed are done in as close to a natural setting as feasible. Neistadt's (1994) and Trombly's (1993, 1995) works have demonstrated that the outcome of using a top-down approach to intervention was more effective than using a transfer training approach. Development of client-centered assessments also has had an impact on how clients choose to focus their occupational therapy in order to improve their ability to care for themselves and to participate in activities they personally value.

Reasoning in the Selection of Activities

As discussed in Chapter 7, the choice of activities must be based on logic and sound reasoning. In occupational therapy, clinical reasoning is the process that underlies logical, contextual choice of activities. *Clinical reasoning* involves several types of reasoning: procedural, contextual, conditional, and narrative (Mattingly & Fleming, 1994). Outcomes of procedural reasoning, contextual reasoning, and conditional reasoning form the basis for the *narrative reasoning* or storytelling process, which is the cumulative impact of the clinical reasoning process that guides in the selection of the right activity for the client. Narrative reasoning in process tells a story about the person receiving occupational therapy and about his or her activity history. The story takes its shape as rapport builds between the practitioner and the client and as the factors, which declare the need for change in how life is lived for the individual who seeks care, emerge or declare themselves in full view of life (past, present, and future).

Procedural reasoning is a process through which the practitioner gathers data about the client: What was the event that happened in the person's life to require services? What were the medical issues (in a medical model) or reasons the person would benefit from occupational therapy intervention (in a community-based context)? The psychological issues? The social issues and concerns affecting the person's general health and well-being? Procedural reasoning generally takes more time for a novice than it does for a skilled practitioner. Once a practitioner gains competence in evaluation and intervention, there is greater proficiency of deductive reasoning based on familiar practice trends. A novice clinician seeks items of evidence to build an understanding of the underlying issues. An experienced, competent practitioner sums up the factors surrounding a case with greater implicit insight and greater speed and anticipates a clinical context more rapidly. For example, a novice clinician will review a medical chart and need time to process meaning about the tests and findings of scans and x-rays. An experienced practitioner will read and process more rapidly, seeking clues to limitations the person may encounter as he or she attempts to engage in normal life tasks and activities.

Contextual reasoning occurs through gaining insight and perspective into how the events that the person has experienced may affect his or her ability to resume life roles with all of the component tasks and activities that make up the person. *Conditional reasoning* is shaping the occupational therapy process context to the client's perceived need for change and desire to work with the practitioner toward change. Practitioners gain insight into the client's perception of his or her functional ability and the issues he or she personally wishes to address in intervention.

Sometimes, a therapist may have potential goals for a client that the client does not have for him- or herself. For instance, if a client has had a hip replacement and has met his goals in therapy, but he continues to require his wife's assistance to don socks, the occupational therapy practitioner should determine whether it is his personal goal to be able to don socks. Although the practitioner may know that the client could don socks independently with a sock aid, if the client wants his wife to continue to do this for him, and she is satisfied with this arrangement, intervention relative to donning socks would not be indicated for this client. The client may instead identify other goals of higher priority to him personally. He may be more concerned with how to resume his sex life, which is a common area of concern to many clients that often is overlooked by the surgery and rehabilitation staff. Sex education may be a more pertinent and appropriate area of client intervention than donning socks. Perhaps the client seeks both interventions. The actual application of activities is personalized case by case and person by person.

Case Scenario

Mr. Brown is a 63-year-old man. He is married to his high school sweetheart and is the father of three adult children. Mr. Brown is a self-employed freelance news photographer. He has recently had his right hip replaced. He can participate in all of his self-care activities independently, except he continues to rely on his wife for assistance with his right sock. He likes having his wife assist him with his sock. He says that having her put on his sock allows them a few quiet moments together at the beginning of the day. He is happy with this system and does not wish to do it independently.

Mr. Brown is a landscape photographer. He frequently stands for long periods because of his specialty in time-lapse photography. He would like to work with the practitioner to develop a system that would allow him to sit while he uses his tripod so that he can take pressure off his right leg when he works for long periods. In addition to photography, the Browns enjoy ballroom dancing. Mr. Brown wishes to conserve his energy during the day so that he can begin ballroom dancing again with his wife.

The focus of intervention for Mr. Brown would change from a focus on self-care activities to a vocational context and its related activities. Mr. Brown wants to go on photographic expeditions. The focus of treatment is to modify or adapt the activity so that Mr. Brown can engage in his photographic occupation. Because landscape photography requires that Mr. Brown change his positioning, the practitioner and Mr. Brown explore the use of a portable seat to allow him to develop greater endurance. Because intervention in this case is limited to the acute-care hospital setting, the occupational therapy practitioner may provide simulated opportunities for Mr. Brown to practice the various tasks involved in taking photographs. On the other hand, if the practitioner saw Mr. Brown in home care, private practice, or community-based practice, opportunity may present itself to go with him into the field and observe actual, in-context participation in the modified activity.

Mr. Brown's occupation of photography is both a vocational (work) and an avocational (leisure) occupation for him. The activities include going into the field to take pictures, taking pictures while sitting, and so forth. A specific task would be taking a picture of the George Washington Bridge at sunset, using a specific technique. An occupation has activities and requisite tasks that relate to those activities, which need to be accomplished for occupational engagement to be successful and meaningful in occupational context.

Activities Selection and Application in the Real World

In the context of occupational therapy, intervention is aimed at helping a person to function within the performance areas of self-care, work, play and leisure, and rest. A balanced lifestyle is one in which a person is able to function across these domains while maintaining this balance across physical, psychological, emotional, and social contexts. Occupational therapy promotes holism and a balanced lifestyle for all people and across the life span. The context of the application of occupational therapy is vast and diverse. Occupational therapy practitioners may use their skills of activity analysis and synthesis to focus on the reality of a person's ability to participate in the roles that form his or her occupational roles. This section of the chapter provides some guidance and suggestions for how activities may be applied in the real world of practice.

Occupational therapy practitioners' use of activities in the real world involves creating the "just-right match" among the client, context, activity, and the service delivery model. The ultimate goal of an occupational therapy intervention is for the client to engage in occupations. As stated throughout this book, one specific valuable tool is purposeful activity. All purposeful activities have two goals: the goals for the client and the goals of the occupational therapy practitioner. Many factors influence the selection and use of activities, including the different abilities, needs, desires, and motivation of the clients; the practice site in which the intervention takes place; the service delivery model and where it is applied; the resources available to support the intervention; and the knowledge and skills of the practitioner. In the following sections, activities are discussed within the circumstances of real-life practice confronted daily by occupational therapy practitioners.

Purposeful Activities That Address the Client's Unique Needs

Occupational therapy practitioners select and use purposeful activities that address the unique developmental needs of the client. Thus, a person's unique needs are always considered when selecting activities for intervention. Beginning with the client's needs, the occupational therapy practitioner learns from the client what activities are appropriate. Working with the client, the practitioner matches the specific purposeful activities to the client's needs.

NEWBORNS AND YOUNG CHILDREN'S PURPOSEFUL ACTIVITIES

Purposeful activities for a newborn usually involve activities done for the child in response to the child's specific needs (e.g., feeding, changing a diaper). These activities take place between infant and adult to provide the infant with needed sensory stimulation. Playful sensory stimulation activities are selected because they provide opportunities for infant–caregiver interaction. Occupational therapy practitioners use their knowledge of normal growth and development and the nature of sensory input to guide in the selection of specific activities.

Case Scenario

A child who is born premature, or one who requires hospitalization in a neonatal intensive care unit (NICU), requires special attention. For these children, stimulation is received passively, and special caregiver and infant activities are needed. Developmental stimulation, provided by the therapist or a trained caregiver—swaddling, holding, gently rocking, and supporting the premature infant in a positional device, within the controlled atmosphere of the incubator and amid monitor wires, pulse oximeters, and respirators—may be the scene. Being held and feeling the heartbeat of another warm-blooded human being may be beneficial as well. Newborns who are born prematurely may not be neurologically ready to receive a bombardment of activity. Often, they have not had time for their nervous systems to mature to the level of a full-term newborn. Feeding can require skill and knowledge of how the ability to suck and swallow can be assisted and facilitated by the therapist or taught to the mother or other caregivers. Recent studies in aromatherapy indicate that an infant in the NICU may be less stressed by the scent of lavender or vanilla (Dunn, Sleep, & Collett, 1995).

Case Scenario

If premature infants in a NICU cannot swallow, they cannot be fed by breast or bottle because they would aspirate into their lungs anything introduced to them by mouth. Aspiration could result in a life-threatening circumstance, aspiration pneumonia. An occupational therapist who works in a NICU, however, would know that these infants could have developmental problems if they do not receive oral stimulation, such as that which comes from nippling. Contextually, the therapist in a NICU would know how to use a pacifier to stimulate the mouth as normally as possible. He or she also would know which pacifier is best for the neonate in this context. For example, some neonates use orthodontic nipples, which may be the nipple of choice for infants who have metabolic disorders and who may have abnormalities in the development of their hard palate related to nutritional issues.

Activity for the infant often is embedded in the care and attention they receive from caregivers. Infants need periods of being held and require someone else's help to sustain their nutritional needs. Someone else has to address their elimination. Interaction, at first, may mean turning one's head toward a rattle or making eye contact or face-to-face communicative contact. Over time and as the nervous system and body develop, infants become more interactive, seeking eye contact or verbal response to their needs. Infants cannot speak, so making noise, cooing, or crying are their attempts to get their needs addressed. Activity participation greatly depends on response from another.

Case Scenario

Developmentally mature infants who are born addicted to substances, such as cocaine, may have neurological reactions to the withdrawal of the drugs. They may require more handling, positioning, and developmental stimulation than full-term infants or other premature infants who were not exposed to chemical substances. Activity for these infants is introduced passively. They respond to the input as they receive and perceive it. Infant massage can promote relaxation and offset gastrointestinal discomfort that many infants withdrawing from substances can experience.

Newborns quickly learn to respond to movement, feelings, and sounds generated by their own movement or action. Gradually, the infant's activities begin to become purposeful or self-directed as the infant interacts and responds to his or her world. Objects, including all kinds of people, in the environment become important as the newborn responds to them. Infants develop an awareness of their bodies as they move and repeat actions over and over. Wearing a wrist rattle gives auditory feedback caused by active movement. Newborns generally see black, white, and red. Often, they are drawn visually to corners of rooms or to patterns that include straight and rounded lines. They begin to actively track visually. Placing black-and-white drawings of faces around the crib can provide various choices of objects to track visually and maintains infants' interest in their environment for longer periods. The sound of a human voice conveys information about the human environment. The sound of a parent's voice and the quality and degree of tactile stimulation influence the interactive environment for the infant.

Infants require another person's assistance to set up and initiate the play so that play may occur. Infants passively play but learn to track visually and fix on objects of interest. Moving objects, such as spinning tops, can be intriguing. Playful activities

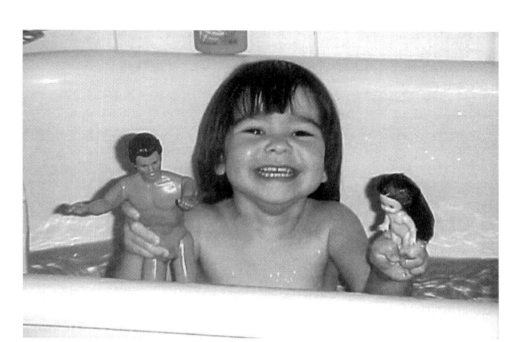

Figure 8.2. The major occupation of children is play. Play carries over to all other occupations as children explore and learn the context and form personal habits. Here a young girl plays with dolls while bathing. Her dolls also are having a bath. Self-care may be learned through the doing as well as through mimicking routine patterns. The exploration, testing of limits, and repetition are the part of play that contribute to learning new skills, new behaviors, and new habits and are a part of the process of becoming occupational beings.

for infants include using rattles and other toys (e.g., stuffed animals, activity centers, cloth books, cloth balls).

Feeding is an important purposeful activity for infants and young children. Children who cannot suck require oral stimulation and manual facilitation to reinforce attempts at sucking. Sucking and swallowing are vital functions. One needs these functions to swallow secretions (e.g., saliva). Additionally, to draw nutrition normally through breast-feeding, an infant must be able to suckle a breast. Activity for these infants also is introduced passively but requires a response from the infant to have a successful outcome. There are instances where something that should have developed naturally needs a hand to overcome developmental delays under abnormal circumstances. Infants respond to the input as they receive and perceive it. Repetition shapes behavior and the ability to respond.

Case Scenario

Parents may require assistance to learn when to discontinue a child's use of a pacifier. It sometimes involves tears and emotional adjustment to assist the toddler to stop drinking from a bottle in favor of a covered drinking cup. Finger foods, such as ring-shaped cereal, can stimulate early self-feeding behaviors. For example, children usually learn to finger feed before trying to feed themselves with a spoon. Learning to adjust or modulate the position of the spoon through the fingers results in less spillage and mess during feeding. A little one-on-one time with a skilled care provider, such as the occupational therapy practitioner, can assist the mother to make the right choices for the baby while stimulating and facilitating skill development.

Case Scenario

Occupational therapy practitioners frequently work with older children who have developed food aversions because they were not allowed to eat by mouth for a while or because of metabolic disturbances. When older children are allowed to eat after years of not eating, it may take a slow-paced, consistent motivational strategy to gain their interest and participation. Children with food aversions may have to be enticed into exploring textures in their mouths. Creamy is very different from crunchy or bubbly (like soda). Spices and herbs also alter taste. Salty is very different from sweet. One strategy may be to create a "Clean Plate Club." When everyone involved in the child's care is aware of the intervention, lots of positive reinforcement can be given whenever the child clears or cleans his or her plate. Over time, children eat because of the reinforcement and because of their eventual joy in eating and actively receiving nourishment.

Initial interactions among human beings, children and other, more mature, people and the nonhuman environment shape one's response to life.

ADOLESCENTS' PURPOSEFUL ACTIVITIES

Because of their developmental needs, adolescents often take part in activities that are physically demanding and involve others of their own age. Social groups of peers often strongly influence their own activity preferences. Purposeful activities for adolescents involve a wide range of activities that vary from community to community, culture, and the adolescent's skills and abilities. When selecting an activity with an adolescent, occupational therapy practitioners must use careful reasoning to guide the adolescent toward an activity that he or she can perform with some competence. Adolescents often are aware that peers and adults are watching and judging them when they engage in activities. Further, it is important that the adolescent does not perceive the chosen activities as infantile, immature, or useless. When engaged in a purposeful activity, the practitioner must address the underlying psychological issues that may arise as the adolescent participates.

Selection of activities with adolescents must carefully consider the limited attention span and concentration of many teenagers in any or all settings. If an adolescent has attention and cognition impairments, the occupational therapy practitioner can work with him or her to improve and maximize study habits, memory skills, sequencing of life skill activities (e.g., instrumental activities in context), and ordering of activity participation and limit setting and redirecting behaviors that are potentially self-destructive. Additionally, many adolescents are self-conscious during attempts to practice self-care activities, especially those activities that are more intimate in nature, such as toileting or skin inspection. In partnership with the adolescent, practitioners can select activities that are both acceptable to the client and therapeutic.

ADULTS' PURPOSEFUL ACTIVITIES

Adults have an extensive range of activity needs, depending on their personal circumstances, such as health status, disability status, developmental skills, life circumstances, or personal desire. As when working with adolescents, occupational therapy practitioners should strive to work in partnership with adult clients and their significant others to verify that the therapeutic activities are acceptable to clients and meet their needs.

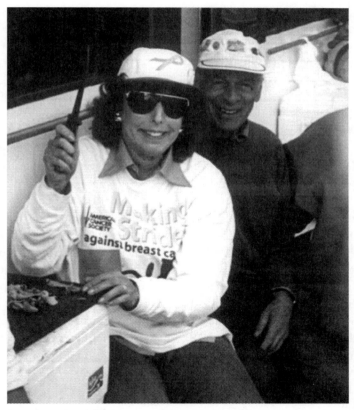

Figure 8.3. Regaining the ability to participate in meaningful occupations after recovery from illnesses can be a means of measuring health status and life satisfaction. In this example, it was possible for this woman to go deep-sea fishing once again with her husband. Deep-sea fishing was an important leisure occupation for them as a couple. The ability to resume her role as a leisure fisherperson improved her outlook and perceived sense of well-being despite her medical diagnosis.

When selecting activities with adults, practitioners often begin with the presenting problem or diagnosis. Based on the problem or area of difficulty and knowledge of the client and his or her needs, the occupational therapy practitioner begins to suggest a variety of activities that would be appropriate for the goals of therapy. Working in collaboration with the client and, in some cases, his or her significant others, the occupational therapist develops an intervention plan that includes those activities that the adult finds acceptable, challenging, and gratifying. With adults, it is crucial that the client understands the relationship between participation in the activity and the long-term therapeutic goals.

When working with adults, adapting activities to address the therapeutic goals may be necessary. For example, clients with orthopedic conditions, traumatic conditions, or burns commonly may have to execute specific actions. In such cases, the occupational therapy practitioner creatively adapts one of the client-selected activities to include the specific actions required for therapeutic purposes. When adapting or modifying activities, again involving the client is important because if activities become too contrived, they may become meaningless and, thus, not therapeutic. Choice of activities and ability to participate in an activity program will depend on the client's interest, ability, and needs. A balance of self-care activities, socialization, and avocational activities can be useful with adults who are not cognitively impaired.

Most adults value their independence in completing self-care activities, such as personal hygiene and grooming-related tasks. Adults have developed habits: automatic behaviors that are organized into complex behavioral patterns and that enable people to perform on a day-to-day basis (Neistadt & Crepeau, 1998). Adults rely on their habits to increase efficiency of participation in occupation-supporting tasks and activities. Habits have made us more efficient and energy conserving, so we might accomplish more routine tasks and be more productive overall. When adults have immobilized limbs or wounds, common objects may require adaptation to allow participation in basic self-care tasks. For other disabilities, occupational therapy practitioners may need to adjust the method the client normally uses in order for him or her to be successful in completing self-care tasks. If a client cannot bathe or groom in the manner to which he or she is accustomed, the practitioner may need to simulate the environment as closely as possible to that at home and have the client practice an adapted bathing or grooming routine, a basic activity of daily living skills. If feasible, the practitioner could practice the actual adaptation with the client during a home visit before discharge to the community. If adults have mobility problems, training in adapted techniques as well as training in and provision of adapted equipment may be the focus of activity participation.

Distinctive Characteristics Drive Selection of Purposeful Activities

Occupational therapy practitioners often select activities for intervention because of the distinctive characteristics of the activity. An analysis of the activity is skillfully used to match the activity and its inherent characteristics to the needs of the client.

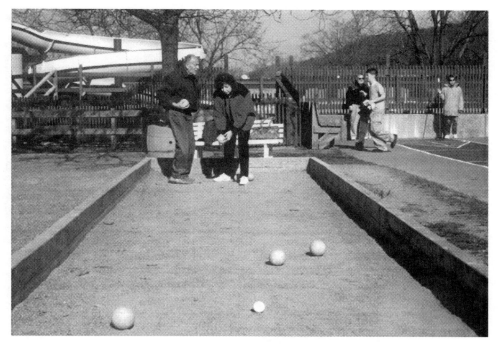

Figure 8.4. Leisure activities, such as playing bocci ball, often can support physical, social, and emotional well-being for older adults.

CHOOSING PURPOSEFUL ACTIVITIES FOR CHILDREN

For children, the choice of activities depends on both chronological and developmental age and the child's intact abilities. Children who are ill still seek interaction with people and toys. Adapting toys to encourage and enable participative play can be a focus of intervention. Further, technological devices and equipment often allow children to interact actively with their environment.

Case Scenario

Children with impairments may benefit from special adaptations to encourage and allow their participation in activities. Children with cancer, such as leukemia, may develop peripheral neuropathy as a result of chemotherapy. Adding switch activation to wind-up toys, for example, may provide opportunities to play actively and manipulate toys despite impairment. Children with heightened sensory awareness and poor sensory modulation may benefit from activities such as parachutes, therapy balls, swings (if they do not have seizure precautions), rocking chairs, bubbles, and balloons that encourage sensory integration.

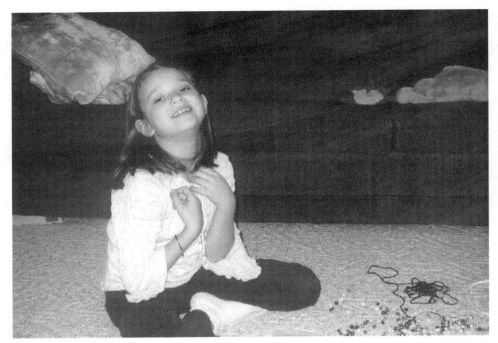

Figure 8.5. Children choose activities that are appropriate both chronologically and developmentally.

Children who cannot interact well with their environment as a result of disease or disability can sometimes gain control through environmental adaptations, such as the use of environmental control units or computerization. A child with progressed muscular dystrophy, for example, can still gain mobility with the appropriate powered mobility device and in the right circumstances. Computers can be operated by adapted switches, mouth sticks, head controls, joy sticks, or sip-and-puff mechanisms. Games may assist the child in gaining mastery over the adapted devices during the training process. Connecting successful outcomes with rewards can build self-esteem and a comfort level for the child in the use of the adaptation. One colleague of mine shared the following story about Joe, a young child with C-6 quadriplegia, and how she had built a docking station for a variety of mouth sticks for Joe.

<hr>

Case Scenario

Joe gained mastery over the mouth stick by playing a game of fish. A variety of objects were placed within reach. There were a few shapes for each adapted terminal end of a mouth stick in the docking station. Joe had to retrieve and replace each stick as needed to fish for all of the objects. The therapist had a matching set of mouth sticks, and she fished for the objects alternately with the boy. Once all the objects are retrieved, the player with the most objects wins the game. This example is just one of how a game can be used as a training activity for adjustment to the use of adapted devices.

Most activities have a specific performance component that is a key aspect of the activity. Accordingly, some activities are considered fine motor, gross motor, or perceptually based on the key performance component of the activity. All activities require skills in more than one performance component. When occupational therapy practitioners select activities, however, they often group them by the dominant performance component. These activities then become associated with a specific goal. As part of daily practice, practitioners select activities because of the dominant performance component.

Case Scenario

A large area of involvement of occupational therapy practitioners in school-based practice surrounds the child's handwriting ability. Children develop hand skills by a variety of means. Benbow (1995) found that a child needs good control of the entire extremity before he or she can achieve skilled writing. A child must first receive proprioceptive input to his or her shoulder to develop body sense of the arm in space. Activities Benbow recommended are writing in overhead planes, such as on a blackboard, easel, or paper taped to a wall. The overhead positioning of the arm provides stimulation to the rest of the body, and the child develops skilled use of the arm in overhead planes. The child's balance is stimulated and gives him or her an ability to develop the use of the arms in multiple contexts. A magnetic drawing board also provides proprioceptive feedback to the arm. Activities with proprioceptive and kinesthetic feedback assist the child in the development of coordinated movement and skill development.

Children learn and enhance hand skill development and develop concentration and prevocational skill through the use of craft activities. Arts-and-crafts activities were, at one time in occupational therapy history, a primary focus. Over time and with an increasing emphasis on working in the medical model, many occupational therapy practitioners abandoned or deemphasized the use of arts and crafts. Engagement in arts-and-crafts activities reinforces hand skill development, builds the ability to concentrate and follow written directions, and fosters values for creativity and effective use of leisure time. It is a mechanism for building a child's self-esteem through the completion of a finished project to keep for oneself or to give as a gift.

Case Scenario

Occupational therapy practitioners often select activities that focus on a child's development of psychosocial skills. Children who may have learning disabilities, such as dyslexia, or who may be dealing with a difficult psychosocial adjustment, such as divorce of their parents, may act out and physically attack others. They often lack self-esteem or may feel guilt or responsibility for the break up. When experiencing the loss of one parent from the home, children may glorify the parent who has left. They may act out and strike out at the parent who continues to be their caregiver. An occupational therapy practitioner can work with the child toward finding more productive ways to express his or her feelings as well as toward developing better interaction with the custodial parent and others under controlled circumstances. If the child is having a problem writing or reading and becomes frustrated, sometimes by 7 years of age, he or she can begin to work with a computer to substitute for the frustrating activity (e.g., writing). Seeing words in a composition can be less threatening. Words with which the child has difficulty can be macrocoded, grouped together in frequently used phrases, and stored for ease of successful use during computer time.

Having children participate in controlled play activities one-on-one with the practitioner can improve their interpersonal skills and ability to engage in parallel and cooperative play in various situations with others. Therapists may need to set goals for the activities chosen with the child, and practitioners may need to set limits on acting-out behaviors during the session. Sometimes a practitioner has an advantage over a parent in getting children to discuss their feelings. A rapport with an impartial third party who works with the child, like an occupational therapy practitioner, may be less fearful and threatening to the child. Truthful sharing with family may generate fear of rejection or reprisal from the family.

Choosing Activities for Adolescents

For adolescents, selecting activities requires an artful match with the activity and the client's personality, social skills, and motivation. Adolescents may have a variety of physical, psychological, and emotional impairments. Problems occupational therapy practitioners see may include dyslexia; vision impairment; physical impairment; and acting-out behaviors associated with anxiety, depression, poor coping ability, personality disorders, or schizophrenia. Adolescents with dyslexia may be involved in delinquent behavior. Many adolescents convicted of crimes in their teenage years have learning impairments. Computer-based programs have been demonstrated to be very valuable with this population. With computer games and access to the Internet, attentional skills can be improved; success can be attained through use of a fun format to achieve successful participation with the written word and media.

Adolescents often need to develop life skills. Life skills programs are currently a topic area targeted for federal and philanthropic funding. A variety of media can be used for life skills training. One group of graduate students in a management and supervision class at Columbia University recently proposed a computer-based life skills program in a drug and alcohol treatment setting for adolescents. The students suggested using key words that promoted acceptance and a sense of belonging as target phrases for search engines to locate the program source. In a hospital setting, a life skills program could have information on how to perform instrumental and basic activities of daily living tasks when living with a variety of impairments.

Adolescents often develop positive behaviors when they are appointed as role models for others. Imbuing adolescents with responsibility instills values about responsibility. Making adolescents responsible and contributing participants in systems works extremely well in positively facilitating behavioral change. Some of the hot topics for adolescents include safe sex, prevention of smoking and drug use, and proactive development of good eating and physical activity habits. Individual activities with a counselor; participation in a group activity wherein participants take turns at leadership; and use of multimedia activities involving film, slide presentations, rap sessions, graphic arts, and performing arts are all media that have been used to develop activities for this age group.

Teens with impairments still may seek out opportunities to be role models to younger siblings. Role-modeling can enhance self-esteem. The perception of feeling valued or looked up to for one's skill, wisdom, and contribution is self-affirming and valuable to both the role model and the protégé. An occupational therapy practitioner can coach a teenager through this process or assist him or her with skill development, if the practitioner is skilled in the activity selected.

CHOOSING ACTIVITIES FOR ADULTS

For adults, selecting activities requires matching the adult's specific performance deficit(s) and the activity that has performance requirements that will address the deficit(s). Although most children learn by repeating activities over and over in the same contextual relationship before they modify the activity or tire of the core activity, adult learners generally learn best when presented with a variety of tasks and activities from which to choose or alternate. Adults tend to do well with repetitive tasks only when they are for improvement of mobility, such as exercise machines or a desire and focus on the ability to walk. Many commercially available items of therapeutic exercise equipment for home use are rote and repetitive, and many adults use them as clothing collectors rather than as something to help them to get in shape. Adult learners require a variety of different types of learning challenges. In inpatient rehabilitation settings, activities often are closely related to self-care and ability to function in the home or community or to return to work. To vary skill acquisition methods, many inpatient rehabilitation settings use group activities to put choice and diversity into the recovery process and retain the client's active interest in participation. Some examples of groups used in inpatient settings include movement groups, strengthening groups, upright mobility groups (focusing on standing ability and mobility in standing or walking), cooking groups, and specific diagnostic category groups (e.g., hemi group or amputee group). Some groups may perform a psychosocial adjustment activity, such as sharing questions and concerns about their condition and anticipated degree of recovery.

When mobility impairments are severe or accompanied by communication impairments, occupational therapists may use technological resources to enable adults. Uses of environmental control units, powered mobility, or computerized adaptations are examples of highly technological resource equipment. In the training phase, once technology is obtained for personal use by a client, the occupational therapy practitioner can use games or other fun activities in the training process as a way to assist the client to acquire the agility and skill to substitute the function of the technology for their own impaired functional ability. The client can play games on his or her own, such as computerized solitaire, or games can be played competitively between the client and the practitioner, a volunteer, or a friend.

When occupational therapy practitioners intervene with adults who work, they may select activities that directly relate to their employment. Adults who work full-time spend 7½ hours a day, 37½ hours a week, on average, at work. Work-related activities generally revolve around the activities that describe the position the person fills. In work environments, the focus of intervention may involve doing a work task in a modified way. People who use strong postural sets to accomplish tasks may be prone to injury because their muscle activity is maximized. Relearning less stressful ways of doing work tasks can be one area of focus in work-related occupational therapy practice.

Case Scenario

The most common injury in a work setting is back injury (Nassau, 1999). Placing objects in the environment that can be used to improve the ergonomics of task performance, through trial and error and at times using commercially or custom-made adaptations, can be a focus of activity. One factor that influences recovery from back injury is smoking. Workers who sustain a back injury and smoke are less likely to return to work.

Case Scenario

The second most common work-related injury is cumulative trauma disorder (Feuerstein, Miller, Burrell, & Berger, 1998). Carpal tunnel syndrome can develop from cumulative trauma disorder of the carpal tunnel. This condition can be treated by changing the heights of monitors, the ergonomic demands of the keyboard, the amount of time spent at computer terminals between rest breaks, adjustment of the position of the keyboard, or adequate ergonomic seating support. Occupational therapy practitioners can teach workers to keep schedules of rest and stretch breaks. Fun activities encouraging changes in posture and gross mobility rather than concentrating on use of the hands, may provide a balance between concentrated clerical activity and a healthful amount of break activity.

Activities also can be used to develop new skills. When people are adjusting to life with impairments, they sometimes are unable to resume all of their prior life roles. Learning new activities can assist their adjustment to a lifestyle after becoming disabled. The old cliché usually is that a client will say, "Will I ever play the piano?" With experience, the practitioner learns to retort, "Well, did you ever play before?" A few years ago, a young man with bilateral hand burns and an interest in jazz asked this question of me. Initially, we chuckled at our dialogue. Several years after his hospitalization, he came back to visit. He sat at the piano in our clinic and proceeded to play an absolutely amazing rendition of Scott Joplin's "Maple Leaf Rag." In retrospect, trying to play the piano as a part of his inpatient therapy could have been appropriate for this gentleman. The activity, although new to him and potentially disappointing to him, could also have been meaningful and motivating. Whenever a client asks this question these days, my answer is different from what it used to be. Activity choice is individual and unique in each case. Being an active listener can be ultimately the best strategy for problem solving and activity choice.

Context Influences the Selection and Use of Purposeful Activities

Activities are selected relative to the context in which they will be used. Occupational therapy practitioners work in a variety of practice settings and with a variety of age groups. Settings include the home, schools, hospitals, long-term-care facilities, day treatment, business and industry, community settings, and institutions of higher learning. Practitioners work with all age groups across the life span: infants, children, adolescents, young adults, middle-aged adults, and older adults. The use of activities in context in occupational therapy will vary case by case and setting by setting. Activities can be valued by one age group in one context and yet be meaningless to another age group in another context.

In all treatment settings, use of clinical reasoning assists the therapist to prioritize the focus of treatment across physical/skilled movement, psychological/emotional, cognitive, and social domains within the following contexts:

- *Self-care*: for example, removing one's own bandage, establishing a sense of control, washing one's face, putting one's clothes on, eating one's meal, performing age-appropriate toileting

- *Work*: for example, studying and writing in the hospital school or with a tutor, using a computer for a school-age child

- *Play and leisure*: for example, testing physical limits; role-playing and pretending; discussing and sharing feelings; expressing fears; coping with fears and pain; gaining a sense of self, privacy, and self-esteem; experiencing success through activities in all levels of developmental groups; making friends; exploring and developing continuing relationships with family; experiencing moments of joy and pleasure; learning cause-and-effect relationships; learning to accept and test social limits; developing coping skills and strategies to manage the impact of illness on life and to instill day-to-day living with a sense of hope so that change can occur to improve quality of life and to work toward the best outcome in treatment, so one has benefit of life and a future.

Rest is also something one learns. As children, we rely on the adults in our lives to structure our naps and rest periods and to determine bedtime for us. Our bodies and minds require rest to assist with processing all that has happened in our lives each day. Without rest, our thought processes become adversely affected. We are less able to concentrate, and our social behaviors deteriorate. Rest is an activity of daily living, as well.

SETTINGS FOR SERVICES TO CHILDREN

Occupational therapy practitioners provide services to children and their families in a wide range of environments, including NICUs, acute care hospital settings, early intervention programs, home care settings, school-based practice, inpatient psychiatry, and wellness-based practice.

Case Scenario

Children who may be at risk developmentally or are developmentally delayed are eligible for early intervention services. Occupational therapy practitioners usually see children receiving early intervention either at home or in a community-based clinic setting. The age group receiving care in this category is children between 0 and 3 years of age. Activities used with infants and young children at risk for developmental impairments should be focused on parent–child interactions. Much of the context of interaction between the occupational therapy practitioner and the family revolves around hands-on demonstration and working with parents and other caregivers on their interactions with their child. Activities include showing parents how to hold their children and promote the child's motor abilities along a developmental continuum. Parents receive education on how to recognize developmental milestones and to promote the child's ability to grow and develop.

Children in the hospital have a role; they are pediatric clients. Play too often is lacking in their day-to-day routine. They experience a lack of stimulating activity, become isolated, and can regress. A child who is hospitalized may seek time and opportunity to play with toys that he or she should have outgrown in a chronological sense. This developmental regression is not necessarily pathological in context. Reverting back to a remembered level of mastery with a toy can be comforting. Occupational therapy practitioners learn to dance with the child's needs for developmental stimulation, ever introducing a challenge here and there throughout play to move the child toward the place that should be more appropriate for his or her age and the sophistication of his or her nervous system at any given moment in time. Recently, I met a 6-year-old who wanted to play with Teletubbies® rather than his model trains and Legos®. The Teletubby fascination resolved when he began to develop trust in the situation and his caregivers. Fear and an illness contributed to his regression.

Case Scenario

Activities that promote self-care for children may all be available within the environment of the hospital room. Most children have clothes and socks and shoes with them, implements to wash their faces or brush their teeth, cups or bottles to practice feeding, and usually some toys (pull toys, favorite stuffed animals or dolls, books, crayons and coloring books or pads). Therapy balls may be readily available and can provide balance stimulation. Playrooms or child life departments may have other toys or experiential learning tools, including computer technology. Several different disciplines may use the same or similar equipment with children for different, noncompeting treatment goals. Interaction with parents or others can be observed during play. Children often offer insights into their understanding of their illness, revealing confidences as rapport is gained with trust. Engaging parents in treatment can assist with carryover of therapy goals.

Case Scenario

Children in acute care hospitals often are admitted for medical or surgical intervention. Those who are referred to occupational therapy have a variety of medical or surgical conditions. The conditions vary according to the specialty departments within the setting. Often, children who are hospitalized regress developmentally. Being ill can preclude engagement in play. Children normally and naturally test limits and explore new behaviors during play. In a hospital setting, all rehabilitation recovery from a child's perspective occurs through play activity. If a child has a burn, for example, he or she may need to maintain range of motion at the joints over which the burn extends. Having him or her reach for a stuffed animal, pull a pull toy, or ride a bike can assist with the child's willingness to move, ability to demonstrate active range of motion within the context of an activity, and participate in play. Using activities to encourage both movement and participation produces a successful recovery outcome. The practitioner must have a double agenda to accomplish effective treatment with hospitalized children. Providing the opportunity to play while working to prevent possible side effects of the medical or surgical treatment that could affect their future ability to succeed is the goal. The possible problems vary according to the disease and its treatment.

Case Scenario

Not all children regress during hospitalization. Some children, despite illness, adjust well and seek out opportunities for age-appropriate developmental play participation. Another recent acquaintance of mine, a 7-year-old girl, had experienced smoke inhalation and exacerbation of her asthma when her family had a house fire. She had learning disabilities premorbid to her smoke inhalation but was experiencing some new balance problems. Despite a need for intermittent oxygen through a nasal cannula and despite hospitalization, when her older brother and sister visited her in the unit, she wanted to come to the play area for a physically challenging game of Twister®. She played, tolerated it well, and seemed to enjoy the challenge. The game was not simple for her, but she perceived it as fun and, therefore, was willing to challenge herself in the attempt to participate in the game activity.

Case Scenario

Occupational therapy practitioners have increased their visibility and standing in schools over the past 20 years. One group of issues addressed in the school system is the mainstreaming of children with impairments into regular classrooms. Practitioners in school-based practice may participate in classroom activities with the children they treat. They may determine whether adaptations in the classroom could facilitate participation and assist a child to meet his or her learning objectives in an individualized education program. Sometimes where the child is seated in the classroom can be very important. If a child has a visual impairment and needs to be closer to the blackboard, the occupational therapy practitioner may recommend modification of this positioning in the classroom. If the child has difficulty responding verbally, the practitioner can work with the child and educational team to enable communication through the use of augmentative communication technology, such as a speak-and-spell board or computerized assistance.

Case Scenario

Children who are inpatients in a psychiatric setting may have a number of issues that have so severely impaired their activity participation that they are hospitalized and separated from mainstream society. Childhood schizophrenia is one problem. Children who have hallucinations from an early age may not respond well to either their own human environment or to external environments, human and nonhuman. Children with schizophrenia may not initiate play or peer interaction. Activities may be used to assist the child in skill development. Basic self-care activities are one aspect. Learning to wash and dress oneself is a way to gain a sense of pride from the ability to demonstrate age-appropriate self-care accomplishments. Additionally, learning to concentrate and to try to do activities from single to multiple steps is gained from skill acquisition and grading of activities with increasing difficulty to support establishment of self-esteem, work- or school-related behaviors, and socially acceptable emotional and behavioral interactions. Crafts and games can be useful tools in this setting. Sensory integrative activities, which challenge mobility and coordination skills, are useful. Activities should be pleasing and fun for the children to encourage willing participation and age-appropriate skill development. Whether it is skipping rope, playing hopscotch, or playing team games or board games, children in all settings must learn to play and relate well to others and feel a sense of participation and accomplishment.

Working with parents and caregivers on strategies to achieve successful participation in play, age-appropriate developmental self-care activities, and self-esteem building can be a focus of treatment. Parents and caregivers may need to learn how to hold a child, position a child, or engage a child in play. They also may need guidance and encouragement to let children try to participate and to repeat attempts or fail in the process of trying. Many children acquire passive behaviors. They do not seek out opportunities to play or participate in their self-care. Occupational therapy practitioners who work in home care often have to practice limit setting with caregivers so that a child is challenged to take the lead in pieces of their self-care, school work, and fun activities.

SETTINGS FOR SERVICES TO ADOLESCENTS

Occupational therapy services are provided to adolescents in a variety of settings, including hospitals, homes, and the community. Adolescents may be hospitalized in acute-care settings for a variety of reasons. Some of the leading causes of hospitalization related to trauma in adolescents are vehicular and sports-related injuries. High-risk behaviors are one causal factor leading to the propensity for these injuries. The injuries may involve head trauma (e.g., concussion, head injury with central nervous system involvement, contusions) as well as spinal cord injuries (all levels, including cervical, thoracic, lumbar, and sacral regions) and fractures (e.g., long bones, pelvis, spine, joints, small bones of the face, hands, and feet). Recovery depends on the constellation of the activities and the ability of involved organs and structures to heal. When adolescents are hospitalized for long periods, they may not be able to attend schools and may have to be tutored. If they have sustained head injuries, their cognitive abilities may have become impaired, and they may have to relearn many life relationships from a low level of cognitive skill. The occupational therapy practitioner uses graded task activities to increase attentional skills and may work together with the educational staff at the hospital and the parents to adjust educational programming to the adolescent's new appropriate skill level.

Often, adolescents who sustain head injuries and cognitive impairments have lost attentional and social skills but may have awareness of inappropriate presentation of activities, which may seem too infantile to them. Attempting to pace the learning experience from a skill acquisition approach may require the unique participation of an occupational therapy practitioner. Many other educational and health care providers do not have knowledge about cognitive and perceptual impairments as they influence neurobehavior and affect performance of activities. Developing a new personality and new socially acceptable behaviors requires plenty of opportunities to try out new skills as they are developed. Activities can be developed, tapping into the adolescent's interests to assist him or her in new role development. For example, being a collector can be a role. Acquiring a collection can be a challenge to one's memory (knowing what one has as well as thinking about what one would like to acquire); ability to sequence or organize the collection; and ability to seek out new information by solving problems about how to find resources, communicating with those resources, negotiating acquisition terms for new items to add to the collection and managing money, recognizing financial constraints, and learning to budget money to meet the goals of building the collection. The collection can be highly individualized.

Some suggestions might be autographs, postcards, e-mail messages and letters from near and far, baseball cards, and memorabilia.

Adolescents also are hospitalized for other general medical and surgical problems. Cancers of the bone have their highest occurrence during adolescence. Amputations as a result of cancer have a great impact on adolescents. Just at a developmental stage where people are most sensitive and aware of appearance, the ability to sustain their lives and to enter a stage of remission depends on their losing a body part. Activities to promote acceptance of their modified body image can be useful.

Case Scenario

Cultivating role models with others who have had amputations or having an opportunity to meet someone else who has had an amputation from cancer and has gone on to live well are other possibilities. One program that may involve occupational therapy practitioners is the Achilles Track Club. In New York City, the Achilles Track Club sends representatives to some hospitals to work with adolescents with impairments who have a desire to participate in track-and-field activities. Members of the Achilles Track Club have participated in and completed marathons, including the New York City Marathon. An adolescent does not need to have been a runner before becoming a person with an amputation to participate in the Achilles Track Club.

Adolescents in home care settings often are in a transitional stage between the hospital and the community. If they are recovering from an illness or injury, home care may provide them with the time to explore community integration. Community mobility is more than leaving one's apartment; it involves crossing streets, entering and leaving buildings (businesses, churches, social clubs, theaters, housing units, and open-air settings such as parks and fields). If the adolescent has impaired mobility, obstacle courses to learn to operate or navigate with a wheelchair or ambulatory device may be a focus. In wheelchairs, learning to pop wheels, using public or private transportation, and participating in volley or team wheelchair sports are all possible activities. Ambulatory adolescents may require adaptations to enable participation in a particular sport. Sometimes, reinventing roles may involve exploring possible activities through searching the Internet or participating in interest surveys or interviews to determine or explore interests, thus setting longer-term goals.

Adolescents in community settings may be coping with social risk situations. Today, single parents head many families. After-school programs often contain activities to teach adolescents effective study habits. Job skills can be developed through volunteering at a neighborhood center or in the community in jobs such as Meals On Wheels, which delivers food to people who are ill or elderly. Volunteering in the spiritual community in ritual activities, such as serving as an altar assistant, is a metaphysical-related spiritual activity and may be instrumental in the adolescent's worship of a higher power and development of community-sustaining values and beliefs. Volunteering in community projects can instill citizenship and influence value development toward the need to sustain and support the community.

SETTINGS FOR SERVICES TO ADULTS

Adults receive occupational therapy services in homes, hospitals, clinics, work sites, and the community. In home settings, activities often are severely limited by reimbursement mechanisms. Activity choices usually are related to basic self-care or the ability to accomplish household tasks. By definition, to qualify for home care services a person must be confined to his or her home. Once a person has gained community mobility, he or she often must transfer his or her care to an outpatient setting. Activities in home care can focus on making the environment as accessible as possible. Home-based occupational therapy often is concerned with self-care instrumental activities of daily living, such as kitchen-related activities. A client at home may need to participate in meal preparation activities. Activity choices are made based on what the client reports to be his or her habit, the way he or she ordinarily does things at home. If activities are chosen in collaboration with clients and are within the scope of standardized occupational therapy scales or measures, outcome data can support the validity of the occupational therapy process. Ability to engage in activities that a client chooses are directly applicable to his or her daily life, are occupation supporting, and are valuable to the client as well as to the other customer in this interaction—the insurer or third-party payer. Focusing in on participation in daily living activities and enabling people to participate again in their own care makes sense from both a personal point of view and a fiscal perspective.

When intervening with adults who work, occupational therapy may use activities beyond concentrating on the specific work activities to include those that would facilitate skills to improve the work social environment and the actual work context. These interventions go beyond changing, adapting, or modifying one activity to enhancing the whole work situation. Creating competitions for workers to imagine how job tasks could be changed can be suggested to employers. Sometimes workers, who are the people closest to job tasks, have greater insight into needed change. An occupational therapy practitioner can use employee competitions to encourage creative problem solving and sharing about the job tasks. Group activities and discussion groups can encourage generation of new ideas. Allowing staff members to perceive that they are partners in the work safety process can be a successful strategy to empower workers to appreciate their role in preserving their personal health and the overall health of their workplace.

Money-related activities are crucial to adults who wish to return to the community with a low level of supervision. Budgeting, writing checks, paying bills, counting change, and using bank machines are all activities that can be useful to this population. Postoperative cognitive impairment often is overlooked. Adults who have had general anesthesia may have mild cognitive impairments that alter their clarity of thought and memory, sequencing abilities, and higher executive functions.

Communication activities also are important. Can the person recall what to do in an emergency? Does he or she know how to call 911? Does the person have vision or auditory impairments that affect the ability to use a standard telephone? Can the person express his or her needs? Using activities or scenarios to encourage function in a variety of circumstances is crucial to safety and the ability to return to the community. People with cognitive impairments often need to have caregivers present in the home at all times. The occupational therapy practitioner and the interdisciplinary treatment team must come to a consensus on a case-by-case basis about these issues.

Traditional purposeful activities in subacute care include basic self-care and individual or group participation in some instrumental activities of daily living, such as cooking activities, that the client will need to do to some degree in order to return to the community. An improvement in ability can move a person closer to discharge or change his or her status to a higher functioning physical unit or assisted living, if he or she will remain within the community to receive subacute care. If adult clients in subacute settings will not be returning home, activities can be used to assist them with their adjustment to institutional living. For example, reviving avocational interests that may have been lost over time, planning and selecting objects from home to decorate one's new living quarters, creating memory books, retrospectively organizing old photographs into a meaningful story-like context, and developing a new style are all strategies that can direct activity choices for occupational therapy in context.

Purposeful Activities Support Health and Wellness

Occupational therapists also employ purposeful activities to prevent disabilities and promote health. Activities that meet these goals can be applied throughout the human life span and are effective if they assist clients in addressing their own interests and goals. The challenge for the therapist lies in bringing together healthy activity choices and arousing client's engagement in these activities because they become fascinated or captivated by the activities.

HEALTH AND WELLNESS IN CHILDREN

Children develop health habits by 7 years of age. They also hear health messages from other children better than from adults. Adolescents and older siblings, in particular, can have a very strong influence on the development of good health habits. Stress affects not only adults but also children. One technique that has been demonstrated to be very assuring and stress reducing for children is massage. The confusion for children about touch is in learning to discriminate appropriate touch. An occupational therapy practitioner trained in infant or child massage can be one vehicle for children to learn tolerance of appropriate touch and to learn about reducing stress from an early age. If stress management is taught as part of habilitation rather than as rehabilitation in adulthood, perhaps more children in our society would be better adjusted and less stressed. Some ways children can receive wellness messages are through activities done with their parents. Mothers and fathers can learn massage techniques, such as infant massage. Aromatherapy has been shown to reduce stress. Relaxing music associated with time to slow down and cool off can support the need to have relaxation.

One of the health disparities that is the focus of the *Healthy People 2010* (U.S. Department of Health and Human Services, 2003) initiative is the rising problem in our society of childhood obesity. In outcomes-based research, Gortmaker et al. (1999) found that children need to learn earlier to be more physically active. We are too sedentary in our society. Many children are too sedentary. A correlation has been drawn between the number of hours that kids watch television and their propensity to be obese. Occupational therapy practitioners work with children to develop activity schedules and prospectively to learn balanced lifestyle concepts as they grow and develop. Mapping out times to be engaged in physical play (team or individual sports), such as martial arts, swimming, pair-teamed sports (e.g., tennis), walking, running, and climbing, can be invaluable in preventing obesity. If children develop good health behaviors, they may carry over these habits into adulthood and live healthier, performing at their own personal best.

Good nutritional behaviors also are essential to school-age children. In our society, many children eat only one meal at home each day. Children can hear messages about balancing nutritional choices and recognizing when to eat as well as what to eat. Occupational therapy practitioners who work in wellness programs with children teach them to select proper foods and to prepare the foods. An occupational therapy practitioner could work with a nutritionist and parents toward the goal of developing good nutritional habits from preschool through graduate school. One component of this program could be aimed toward assisting children to learn to love their bodies as they are. Early detection of food and eating disorders could occur prospectively. Additionally, pro bono participation with children's sports teams may reinforce good eating habits and thwart misconceptions about starving or purging oneself to participate in sports, such as one-to-one contact sports, that traditionally overfocus on weight control.

HEALTH AND WELLNESS IN ADOLESCENTS

Adolescents often engage in risky behaviors and test the rules given them for life and living. However, at times adolescents can accept the challenge of being role models for younger children. They can be effective communicators and role models if they are given information to use to influence younger siblings or friends. This is a proactive application of information and a therapeutic and educational strategy from a health promotion perspective. Some of the activities that create risk of injury, and about which one can give health messages, are sports activities such as bicycling, rollerblading, and water sports where the use of helmets and protective gear can prevent injury or death. The use of helmets is controversial. Helmets protect the cranium and may lessen impact to the skull. Bicycle helmets are constructed of firm foam but do not cover the face. Motorcycle helmets engulf the head and protect the face but terminate at the cervical spine. Survival from a motorcycle accident may result in traumatic brain injury, spinal cord injury, or both. Prevention of injuries through safety messages and instilling safety as a value can be of lifelong benefit.

In addition to helmets, when rollerblading, additional protective gear for the limbs also is indicated to prevent blunt trauma to the arms and legs. Awareness of the surroundings where one plans to skate and taking time to inspect the scene for possible injury hazards can be helpful prospectively in preventing an injury. Adolescents can take a leadership role to prepare and deliver safety messages while gaining value for these messages in their own lives.

Water sports can result in spinal cord injuries, thermal injuries, and drowning or near-drowning hazards. Safety messages about proper methods to use when diving, boating, and swimming can be straightforward and useful. Again, adoption of principles about safety can influence value development for the adolescent.

Preparation and participation in sports activities have become so closely aligned with the need for medical intervention that sports medicine has become a specialty area of practice in medicine. Contact sports are characterized by injury potential. Occupational therapy practitioners also may specialize in sports medicine. Activities related to sports can include coordination and strengthening tasks before playing a sport for the actual sporting season. Additionally, designing and implementing the use of protective strategies can avert potential injury while engaging in the sport. Occupational therapy practitioners can design programs and strategies for prevention of injury during sports activities. Designing adapted devices and fabricating them from composite materials are part of occupational therapy practice. Use of visualization and guided imagery has been demonstrated as effective with figure skaters as well as with other athletes. These tools are complementary medical techniques that require occupational therapy practitioners to receive further training beyond the basic education and training received in entry-level professional education.

Adolescents tend to abuse substances such as tobacco, alcohol, and drugs (prescription, over-the-counter, and illicit). A study done in Boston in which adolescents were given positive messages to prevent tobacco use resulted in a decrease in the incidence of starting to smoke in the neighborhood where it was piloted (Hunt et al., 2003). Using health promoting groups, such as SADD (Students Against Drunk Driving) and DARE (Drug Abuse Resistance Education), can help to teach adolescents positive refusal behaviors so that they will not be influenced by peer pressure surrounding the push to use illicit substances. The "Just Say No" campaigns have been supported by the federal government and have been effective in this respect. Values in American society are strongly influenced by media and advertising. Anti-tobacco advertising has been demonstrated to be effective in assisting people to quit smoking. When advertisements compete for use versus avoidance of use, the competition is tough. As health educators, occupational therapy practitioners can use health promoting activities with groups and individuals to influence positive health choices.

Adolescents also may develop maladaptive behaviors through peer pressure and ineffective socialization or demoralizing, impoverished experiences. Occupational therapy practitioners can act as positive role models and assist teenagers to develop life skills. Life skills with mentally impaired, chemically addicted populations are currently one of the primary priorities in philanthropic funding for behavioral disorders. Creating positively oriented Web pages that teenagers can access to learn everything—from doing laundry, to budgeting funds, to developing realistic and affordable leisure activities in the community—can be part of life skills programming. With the dissolution of extended families, adolescents have fewer closely related and accessible adults after whom to model themselves and their behaviors.

Occupational therapy practitioners can coach adolescents and their parents or guardians toward exploring the resource opportunities relative to these initiatives. Coaching implies acting in a capacity through which individuals learn to set goals and identify or explore potential opportunities. It does not necessitate expert skill or knowledge attainment to coach, merely the skills necessary to solve problems and resource opportunities. Activity analysis and synthesis and an awareness of social and cultural context are used in this process.

Finally, teenagers can respond positively to encouragement to speak about psychological and social stress that they may experience. Adults who are positive role models for teenagers encourage them to discuss stress, such as exam stress, individually and within a support group setting. Sometimes the experience of this stress is related to other issues, such as undetected dyslexia. However, stress often is related to irrational or rational fear. Fear and stress can be well managed with stress reduction techniques, such as guided imagery and visualization, hypnosis, or conscious relaxation. Additionally, knowing that others can listen to their fears and support them through resolution of problems can change values of belonging and being valued as a member of a social group or family. When adolescents do not develop skills for effective and proactive management of their stress, they act out. Acting out can result in violent behaviors, such as suicidal ideation or attempts or commission of violence or abuse of family members and others.

HEALTH AND WELLNESS IN ADULTS

With adults, as life patterns emerge and responsibilities broaden, they often overlook their own needs in favor of meeting the needs of their families. Adults who are parents often are so invested in supporting their children's efforts in activities—acting as chauffeur as well as cheerleader and financier—that they do not plan or participate in physical activity for their own benefit. Adults in middle age often develop conditions that can be tied to the development of pathology in later life.

One common diagnosis that responds well to wellness initiatives is hypertension. Adults with hypertension often can control their condition through diet and exercise. Occupational therapy practitioners can work with at-risk populations, such as healthy adults who seek the opportunity to improve their health. Setting up a schedule that encourages personal investment in one's own health can be a focus of occupational therapy. Configuring time to encourage a balance of self-care, work, play and leisure, and rest is the definition of a balanced lifestyle in occupational therapy terms. Occupational therapy embraces the value that health is promoted through a balanced lifestyle. Working with people toward the achievement of successful participation in meaningful activities is the method through which people occupy their time within the constraints of their life roles and responsibilities.

Changing habits to promote better health also is a wellness strategy. One of the habits occupational therapy practitioners can assist adults to change is quitting smoking. Changing habitual routines in which one may experience a desire to smoke is a strategy that one can use. In 1999, the AOTA Representative Assembly adopted a smoking cessation policy (Policy 5.9; AOTA, 1999). The Agency for Healthcare Research and Quality's four-step process has been demonstrated to be effective through research, and its application is straightforward in an occupational therapy context.

Decreasing stress is a major wellness initiative. Stress can influence the development of cardiovascular disease. Occupational therapy practitioners can use mind–body techniques to promote conscious awareness in preparation for activities. Some techniques that practitioners use are based in movement (yoga, tai chi, qi gong, Alexander technique), meditation (e.g., guided imagery, transcendental technique, neurolinguistic programming, prayer), and other miscellaneous techniques (e.g., aromatherapy, massage, acupuncture, traditional medicine techniques). Use of these techniques requires additional training beyond the basic level of occupational therapy education. Clients may be interested in techniques that are congruent with their socialization and are presented in an appropriate cultural context.

Culturally based mind–body techniques can be very meaningful and more comforting to commit to for some clients. One recent trend in the United States is the move toward traditional Native American ceremonial activities. Ceremonial drumming and dancing are spiritually meaningful and draw on both existential and metaphysical aspects of spirituality through participation. These activities are occupationally based and in a context that can be embraced within occupational therapy practice (AOTA, 2003).

Adults often are referred to as "weekend warriors" in specific reference to participation in sports. There is a high potential for injury when people attempt to push their performance to the limits. Without the advantage of consistent training in preparation for such a demand on the body, these people are prone to injury. Activities can include exploration of interests that the person has about sports and, after assessment, opportunities for the person to do warm-up exercises or train for the sport. If an occupational therapy practitioner is not competent in a sport, he or she can coach clients through the process of identifying training centers through resources such as the Internet, local newspapers, or networking within communities. The practitioner also can assist adults who wish to do more physical activity to choose sports that are challenging but within the realm of possibility of participation for the client. If the client has an area that warrants protection, the practitioner can work with him or her to develop a system of protective strategies or devices to allow participation with consideration for safety and injury prevention.

Selecting Purposeful Activities for a Client's Therapeutic Needs

Sometimes the choice of activities is defined by the circumstances of the client's condition; hence, the occupational therapist develops an intervention plan that includes activities that are therapeutic but may not be within the acceptable or usual culturally appropriate criteria that practitioners most often use to ensure that the ultimate goal of the client to engage in occupations is achieved.

Case Scenario

In pregnancy, some women are restricted to bed rest for months before giving birth. It is difficult for healthy adults to accept the confinement of bed. Occupational therapy practitioners can use activity interest inventories with this group of healthy adults and design an activity program for effective time use while on bed rest. Leisure time can be used to participate in craft, reading, and paperwork activities. When one has mobility restrictions, it often is helpful for "mommies on bed rest" to have adapted devices for activities of daily living that require reaching one's feet or retrieving items from the floor. Avoiding excessive strain on the pelvic floor can assist with sustaining an at-risk pregnancy.

Case Scenario

Children who have cancer may have visible appearance issues and precautions for activity involvement. Alopecia (loss of hair) and peripheral neuropathy (a chemotherapy-associated side effect) are transient, resolvable problems. When a child is experiencing these problems at school, other children may tease him or her and not support the child psychosocially. Children who are receiving chemotherapy on an ongoing basis may have indwelling intravenous lines, catheters, or ports. It can be dangerous for the child to have any trauma or contact with the lines because the lines could dislodge, causing complications, or could place the child at increased risk of infection through the line. Social isolation can make a child less willing to be in school and less willing to participate or try. Occupational therapy practitioners can work one-on-one with these children in the classroom to adapt activities as needed and, therefore, allow participation in class. Additionally, practitioners can assist the child in the situational context to experience success at activities and to ease social reintegration with peers. Again, occupational therapy practitioners are skilled in both the medical model and school-based practice. They are aware of and can collaborate with other professionals to determine how adaptations can be made to allow participation. They also are potentially invaluable in school-based practice because of their ability to treat holistically and use activities that are challenging and fun to achieve the goals of classroom reintegration, even in the face of impairment or disability.

Case Scenario

A 6-year-old boy who had received chemotherapy for his leukemia and has had hair loss and peripheral neuropathy might find, through working with an occupational therapy practitioner, a new personality for himself in the classroom. He finds a cool hat. His splints that support his wrists during classroom activities are the newest shade of neon. He has covered his splints with Star Trek® stickers. He invents a Star Trek personality for himself. He gets to write using a special multicolor pen grip. Maybe he has a laptop computer that allows him to share with the starship Enterprise's mainframe about what the class is learning each day. Using play and reestablishing a special role in a familiar situation are activities that can build self-esteem and peer acceptance of a child who is different but who wants to belong.

Case Scenario

Some occupational therapy practitioners work with children who are recovering from trauma or illnesses and who may need some follow-up care relative to their medical or postsurgical conditions. One group of children who may deal with issues of resocialization in the classroom are those who are recovering from burns. Burns may result from a variety of causes: playing with matches; house fires; accidents around hot water sources and kitchen activities; and crimes where fire, hot substances, or chemicals are used as the force of assault. Often, dolls are used to demonstrate the appearance of pressure garments the children will wear to control the scarring while they recover from the burn. Additionally, they may be shown pictures of burn scars and may have questions about whether the scars will ever go away, whether they will experience physical pain, and so forth. When the child returns to school, he or she may require assistance from school-based occupational therapy practitioners for range of motion and exercise activities to encourage mobility and redevelopment of coordination or dexterity. School-based practitioners also may be involved with compliance with pressure garments and other scar management devices or splints. Facial and hand burns can be particularly difficult for children. Peers may not like to look at them or to touch their hands as children always do in play. Conversely, they may be too curious to touch, but touch in the remodeling phase of a scar can be painful. Additionally, some games may involve too much risk relative to contact with graft sites and healed burn sites. The occupational therapy practitioner, being the most experienced service provider in the medical model, may need to work with physical education teachers, for example, relative to choice of appropriate activities or modifications to activities to allow the student to participate in gym class.

Case Scenario

Adults who have acute medical problems may be too ill to move around well and may become physically deconditioned. Fatigue is a major limiting factor related to activity tolerance. Many hospitals have formed fatigue committees that strategize about how to keep adult medical inpatients active, in an effort to overcome development of deconditioning that can result from inactivity associated with the fatigue. Some of the medical issues affecting middle-aged adults include heart disease, cancer, kidney disease, hematological conditions, impaired immunity (immune deficiency syndromes), and infectious disease (e.g., hepatitis, tuberculosis, malaria, severe bacterial or viral infections). Pacing activities and developing daily activity schedules and self-care routines can be beneficial approaches to configuring activity to avoid fatigue. Occupational therapy practitioners can be valuable team members on fatigue committees because they practice logical graded application of activity to enhance daily life.

When people are febrile (feverish), they may have decreased tolerance for activity. Occupational therapy practitioners can work with the person or caregivers to better arrange the environment and to provide education about energy conservation and work simplification. Additionally, coaching people to keep up their abilities by doing their daily self-care can be an issue. Fatigue is a side effect of many medical conditions. Fatigue is costly to remediate; prospective intervention to prevent long-term deconditioning resulting from activity avoidance caused by fatigue can save costs and support the need to decrease the length of inpatient hospital stay.

How Activities Are Therapeutic in the Long Term

Activities are a means by which people can be motivated to participate in their daily occupations, the process of living. To do activities, one interacts with other people (human environment) and other things (nonhuman environment). Within the context of occupational therapy, activities are the tools used to acquire skills, to complete tasks, to resume participation in meaningful occupations, and to fulfill life roles. The number of possible tools that can be used is as vast as the known universe and goes beyond that to the unknown areas of life we have yet to explore, create, or interact with.

In choosing activities to use in clinical practice settings, the occupational therapy practitioner must collaborate with the client and caregivers. Obtaining an occupational profile is the focal point of any occupational therapy evaluation. Who the person is, why he or she is seeking services, what circumstances have caused a change in his or her ability to do occupations, what his or her priorities are, and what his or her occupational history has been all give the practitioner a baseline for establishing context for the client. Through an appreciation of the person who will take part in the occupational therapy process, activity choices declare themselves as meaningful in context to each client's life, experiences, hopes, and dreams. The challenge for occupational therapy practitioners is to grow and continue to learn about activities while remaining mindful of the client's role in choosing activities to work toward their personal goals in the therapeutic process.

Through analysis of a client's occupational performance of each activity and synthesis of information from the occupational profile about how the activity can be performed in a context appropriate to the client's life, an occupational therapy practitioner can assist the client to acquire the skills he or she will need to live life to its fullest. Some activities are old and familiar and have great personal meaning privately or publicly. Others can be newly acquired and produce new meaning and life satisfaction as life roles shift and new occupations are explored. Being occupied is generally life satisfying and life supporting. The more personally valuable and meaningful the role that the person fulfills through his or her occupations and the activities that comprise them, the greater the value of the therapeutic intervention that enables living life to its fullest.

Summary

Activities are part of everyday life. As a rule, we all engage in activities we choose or must do to support our occupations. We take care of ourselves and our families and participate within groups of which we are members and within the populations in which we live. In real life, we only break down activities into component parts of related tasks when we develop or learn them as novices or when we teach them to others. Most of us never stop to think about how the things we do day in and day out frame the ways in which we spend our time. Although occupation is originally a 19th-century–early-20th-century concept, technological advances within our society will become more precious to us. Through occupation our lives become meaningful. We assume roles (socially accepted norms of behavioral patterns [Christiansen & Baum, 1997]) associated with and based on our occupations. Interaction with life and with people through the process of doing and sharing supports our feelings of connectedness to a whole. We do not need to feel isolated or inept. Regardless of functioning, disabilities, or health status, we can be enabled to do activities, to participate, and to make an impact on the process of life and living. ∎

Acknowledgment

I thank Jody Weitz Shoenhaupt, OTR/L, for sharing her story about Joe as a case scenario for this chapter.

References

American Occupational Therapy Association. (1999). Policy 5.9: No smoking. *American Journal of Occupational Therapy, 53,* 626.

American Occupational Therapy Association. (2002). Occupational therapy practice framework: Domain and process. *American Journal of Occupational Therapy, 56,* 609–639.

American Occupational Therapy Association. (2003). AOTA White Paper on complementary and alternative medicine. Adopted by the Board of Directors of the American Occupational Therapy Association, July 15, 2003, Board Motion BDM33-62203.

Benbow, M. (1995). *Kinesthetic fine motor activities* [video recording]. Albuquerque, NM: Clinician's View.

Christiansen, C. H., & Baum, C. (Eds.). (1997). *Occupational therapy: Enabling function and well-being*. Thorofare, NJ: Slack.

Dunn, S. C., Sleep, J., & Collett, D. (1995). Sensing and improving: An experimental study to evaluate the use of aromatherapy, massage and periods of rest in an intensive care unit. *Journal of Advanced Nursing, 21*, 34–40.

Feuerstein, M., Miller, V. L., Burrell, L. M., & Berger, R. (1998). Occupational upper extremity disorders in the workforce: Prevalence, healthcare expenditures, and patterns of work disability. *Journal of Environmental Medicine, 40*, 545–555.

Gortmaker, S. L., Peterson, K., Weicha, J., Sobol, A. M., Dixit, S., Fox, M. K., et al. (1999). Reducing obesity via a school-based interdisciplinary intervention among youth: Planet health. *Archives of Pediatric and Adolescent Medicine, 153*, 409–418.

Hunt, M. K., Fagan, P., Lederman, R., Stoddard, A., Frazier, L., Girod, K., & Sorensen, G. (2003). Feasibility of implementing intervention methods in an adolescent worksite tobacco control study. *Tobacco Control December, 12*, 40–45.

Mattingly, C., & Fleming, M. H. (1994). *Clinical reasoning: Forms of inquiry in a therapeutic practice*. Philadelphia: F. A. Davis.

Nassau, D. W. (1999). The effects of prework functional screening on lowering an employer's injury rate, medical costs, and lost work days. *Spine, 24*, 269–274.

Neistadt, M. E. (1994). The effect of different treatment activities on functional fine motor coordination in adults with brain injury. *American Journal of Occupational Therapy, 48*, 877–882.

Neistadt, M. E., & Crepeau, E. B. (1998). Introduction to occupational therapy. In M. E. Neistadt & E. B. Crepeau (Eds.), *Willard and Spackman's occupational therapy* (9th ed., pp. 5–12) Philadelphia: Lippincott, Williams & Wilkins.

Pierce, D. (2001). Untangling occupation and activity. *American Journal of Occupational Therapy, 55*, 138–146.

Trombly, C. A. (1993). Observations of improvements of reaching in subjects with left hemiparesis. *Journal of Neurology, Neurosurgery, and Psychiatry, 56*, 40–45.

Trombly, C. A. (1995). Occupation: Purposefulness and meaningfulness as therapeutic mechanisms, 1995 Eleanor Clarke Slagle Lecture. *American Journal of Occupational Therapy, 49*, 960–972.

U.S. Department of Health and Human Services. (2003). *Healthy people* 2010 Web page. Retrieved on November 31, 2003, from http://www.healthypeople.gov/About/goals.htm.

9

Designing Group Activities to Meet Individual and Group Goals

Mary Donohue, PhD, OT, FAOTA
Ellen Greer, PhD, OT, CPSYA

People by their nature function within groups from birth: within the family, at school, in religious centers, in sports, in clubs, and in volunteer or professional organizations. A group is a gathering of three or more people for a joint, face-to-face purpose over a continuous period. Group activities consist of tasks of work or play actions in which all members engage. The earliest group activities for infants and toddlers include family meals and family play. Later, children participate in family food preparation, travel, and cleaning as a group. Many occupations are carried out within groups. To engage successfully in many occupations, a person must have good social skills and be able to interact with others in a mutually rewarding manner.

The challenge to the occupational therapy practitioner in designing group activities is to target the needs of the individual and of the group. This chapter describes how the occupational therapy practitioner identifies individual and group needs, goals, and activities. We describe the dynamic nature of the person and groups as they interact around activities. We highlight therapeutic actions of the practitioners and adaptation of the group activities. Finally, we discuss the role of occupational therapy practitioners in assisting clients to use their developing social skills as they transition into community settings.

Activity Contexts in Occupational Therapy Groups

Occupational therapy practitioners' use of activities in groups is unique. We use activities within the group context to create therapeutic environments. When providing therapeutic activities, practitioners attend to five major components: (a) the activity, (b) the occupational therapy practitioner's therapeutic use of self as a leader, (c) the group members as participants, (d) the group's process or interactions, and (e) the group's culture and physical context. The combination of these components enables occupational therapy groups to offer a unique, reality-based treatment opportunity. The challenge to the occupational therapy practitioner in designing group activities is to target the needs of each client as well as the needs of the group as a whole. Occupational therapy practitioners use the dynamic nature of the person and the groups as they interact around activities.

The unique expertise of the occupational therapy practitioner is in designing and adapting each activity presented in the group so that it meets the therapeutic needs of each client and the group as a whole. For example, if the activity is a joint, all-group mural with everyone performing the same task side by side, the design or format can foster cooperative interaction across the whole group. If the joint activity is making brownies that involves shelling and grinding walnuts, measuring sugar, sifting flour, cracking eggs, greasing a pan, turning on an oven, pouring batter, and setting a timer, group members assume and can learn a variety of roles to work together as a team. The group interactions around the making of the food and the end-product can be an enjoyable experience for all members.

Occupational therapy practitioners also modify materials used during an activity to meet the therapeutic needs of the clients and the group goals. For example, if the mural is being drawn with permanent markers, the practitioner can deliberately distribute a minimum number of boxes of markers to foster sharing, thus further enhancing an atmosphere of group interaction. If group members and the practitioner discuss the brownie baking ahead of time, members can be asked what job they might like to do or might do the best, thus highlighting individual skills and contributions within the group environment. Likewise, if a discussion precedes the role-playing concerned with which members need to practice listening, which need to be assertive, or who needs to try other behaviors, the occupational therapy practitioner can modify the activity, materials, or the environment to ensure that the role-playing activity addresses these needs. By modifying activities or the methods of engaging in activities, therapeutic goals of individual members and groups as a whole can be worked on jointly.

People Participating in Purposeful Activities Within the Group Context

Social aspects of a group support a person's learning of new skills and behaviors. Learning within a group context allows people to support one another's learning styles and fosters a cooperative learning environment. Group leaders play an important role in helping group members to support and motivate one another. Role-modeling and the camaraderie developed from seeing others carry out and participate in the activity are important aspects of a group activity.

Characteristics and Contexts of Activities

Before selecting and planning group activities, occupational therapy practitioners take into account the group members' needs and goals, the activity's characteristics, and the context of the group. First, they consider each group member's individual and the whole group's needs and goals. Simultaneously, they consider specific characteristics of the activities to decide what activities would be appropriate to meet these needs and goals. Some characteristics of an activity are the length of time for completion; the degree of structure, creativity, and flexibility; the objectives of the activity; and the levels of cognitive ability, social interaction, and manual dexterity required to perform the activity. Last, practitioners consider the context of where the group meeting will take place. The context of the group includes the location of the activity's usual venue; its simulation in a center's setting; its time of day; its length of time for completion; and its emotional atmosphere of work, play, relaxation, study, and discussion. The environmental context may require physical movement, provide musical or other auditory stimulation, expose members to food or chemical aromas, engage them in psychosocial interaction, or challenge their cognitive abilities.

Exercise 9.1—Personal Groups

Think about the activity groups that you participate in daily. How do these groups meet your personal needs and goals? How do the activities vary based on social inter-

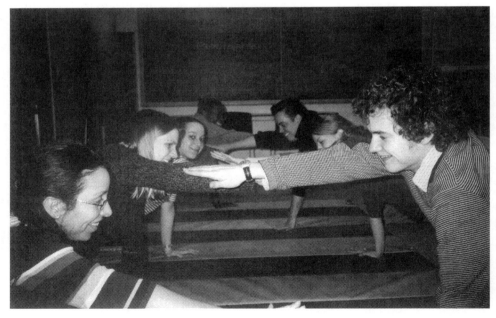

Figure 9.1. This physical activity encourages playful group interactions for young adults.

action, dexterity, and cognitive skills? How are these groups a core to your occupations and the activities you choose to participate in?

_____

Referral to an Activity Group

Activity groups are different from verbal groups and general community or unit groups because they require that a person be actively involved in a therapeutic activity. A person may become a participant in a therapeutic group in many ways. Some common methods are as follows: A person is assigned to a required group, a person requests to participate in a particular group, or a person is recommended to a specific group based on a staff member's evaluation of the person's needs or strengths. In occupational therapy activity groups, a significant aspect of the group is the ongoing discussion or processing of the interactions around the activity. Additionally, at the end of each activity group, the practitioner leads a discussion of group members' interactions and feelings.

Required Groups

In some instances in a hospital unit, as soon as clients are oriented enough to focus on an activity or to tolerate the presence of others in a group, the occupational therapist places them in a generic unit group for observation and evaluation. Clients who are not yet ready for a group may need individual intervention until they are ready to participate in an activity group. When clients are able to attend groups, the occupational therapy practitioner operates within the existing structure of the activity group program. This structure involves evaluating the needs, goals, abilities, and experiences of the members and treating them within the group as far as possible by adapting the activity to most of the group. Practitioners select activities and methods of involvement designed to suit or engage the clients attending that day. On some units, the activity group setting is in a room with cupboards containing general supplies for games and arts and crafts. In this type of setting, the practitioner can invite each client to select an activity of his or her choice for one of the sessions of the day.

When groups are provided in schools, children often are assigned to them on the basis of their skill levels or specific tasks that need to be done. In some instances, children may be required to attend special groups to address specific deficits. In clinics for adults with physical disabilities, clients may be assigned to a group designed to address specific deficits (e.g., cognitive skills group). In these groups, practitioners may offer groups that are designed for specific therapeutic needs, such as developing cooking skills, or treatment may be conducted in the same area with one specialized practitioner (i.e., all the clients with arthritis may be working at the same table). To maintain an interactive dynamic in these required groups, the practitioner needs to elicit the cooperation and motivation of the group participants by individualizing interventions and discussing the goals of the group with all present. A practitioner can increase group participants' involvement by including them in the selection of the activity and asking them for ideas for activities. In school settings, children can be asked about preferences for reading topics or types of games. Similar circumstances can be applied in required adult literacy groups or nursing home geriatric groups. Practitioners continually explore new activities to increase their repertoire. Often, meeting the needs of clients requires that practitioners provide a variety of activities that change daily.

The dynamic of interaction with the practitioner, the activity, and the group members is naturally influenced because clients are required to attend the groups. Activity selection in groups with required attendance may need to come initially from the practitioner. By the end of the group session for the day, the practitioner may ask the group members how they liked the activity and what other activities they would like to select for the rest of the week. Client participation is improved when practitioners offer the group members choices within the group so that the required attendance is not a burden.

Personal Referral

Some people choose to join certain groups for personal reasons related to their needs or goals. Others join groups for a variety of reasons, often with predetermined personal goals. They may select these activity groups from a list presented on a brochure or handout provided by the center or hospital. Within these kinds of groups, the participants may have a greater role in determining the activities and the focus of the group.

Personal contact through conversation and friendly interviews with prospective group members is one approach to evaluating membership for any type of activity group. The activity group leader should, through an interview with the prospective member, ascertain whether the group is appropriate given the client's specific needs and goals. Group membership criteria for self-selected groups must be clear so that potential members can understand them. Protocols and handouts explaining group goals, activities, and methods also need to be specific in criteria for group membership.

Professional Referral

School or team professionals also may refer a client to a group. These personal referrals can be made one on one with other professionals, or they can be made in a group team meeting through joint discussion of what the client has requested or appears to need in terms of a specific activity group designed to achieve some individual goal. When clients are currently unable to speak for themselves, as in some cases of depression, stroke, dementia, or autism, family members can sometimes provide information regarding what activities have been appealing to the client in the past that would relate to some group offered on the unit, at the school, or in the community center.

Professionals often refer clients to groups with expectations about what the group can offer. Specific criteria for group membership should be clearly stated in

protocols and handouts. When the group is an activity group, the referring professional should either speak to the occupational therapy group leader or fill out a referral form. A referral form indicates potential goals for the client and documents
important information about the client's unique case. In mental health settings where
attendance at groups is not required, a practitioner may need to use personal contact
through conversation and friendly interviews with prospective group members to
influence these clients to attend appropriate activity groups.

Referral to Activity Groups Based on a Specific Assessment

An occupational therapist may base referral to a particular group on the results of an
assessment. For example, the Allen Cognitive Level (Allen, Earhart, & Blue, 1992)
leather task assessment or Contextual Memory Test (Toglia, 1993) may assist in indi-
cating the cognitive group performance level needed for an individual client. Allen's
Routine Task Inventory (Allen et al., 1992) may point out the cluster of activities or
daily skills needing a specific group for independent-living-skills training. A lack of
balance in a person's time use results on the Barth Time Construction (Barth, 1978)
tool could indicate a need for a time management group. The Coping Skills Inventory (Zeitlin, Williamson, & Sczepanski, 1988) can assist in determining the individual social interaction abilities of preschool children. The Sensory Profile (Brown &
Dunn, 2002) may indicate needs within a group for balancing types of social participation styles, for example, in an assertiveness training group. The Group Profile
(Donohue, 2003) can assist in answering the following questions: At what level of
group performance is this person? At what level of group performance is this group as
a group? This scale, based on Parten's (1932) and Mosey's (1986) five levels of group
interaction, can assess whether the individual as well as the groups available are at a
(a) parallel, (b) project or associative, (c) egocentric cooperative, (d) cooperative, or
(e) mature level of group interaction skill.

Activity Goals in the Group

Before developing goals, occupational therapists evaluate clients through interviews
and performance of specific activities to ascertain functional abilities and skills. After
assessing the client's performance and determining probable needs, the client and
therapist together establish therapeutic goals. When establishing therapeutic goals
related to participation in an activity in a group, several goals may need to be developed. Therapeutic goals may address the client's goals to be worked on in a group,
general group goals, goals of the activity, goals set by the therapist, and goals of the
other group members. These goals are interrelated. Sometimes one takes priority over
another, depending on circumstances and the client's disabilities.

Group members and practitioners jointly select activities that provide clients
with opportunities to practice their activity goals within the group. The group members and the practitioner refer to a client's activity goals during the group to stimulate

participation. The practitioner routinely asks each group member as he or she enters the group, "What are your personal goals in the activities of this group?" This repetition is necessary so that the client states a commitment to the activity goals to the group as a public contract of intention. If the client's goals are unrealistic, the group members will respond by asking the client how he or she intends to achieve that goal. Other common practitioner questions are, What activities can you work on this week to accomplish your goals? What do you think would be the first activity to achieve your goal? In both questions, the practitioner is asking the client to set a more manageable, realistic, short-term goal. Through this process, the client continually refines goals by examining whether they are "doable" in the group through the activities available.

As a client enters the group and begins participating in the activities, the other group members and the practitioner can provide him or her with constructive feedback about the appropriateness of his or her goals. Problems in working on the activity or with group members may suggest other goals that are more essential. At this point, the client, the group members, and the practitioner may jointly "go back to the drawing board" to reexamine the goals of members and of the group. Previously unstated goals may now be stated. Group members may jointly agree on new goals that are important to individual clients in the group. What applies to one client also may surface as applicable to several others in the group. Often, these goals emerge from the difficulty that group members have participating in an activity. Recognition of these areas of difficulty leads to a new group goal.

When interacting with one another around an activity, group members reveal ineffective interpersonal styles that they may have used with family or friends. Likewise, some group members may expose dysfunctional, nonproductive activity achievement patterns when engaged in an activity. The occupational therapy practitioner points out to clients when they need new goals to deal with ineffectual social interaction or dysfunctional activity efforts. The artful practitioner also points out to the client how the new activity goals relate to previous goals.

——— ⊞ ———

Exercise 9.2—Group Feedback

Based on the occupations that you identified in Exercise 9.1, think about your participation in these groups. How did you enter the group? How does participation in the group provide you with feedback about yourself and your performance? How have you adjusted your personal goals based on feedback during participation in an activity?

———————

Cultural Context of Groups

Occupational therapy practitioners must respect and acknowledge their client's values and beliefs. Shaping self-awareness of one's culture, beliefs, assumptions, and biases regarding other cultures and lifestyles is an essential aspect in developing a therapeutic use of self, bringing about change in self and others. Increasing self-awareness provides practitioners with the knowledge and skills needed to work with people with varying backgrounds. Cultural competence provides insight that is necessary for an effective goal-setting process and a knowledge based on which a practitioner can select activities that meet the cultural needs of a group. When practitioners view their own culture from a multicultural model (Locke, 1992), they have a fuller appreciation and respect for the wide diversity of cultural experience and can relate this knowledge to activities for members in a group.

Case Scenario

Wanda, an occupational therapy assistant, accepted a position at a local long-term-care facility with a diverse population. During a supervisory session, she discussed with her supervisor how insensitive members of the group were to cultural differences. She observed members of one cultural group addressing ethnic slurs toward people of other cultures. She was upset that by not intervening she was perceived as condoning this behavior. She decided to implement a multicultural holiday group and to integrate new activities from different cultures. The group goal was for members to become sensitive to the cultures of others and to be able to describe and share their own culture with each other. Holiday songs, videos of ethnic dances, and storytelling were the activities designed to heighten self-awareness, challenge old beliefs, and bring about new knowledge of one another's cultures.

Culture is the result of socially acquired and transmitted patterns of behaviors. Culture is grounded in symbols, customs, beliefs, institutions, and objects (Locke, 1992). A person's culture specifies his or her activities, social relations, motivations, perceptions of the world, and perceptions of the self (Steward, 1972). These components are important to consider when determining which goals are appropriate for the client and when selecting activities. Some questions to consider are, How does the individual approach activity? How important are goals in life? How are roles defined? What is the achievement orientation of the culture? What is the predominant worldview? How is self defined? What kinds of people are valued and respected? All of these questions can be part of the open-ended interview.

When practitioners are aware of and responsive to the cultural background of group members, they can create activities that move the group toward defining its own group culture. Each client's cultural norms become incorporated into the collaboratively established norms of the new group. When clients begin to care about belonging to a group, they may set aside their cultural patterns in order to cooperate with the new group. Each client and the practitioner need to give up some cultural behavior in order to create new norms that will meet the needs of everyone in the group (e.g., experimenting with degrees of disclosure with cultural others, starting work tasks on time).

Client Group Activity Needs

Clients come to an activity group with their individual needs in mind. They may be thinking, "What is in this for me? How can I receive treatment along with others at the same time? Will I like the activities here? Will my needs fit into the group needs?" All of these questions are legitimate. Occupational therapy practitioners keep in mind that some people are not comfortable in groups. One way to create an environment where clients feel welcome is to ask them to share what activities they enjoy doing. The client may need guidance in suggesting appropriate activities for a particular group. For example, a group member in a prevocational group who says that he or she would like to be an attorney needs help with examining what preparatory steps are necessary to become an attorney (e.g., admission, education, examinations). A practitioner might suggest volunteering at a law office as a more appropriate goal. The group might discuss activities related to developing the skills needed to complete the filing, operate a copy machine, or do computer data entry. During these goal-setting discussions, a practitioner must be careful not to criticize the client's aspirations and demoralize the client. Setting realistic and achievable short-term goals related to the client's activity desires often assists in this process.

Exercise 9.3—Adolescents Set Goals in Individual Contracts

Adolescents find goal setting particularly difficult. Perhaps they find goal setting too abstract, or they cannot think in terms of the future, or goals are associated with adult wishes for them, or their peers jointly devalue goals in groups where attendance may be mandated. In any of these instances, writing a contract with the adolescent jointly with a team of professionals and the parents is helpful. This strategy may be essential to counteract the strong influence of the adolescent's general peer group. Working with a group of adolescents who have signed contracts to achieve certain activity goals strengthens the likelihood of their adopting the norms of their new group. Answer the following questions: What are the favorite group activities of adolescents? What are their typical activities? What unique activities do adolescents enjoy?

Activity Group Orientation

Before joining a group, each client needs to be informed about the purpose and goals of the group. This orientation to the goals of the group may be done verbally or with a brief handout. A written statement of goals of an activity group can provide details about the group's cognitive, motor, sensory, psychological, and social aims. A written handout, which has the advantages of visual impact, acts as a semicontract and provides an added value of being a permanent reminder of the group's therapeutic activity goals. When a client first joins a group, the group leader orients him or her to the group and explains the general goals of the group. General goals are each client's expected level of interaction within the group and the expected level of participation in the group activities. Joint group activity goals may not be obvious to group members, so they need to be clearly established as a new member enters the group.

In occupational therapy groups, the practitioner reminds the group of the activity goals. At each session, the practitioner states the daily goals of the group and relates them to the client's daily life. When the goals are abstract, such as in cognitive skills training, the practitioner connects the activities regarding improvement of memory to the particular daily skills of list-making to eventual greater independent living. In another example, a negotiation group devoted to assertiveness training, by its very nature, calls for an orientation to what assertive behavior is in contrast to aggressive or passive behavior so that all members understand the stated goal of the group.

The practitioner working in activity groups must balance the goals of the individual clients with the goals of the group. As each group member enters the activity group, the practitioner routinely asks, "What are your personal goals for the activities of this group?" In this way the practitioner connects the client's goals to the group's activity goals. After the group has completed each activity, the practitioner leads a follow-up discussion to review the group goals. During this discussion, the practitioner asks members to reflect and examine how they addressed their individual and group goals during the activity.

Goals of the Activity

Some goals are inherent in the context of the specific activity group. For example, the major group goal for an assertiveness training group is clear from its title. In another example, a prevocational work habits group may imply a focus on the goals of daily attendance, arriving on time, and keeping to a schedule. Or a group in activities of daily living social skills implies a goal of learning how and when to greet neighbors, friends, storekeepers, servers, doorpersons, bus drivers, and potential friends.

During participation in the activities, the practitioner reinforces each client's goals by encouraging his or her optimal performance of each task and completion of the activity itself. The practitioner facilitates positive behavior using therapeutic use of self and the group process. Should a client have difficulty joining the group's activity, the practitioner adapts the expectations of the group or the activity to ensure that the client can participate at his or her level of functioning. Sometimes, the client's reaction to the activity may be resistance, which can be resolved through exploration during the group processing discussion. At other times, the practitioner may determine that a particular group is not therapeutic for a client and may refer the client to a more appropriate group.

Case Scenario

A practitioner may observe within a group that one member needs to temper his aggressive style of interaction with others because he intrudes on other members' space by taking their materials. The practitioner can encourage other members who passively permit this person to take their supplies without objection to work on the goal of assertiveness with people who ignore their rights. By setting up an activity such as making a brochure or decoupage using shared magazines, the practitioner gives the members an opportunity to practice the goals they need to work on in this social interaction laboratory called an activity therapy group. In another session, the practitioner can plan to engage the group in an activity of role-playing appropriately assertive behavior by asking which individuals need to practice which roles. In a group that goes out on a trip weekly, the practitioner can foster a discussion in an advance meeting for members to speak up to negotiate for their choice of a destination for the trip that week. If a passive member complains to the practitioner that he or she wants to go to a certain place next week, he or she can be told to negotiate for his or her choice of community activity location (e.g., zoo, museum, pet shop) at the planning meeting the following week.

After the client enters an activity group and begins to indicate a need either to change behaviors or to practice another level of activity performance, group members and the practitioner adjust their goals or recommend that the client move to another group. These adjustments are a natural aspect of the dynamic nature of goal setting. Changes in goals accommodate the contextual factors and daily dynamic needs of the group. While they are engaged in activities, group members' performance and behaviors may reveal other necessary goals. At this point, the individual client and practitioner may jointly reexamine the priorities of all the goals.

Activity Group Levels of Participation

Part of the process of evaluating clients' and groups' participation behavior includes examination of the degree to which the client has the capacity to interact with others. If the group members have the ability to be present with others only in a parallel manner, that is, being engaged in a task or activity without social interactions (parallel level), they would only be able to share supplies minimally and communicate in a dyadic manner. Table 9.1 identifies group levels of functioning, interaction characteristics, and activity functioning.

In conjunction with identifying a group with the appropriate level of participation for clients, questions arise such as, "What approach can I take when group members wish to select unrealistic or inappropriate group levels or activity goals?" A wide range of groups exists for members at various stages of cognitive or psychosocial readiness. Some groups involve people with specific conditions (e.g., developmental disabilities, cerebral palsy, schizophrenia, depression) or specific disabilities (e.g., motor impairments, attention deficits, learning disabilities). Activities for all these groups are selected with attention to the client's needs and the group's goals. Both the client's and the group's goals can be achieved if the activity is relevant and well planned.

Table 9.1.
Group Levels, Interaction Characteristics, and Activity Functioning

Group Level	Interaction Characteristics	Activity Functioning
Parallel	• Does not interact with others • Tolerates the presence of others • Makes no spontaneous verbal interaction • Uses dyadic communication	• Minimal sharing of supplies
Associate	• Interacts with other participants for a short time • Seeks out others who like the same activity • Enjoys carrying out brief projects with one or two others	• Short-term activity or project • Activity emphasized over relating to others • Some sharing of materials
Egocentric Cooperative	• Cooperates with others in longer, ongoing activities • Tries a variety of roles for interaction with others • Begins to problem solve as a group	• Clear norms, guidelines, or rules to direct participation • Group choices • Respect for one another's rights
Cooperative	• Builds camaraderie with others by sharing feelings, thoughts, and mutual need satisfaction • Expresses caring for each other	• Emphasis on verbal and emotional interaction
Mature	• Takes turn leading • Assumes a variety of roles	• Balanced focus on activity and interpersonal interactions • Turn taking with sharing expertise across numerous activities • High-level end-product

When presenting activities, the practitioner must be constantly aware of the goals each client has for others in the group because these expectations can foster or impede achievement of activity in the group.

A common problem in working on a group goal is client resistance. Once the practitioner understands what the resistance to treatment is and believes that the client is in the appropriate-level group, the practitioner works on giving the unmotivated client an opportunity to address these issues during the group activities. When a practitioner exposes a client with resistance to other group members engaged in activities, the client will join in parallel to others engaged in the activity. At times, the practitioner may pair experienced with inexperienced group members to motivate participation and bring the client with resistance up to the expected level of participation. Frequently, the practitioner can engage a client in the activity by finding an aspect of the task that offers choice of an interest, ability, or preference to entice the client's participation. This choice satisfies the client's expertise through recognition of strengths or skills and gives support to the client needing encouragement to undertake an activity. In this way, the practitioner can assist the client individually by moving him or her from the known and attractive activity toward motivation for participation in the group.

Activity Group Process Modality

In occupational therapy groups, activities and group process are used together to meet the specific needs of clients. Activity group process is an effective therapeutic modality. Activities provide the means around which group process takes place.

Group activities are essential for learning social, play, and psychological interactions of a developmental nature. For example, the practitioner selects play activities because of their learning potential for the individual child as well as for the group of children. Presenting a variety of activities in a group for the children is essential to achieve the children's therapeutic goals and facilitate generalization. Children also learn social behaviors from the role-modeling of the group leader and other members. Aspects of the activity address each child's personal and social needs in varying degrees, as much as each child can make use of the activity. Play or leisure needs in a group also can be appealing to adults, whether within a game of bingo, dancing to music, or at a shared meal.

Most work settings employ persons in groups. People with and without disabilities need to be able to function in groups. Whether the groups involve people performing the same activities, such as working behind a fast food counter, participating in a computer office pool, stocking supermarket shelves, or recording and filing medical records in a large medical practice office, they need to know the social work skills appropriate to the setting, to the office policy, and to a particular supervisor. These skills include learning the group's social interaction tone of work information, exchange of banter, and the time acceptable to talk to others around the task without disturbing the demands of the work. Persons involved in rehabilitation need to learn or relearn these skills so as not to be a misfit by engaging in inappropriate greetings, interpreting remarks in a paranoid manner, or remaining silently aloof. Many clients who are referred to occupational therapy for activities of daily living or prevocational skill development need activity group process to assist them in developing their social skills.

Selecting Group Activities to Meet Goals

What are the preferred activities used as interventions in occupational therapy groups today? A survey of mental health practitioners conducted by the American Occupational Therapy Association's (AOTA's) Mental Health Special Interest Section indicated that the most regularly used activities in groups consisted of training in daily living skills, assertiveness, behavior management, coping skills, self-awareness, social skills, and time management (Bair, 1998). We can see that these activities are both realistically related to goals for people with psychosocial learning needs and simultaneously attractive because they provide an opportunity for growth in these areas. Many of these group activities fall into the category of psychoeducational activities and are described in current texts about activity groups in occupational therapy (Bruce & Borg, 2002; Cole, 1998; Early, 1993; Posthuma, 2002; Stein & Cutler, 2002).

Nine types of groups frequently offered by occupational therapy in the treatment of group members are exercise, cooking, tasks, activities of daily living, arts and crafts, self-expression, reality-oriented discussion, sensorimotor, and educational (Duncombe & Howe, 1985). These types of groups provide the beginning practitioner with examples of common group activities. With experience, practitioners develop groups that combine the element of enjoyable, appealing activities with what is needed according to the goals of the clients in the groups. As an approach to therapeutic intervention, some occupational therapy authors (e.g., Allen et al., 1992; King, 1974) have emphasized the need for activities that attract the group members and even distract them from the treatment aspects of their involvement.

Food-Related Group: Daily Living and Social Skills Training Activities

Over the years, food selection, food preparation, and food sharing have been time-honored activity favorites of many clients and practitioners. Many clients are eager to join in a food-related group. Purposeful goals of food selection include learning to make economical choices that also are easy to prepare. This demands the cognitive ability to know what is available, make price comparisons, and assess ease of preparation. Purposeful goals of food-sharing activities include the psychological readiness to cooperate with others and the social skills to relate to others during a meal, snack, or party.

The enjoyment of the food can be enhanced with music, decorations, and placemats made by the group members. Conversations while planning, preparing, and consuming the end-product can provide significant therapeutic opportunities. The cognitive aspects of food selection also can incorporate educational group sessions devoted to the activity goal of learning what type of diet is nourishing and appealing.

Senior groups who need to watch dietary restrictions have been inspired by an herb-growing, preserving, and cooking group.

Self-Esteem-Building Group: Self-Awareness Activities

Many versions of self-awareness activities exist, and all build esteem for members in a group, thus meeting a basic psychological goal of mutual respect for other group members. In some cultural groups, being "dissed," or put down by others, is a great concern. Many people have low self-esteem while in rehabilitation and feel discouraged and depressed because of their disability.

In one version of this activity, the occupational therapy practitioner requests that all group members write three positive characteristics about themselves, one on each of three index cards, without giving their names. By way of introduction, the practitioner encourages the group members to overcome tendencies to think modestly of themselves. The practitioner guides the group's members to think positively and to write down their traits that they believe are their strengths. The group leader then instructs the members to place their cards in a box. A member mixes the cards, and another pulls out one card at a time. The group member reads the trait aloud, and the practitioner says, "Who in this group do you think has this trait?" A good follow-up question is, "Why do you believe that this person has this trait?" Then the practitioner asks, "Who else has this trait in this group?" After they have identified several people with this trait, the group leader then asks, "Who originally wrote this trait about themselves?" If the group members had not previously identified that person as having this trait, the practitioner says, "Why do you think that you have this trait?" In this way, answering questions becomes a group activity.

This procedure continues for as long as there is time, ending with a discussion of positive traits and strengths in general, how people perceive themselves, how we can all think more positive thoughts about ourselves, how people felt about being identified as having a positive trait, and how this changed the climate of the group. Although the major "activity" of this group is discussion, it meets cognitive, social, and psychological activity goals for the group and for the individuals in the group and usually leaves the group with warm feelings of positive regard for each other.

Sensory Relaxation Group: Coping Skills Activities

Learning how to relax and relaxing in a group make up another favorite activity. Some group members need to be taught how to relax. Group instruction in meditation and following the breath and the movement of the lungs— the rhythmic regulation by the diaphragm in breathing—make up a revitalizing experience that the group members can ponder on and feel physically. In another relaxation activity, cognitive control of muscles through behavioral regulation of arm, leg, stomach, back, and facial muscles gives a sense of mastery over feelings of tension and anxiety. Carrying out these activities in a group is supportive of the activity and provides the practitioner an opportunity for coaching as the activity is under way.

Activities identifying scents and associating them with memories incorporates cognitive and sensory components. This activity can be achieved by first wrapping bottles or cans of spices, colognes, or perfumes in paper, then having group members explain what they associate with that scent. After most of the members have talked about their memories, they can then identify the scent. This group activity operating at the basic level of use of the sense of smell imbues the group members with an altered state of reminiscent relaxation.

Work-Related Group: Daily Living Skills Activities

Many group members are ready to take on the challenge of work-related activities and find these activities gratifying as they meet each member's esteem needs. Completing tasks in computer, clerical, wood, greenhouse, ceramics, food preparation, and other work skills builds habits of timeliness, attendance, and cooperation. Task groups enable their members to learn how to relate to a boss, how to relate to others around the task, and how to carry a project through to completion or to complete the assigned task or project. Vocational skill groups are popular because they permit the members to experience feelings of competence for a job situation.

Music-Based Group: Semisocial Activities

Listening to music is a frequent favorite. Occupational therapy practitioners can structure music listening in many ways. The practitioner provides the initial tapes or compact discs if the group is on an inpatient unit. In a day hospital or outpatient setting, group members can bring in their favorite tapes or compact discs, which provides the opportunity for further participation. When bringing in music is not feasible, a preliminary discussion about the types of music members like adds an aspect of negotiation and collaboration before the practitioner brings in tapes or compact discs.

Music combines group activities of listening, movement, and discussion. Art projects done to music are two-dimensional activities, combining two enjoyable spheres to enable the group members to be pleasantly enriched and distracted from serious concerns. Group members can share and describe feelings that arise during music listening. Thus, music can incorporate factors of social interaction through discussion and observing others enjoying the music, the psychological experience of relaxation and stimulation of moods, motoric expression of rhythmic movement, cognitive recognition of music development and performance, and the sensory activity of listening pleasure.

Physical Disability Activity Groups

For a number of years, treatment settings in physical medicine and rehabilitation have been using activity groups to treat people after stroke, head injury, or other physical injury (A. L. Lim, personal communication, April 1, 2003). Efficiency and economy of treatment for large numbers of clients have prompted life-oriented activity groups:

home, kitchen and food planning, daily living skills, and life skills. The groups may be modified for pediatric, adolescent, and geriatric clients.

Group Process and Participation in Purposeful Activities

During a group session where purposeful activities are used, the "doing" of activities may need to be adjusted, adapted, or changed. Perhaps the group needs a longer warm-up, a more detailed explanation of directions for the activity, or a step-by-step demonstration of the activity. Or, perhaps, only some people in the group need this extra attention. The practitioner is ready to be flexible in carrying out the activity if the abilities of the group or people demand it. It may be that the practitioner underestimated the length of time to complete the activity. The activity may then need to be continued a subsequent day.

Even more difficult is the need to slow down the pace of a group that wishes to rush through an activity rather than relish its performance. In this case, if group members have low attention spans or are unable to tolerate an activity, the practitioner may suggest to the group members how to elaborate on the activity to obtain full benefit from it. On the other hand, if an activity totally falls apart, if it rains on an outdoor ball game, or if the van for the outing is out of service, the practitioner role models the expression of some disappointment while providing ideas for an alternate plan for the day. If some unforeseen occurrence happens, such as an emergency, sudden illness, or death of a group member, the practitioner sets aside the planned activity and addresses the issue in a discussion appropriate to the level and interest of the group. The process within a group is discussed later, looking back on how the group dealt with the issue.

Practitioner's Role as Clients Participate in Group Activities

Occupational therapy practitioners plan their actions to ensure the best outcome for group members. Once the therapist verifies the group's and individual client's goals, he or she selects a frame of reference (i.e., model for practice, guideline for intervention, practice paradigm) to guide the activity selection. The frame of reference describes how the practitioner will present and use activity in the group. The approach also specifies how the practitioner will respond to clients and run the group. Common approaches or frames of reference that occupational therapy practitioners use when working with groups have been proposed in the literature (Borg & Bruce, 1997; Bruce & Borg, 1993; Cole, 1998; Howe & Schwartzberg, 1995; Kielhofner, 2002; Olson, 1999; Posthuma, 2002; Stein & Cutler, 2002).

Practitioner Expectations

An important aspect of an intervention approach or frame of reference is the guidelines on how the practitioner will respond to the client's behaviors. The practitioner is a critical person for creating a positive environment for change. Thus, practitioners need to examine their own behaviors and expectations of group members. The expectations of the beginning practitioner may be unrealistic for some group members. Practitioners' projections for the group members could range anywhere from optimism to bias related to the potential ability of group therapy to bring about change. Practitioners need to be aware that low expectations for group members could set up a barrier to progress in rehabilitation. Another caution is when the practitioner becomes too attached to "star" clients who are successful in using group activity therapy and then wishing that they would remain as group members. Unconsciously, a practitioner might inhibit the growth of the client and give nonproductive messages to the group.

A significant challenge for the occupational therapy practitioner is to balance his or her own expectations for the end-product of the activity with achieving the therapeutic goals for the group. Poorly produced arts and crafts, slipshod food preparation, or inattention to skills in games undermine the value of the activity. Practitioners who avoid intervention or omit discussion of the goals and meaning of the activities deprive the group members of the full therapeutic benefit of the activity. Both performance and the process of awareness of the group members' interaction with one another and with the nonhuman environment are rich sources of recovery and human growth potential. Both ought to be intertwined, not on a 50/50 basis every session, but over time, with some proportional balance of product and process. In attaining a balance between product and process in activity groups, the aspect of practicality also needs to be kept in mind. Perfectionism in the performance of the activity or the end-product is counterproductive to the group therapeutic process if the group member never completes a goal. The lesson is that the activity goals and the need for practicality serve as opportunities to address a member's tendency to be obsessive, a quality found in a number of people in need of therapy.

Nature of Interventions in Groups

As with all aspects of treatment in occupational therapy, assessing incremental or graded aspects of an intervention is essential. First, intervention should use the approach appropriate to the activity context. In general, if an activity is work oriented, the interventions or guidance should be of a business-like nature. For example, although some humor is always helpful in relaxing group members, too much humor in a prevocational group would be contraindicated, teaching behavior that might distract members from their tasks.

The occupational therapy practitioner frequently reminds the group members of the group goals and the goals inherent in the activity. For example, if the activity is a type of sport, dance, or movement, the practitioner reminds the group of the benefits of physical activity for building muscles, increasing lung capacity, and stimulating endorphins. During a movement activity, the practitioner reminds group participants of how the coordination of movement is achieving the goal of a more cohesive group through awareness of the parallel movement of others.

When a client's behavior is in conflict with his or her individual goals, the intensity of the intervention needs to be proportionate to the negative behavior and the therapeutic goals. When a practitioner has repeatedly reminded a client of the therapeutic goals, the group interventions may need to be adjusted in a graded manner (see Table 9.2). For example, if two members always pair up and never mix with other members in the group during activities, the practitioner may need to set a goal for and with the pair to interact more with others. If the pair sits together as the group assembles on a given day, the practitioner would initially ask the two to sit near others in a direct behavioral intervention. Then, if later during the activity the pair is seen spending long periods together, the practitioner can remind them that their goal is to build social skills with many people. Finally, in the discussion section of the group, if the pair offers to carry out the group's goal of preparing a meal the next day by volunteering to shop together, the practitioner again would remind them that one goal of the group is social interaction. This reinforces the pair's goal, linking it to the group's goal. Furthermore, the pair could be told that being together too frequently could weaken the group's cohesion and represent loss of an opportunity to try out new behaviors.

When interventions are not effective for a member, a contract may need to be developed that outlines the specific changes in behavior that the client must demonstrate. When a more serious, personal intervention for one group member needs to be made, the practitioner may talk to the client outside the group.

Processing in Activity Groups

Group process is always going on whether the group and practitioner choose to focus on it. The elements of group process include goals of the group and of the group members; attraction toward the activity and the group members; power assigned and assumed; roles of task organization, maintenance of the group, or individual resist-

Table 9.2.
Practitioners' Interventions in Activity Groups, in Graded Order of Use

- Ask a question about the behavior
- Use humor if appropriate
- Remind the member of his or her goal
- Give a direct instruction
- Raise observations of behavior in processing period
- Set up a contract with written goals
- Carry out all the above in a caring manner. Be yourself. Use your own style.

ance to the group; cooperation or climate of the group with respect to goals of the group and members; communication patterns of quality, quantity, and direction of speech; norms of the group's members individually and as a whole; and nature of the long-range and daily activities. Many books discuss the factors of process in groups (Borg & Bruce, 1997; Bruce & Borg, 2002; Cole, 1998; Corey & Corey, 2002; Howe & Schwartzberg, 1995; Kaplan, 1988; Posthuma, 2002; Riley, 2001; Ross, 1997; Stein & Cutler, 2002; Yalom, 1985).

Processing is the heart of the therapeutic nature of activity group process. Without processing, the group would be a social club, a team, or a class, but it would not be a therapeutic group. Good things may happen in these groups, but they do not represent focused therapy. Processing takes time and can be emotionally challenging and scary to some, but if carried out as described here and by other authors, it should result in the emergence of the curative growth process (Yalom, 1985). For occupational therapy practitioners, understanding the structure and key components of processing are fundamental to being able to lead a therapeutic group. It is the processes of the group's session that makes the practitioner a reflective practitioner engaged with the group in a meaningful activity. Practitioners need to be comfortable asking such questions as

- How do you feel about what happened today?

- How do you feel about the nature of the activity?

- How do you feel about the exchange of emotion?

- How do you feel about the time devoted to each part of the activity?

- How do you feel about the effort to achieve the goal?

- How do you feel about the cultural norms manifested?

They also can ask:

- Did you (we) achieve our goals through this activity?

- What emotions did you see in the group today?

- Can you tell the group why you wanted to leave?

Here, the occupational therapy practitioner's judgment is needed to evaluate what questions are most pertinent by first asking him- or herself the following questions:

- How much can the group absorb today?

- What are the group members ready to deal with?

- Do the group members need a gentle or direct push in a particular direction?

- How much time do we have?

- What should have first priority among the interactions or factors manifested today?

- What issue relates to the largest number of members or neediest subgroup?

- What was the strongest emotion manifested today?

In engaging group members in processing, the occupational therapy practitioner may expect some resistance, as was previously indicated. However, certain groups with limited cognitive skills, such as children or people with dementia, may need a modified expression at their level of vocabulary. Group members with limited emotional capacity, such as those with chronic schizophrenia, need examples on a basic level of what emotion is. Thus, the degree of processing that can be expected of any group member is influenced by his or her unique needs and abilities.

The best way for a practitioner to learn about group processing is by doing it and discussing the process in supervision. In supervision, the practitioner looks at the group process factors, the segments of processing, and his or her resistance and transferences as well as those of the group. Like any therapeutic skill, the more the practitioner does it, analyzes it, and works at it, the better he or she becomes at using it as a therapeutic tool. When a practitioner enjoys it, he or she then knows that he or she has learned it.

Collaboration

Collaboration is the process of people working together on an endeavor. In individual and activity group therapy, the collaborative process may be viewed through a therapeutic lens used to set therapy goals. Practitioners' expectations for collaborative goal setting take into consideration the client and group level of function. When the beginning relationship is fragile or ambivalent, establishing a therapeutic relationship will be most successful when the practitioner can foster a cooperative environment that is based on the needs of the individual or group. How does a cooperative goal-setting environment occur, and what tools must the practitioner use to establish it?

First, every practitioner must be aware of transference (Yalom, 1985). When an individual client or a group has a transference to the practitioner, feelings, reactions, and processes are experienced in relation to significant people in early life, and these emerge toward the practitioner (Bollas, 1987; Freud, 1912; Yalom, 1985). The importance here is that clients cannot always tell us about their past, but they can communicate their history through transference (Bollas, 1987; Yalom, 1985). How does the beginning practitioner know transference is occurring? Sometimes the practitioner becomes aware of a particular feeling, a pattern of interaction, or nonverbal communication coming from one client or the group.

Case Scenario

Celia, a practitioner in a geriatric setting, noticed that whenever she worked with Mr. Brown, who had a reputation for being taciturn and withdrawn, he seemed to respond to her like a loved one, with tenderness and warmth. There was no objective reason for his reaction to Celia because they were just getting to know each other. Celia learned during a group activity when residents were sharing their reminiscences that she resembled the woman he loved in his young adulthood.

In response to the client, the practitioner will have feelings and attitudes related to the client's transference, which is called a countertransference (Sandler, Dare, & Holder, 1995). In her collaborative goal-setting sessions, Celia was aware that she looked forward to working with Mr. Brown, even though her colleagues were all complaining about his behavior. This contrast indicated to Celia that her unique feelings were important in getting to know Mr. Brown. Her countertransference feelings were critical in establishing a collaborative therapeutic relationship. The positive transference–countertransference condition would ultimately empower Mr. Brown to work toward his therapeutic goal of developing interpersonal skills in a hobby exploration activity group at the nursing home.

When occupational therapy practitioners are aware of countertransference in relation to the individual or group, they have a rich source of data to assist them in facilitating the growth of those with whom they work while the client engages in purposeful activity. Staying close to one's intuition and countertransference feelings that emerge in the therapeutic collaboration assists in choosing the frames of reference that best serve the process of goal setting and creating contexts for the attainment of goals.

Case Scenario

Timmy, an energetic and impulsive 9-year-old, was having difficulty concentrating and focusing in the classroom. Mina, his school-based occupational therapist, was aware that Timmy wanted to please her, although he could not control his behavior when working with her. Using her intuition that Timmy needed structure, modeling, and positive reinforcement, Mina was aware of her countertransference of wanting to play with Timmy and just have fun together. Reflecting on this awareness with her supervisor, she chose frames of reference based on a sensory, interpersonal, and behavioral theory to develop a treatment plan to help Timmy gain mastery over his impulses that interfered with learning. Consistent with the frames of reference, Mina selected activities for Timmy that allowed him to discharge energy constructively, such as beanbag throws from a swing apparatus, trampoline jumping, and obstacle course play. Mina helped Timmy to select specific activities as part of the goal-setting process. As part of the plan, Mina and Timmy agreed that he would be rewarded with a star on his score sheet when he achieved a goal.

The successful implementation of a frame of reference relies on the occupational therapy practitioner's therapeutic use of self (Mosey, 1996; Posthuma, 2002; Yalom, 1985). Therapeutic use of self, finely tuned, enables practitioners to understand what the client or group wants and, ultimately, leads to the necessary questions that help the client and the group to identify personal and group goals. When Mina recognized that she wanted to "horse around" with Timmy, she was able to use this insight to redirect herself. Through the therapeutic use of self, Mina was able to ask Timmy questions about what kinds of activities were satisfying for him and what created a structured environment that was therapeutic, not recreational. When clients feel understood, they can tell the practitioner what they really need.

Beginning practitioners require ongoing supervision and a group of peers to discuss their own reactions and feelings toward what happens during group activities. This supervision and peer support facilitate the practitioner's development of skills that are essential to the therapeutic use of self. With increased experience and self-reflection, practitioners develop skills suited to meet the specific and unique needs of the clients. Mina, for example, was able to express in supervision how overwhelmed she felt when working with Timmy. She realized that she just wanted to throw rules out the window and play with him. She knew from her professional education that Timmy needed a structured environment to control his impulses. She also knew that she was an important aspect of the therapeutic environment. Mina and her supervisor explored the pros and cons of various frames of reference, and through dialogue, they collaborated and arrived at a plan to use a frame of reference based on behavioral theories. Even the master clinician, who is very comfortable working in multiple frames of reference, uses collaborative supervision to sort out the web of feelings that are used constructively in complex therapeutic interactions.

Transference and Resistance

Transference and resistance emerge and are used in the dyad or activity group. Resistance "embraces all of the forces that prevent the patient from functioning...in an emotionally mature way. It is the main form of communication of the patient's conflicts, life history, and character structure" (Rosenthal, 1985, p. 167). Often, beginning practitioners have personal beliefs and assumptions that underpin a philosophy of practice that aims to empower clients to find meaning in engaging in occupations. When collaborating in a new therapeutic relationship, both the practitioner and the client bring their own unique character and patterns of response to the therapy process.

Case Scenario

Drew, a recently graduated occupational therapist, wants to empower his new client, John, to identify independent therapy goals in preparation for entering a problem-solving group at a day hospital. In the first goal-setting session with Drew, John could not put into words what he wanted or needed in group treatment. John's history suggested that he allows others to think and make decisions for him about his activities. Drew found himself becoming irritated by John's passivity. Drew realized that he was creating goals and leading John to think from his perspective. In supervision, Drew discussed the pattern that was emerging, which was John's resistance to think and transference to get Drew to think for him. Drew reflected on John's and his own behavior in the problem-solving group. John passively sat in group while Drew continually cued him to become involved in the time management activity. This interaction seemed to increase John's resistance to verbalize his ideas during the group session.

————————

In such interactions, the client or group is doing the best they can. The practitioner's actions are not therapeutic because they enact a conflict with the client within the group (Yalom, 1985). The new practitioner can be assisted in this situation by always asking, "What is going on here?" Drew's reflection on the situation in supervision made conscious the unconscious through disclosure of underlying assumptions, thoughts, and feelings, paving the way for newly gained critical knowing (Irwin, 1995). Thus, Drew was able to adjust his behavior to empower John in increments, grounded in John's capacity to participate in making decisions.

When a stalemate in goal setting or inadequate participation in the therapeutic process occurs, the practitioner also must ask, "What kind of resistance is operating in the client, the group, and the practitioner?" Resistance, found in all professional relationships, is embraced by the practitioner and should never be viewed as something bad or wrong (Laquercia, 1990; Sandler et al., 1995). In supervision, when Drew recognized John's resistance, he could accept his negative feelings about being a bad practitioner who cannot help his clients. Instead of continuing to intrude on John during the problem-solving group, Drew embraced John's resistance by not making any contact with him unless John asked. Eventually, John got tired of his own passivity and being ignored by the group and the leader. He slowly began to interact with others. When Drew believed that John was ready to say what was on his mind, he adapted the group to incorporate role-plays of vignettes that required time management strategies for success in daily life activities (occupations). Drew's understanding of the transference, awareness of his own negative reactions, embracing of the resistance instead of opposing it, patience, and adaptation of the activity to meet the needs of John and the group were all important aspects of creating a therapeutic environment for John and the group.

Treatment of Destructive Resistance

Sometimes clients or groups fear the success that goal setting brings and find ways to destroy the effects or purposes of therapy. Such attempts are called treatment destructive resistances (Spotnitz, 1985). They happen in subtle ways. A client may not show up for the goal-setting session, come late, want to leave early, or refuse to consider constructive goals. Another client may drop out of a group, sabotaging the cohesiveness of the group; come late or monopolize the group; or behave in a manner that drives others out of the group.

The practitioner's reactions to these destructive resistance behaviors may form a counterresistance. When feeling discouraged by these behaviors, the practitioner may collude with the client or group by canceling a group or individual session, coming late, forgetting to bring supplies for the activity, daydreaming instead of listening to clients, talking too much, responding without empathy, or attacking the client or other group members. All of these subtle behaviors can occur and work against the collaborative process. Working collaboratively does not mean it will always be a pleasant experience. Sometimes, both practitioner and client may be stressed by the client's illness, disability, or emotional barriers to performance. In such cases, the practitioner chooses appropriate therapeutic activities. Some activities like drama games, journaling, and letter writing may allow clients to recognize their feelings. Other activities like role-play provide opportunities for clients to express emotions and deal with the many aspects and pressures of their personal situations (Dayton, 1994). Throughout this process, it is critical that the practitioner engages in a process of self-examination and reflection during supervision.

Practitioners often have opportunities to work with family members, caregivers, or significant others. Sometimes family members are appreciative of the practitioner's attention and are eager to engage in goal setting. At other times, family members, caregivers, or significant others may be stressed and expect the practitioner to do all the work. In some cases, the family members, caregivers, or significant others also may want to be taken care of by the practitioner. Thus, the practitioner may have to cope with the multiple transferences of these individuals. Likewise, the practitioner needs to examine his or her own countertransferences.

Case Scenario

The mother of twins with developmental disabilities is coordinating therapy services, carrying out necessary interventions, working, and doing all the other tasks of a new mother. With one child on a ventilator, her family life is dominated by medical procedures. As part of the intervention plan, the mother has been asked to join a group for mothers with young children with disabilities. Although she attends regularly, the team is concerned with her apparent level of stress and underlying depression.

A mother in this circumstance may feel desperate about her children with all their needs. She may want the practitioner to do something about it and to teach her what she needs to do. Her concern may be focused on her children's needs and not her own. Under this stress, the mother may become demanding. During the groups, the practitioner may be overcome by the powerful feelings of hopelessness in the family and wish to withdraw from the case. Practitioners must identify these personal feelings and explore with group members realistic and achievable goals and objectives. Activities that address natural events in the home often are most therapeutic and meaningful for these clients. Family members, caregivers, and significant others can engage in and plan for events in the home, such as cooking and eating meals together, going shopping, or attending medical visits. During all these activities, practitioners must attend to transferences and their own countertransferences.

Collaboration With the Team

Team members and the ways that they function vary depending on the service delivery model and the location of the intervention. Occupational therapy practitioners who work in home care may have little contact with a structured team, whereas in a hospital, school, or long-term-care setting, a practitioner may be a member of a structured team with specific functions to perform. In all cases, each team member brings to the conversation a particular perspective. Whether the occupational therapy practitioner is working with the team over the phone or in a conference room, the same principles of transference, countertransference, and resistance are operating. Practitioners meet the best interests of the clients and groups when a team functions in a mature, cooperative manner. Open communication among team members develops out of a willingness of each member to clarify feelings. When team members' interactions are oppositional, hopeless, or competitive, they should spend time dealing with these issues. Teams that work cooperatively are important vehicles to creating interventions that move the therapy forward for the clients.

Dynamics of Implementing Goals in the Group Process: Resistances

As an activity group forms, individual members initially look toward the practitioner rather than one another for interaction. Progressive engagement among group members is a process that the occupational therapy practitioner facilitates by the activity selected to achieve the group goals. Group interaction among members is desired in order to teach members how to help one another meet their individual goals, instead of relying on the practitioner.

Case Scenario

One activity group had a group goal of increasing empathy in social interaction between members. This group decided to use role-playing techniques to explore the range of possible responses. Each member had an individual goal that represented working through a particular obstacle in responding to others with empathy. One group member, who always felt shut out, wanted to know how it felt to be in the others' predicaments. Another, who frequently cried, wanted to have more control over showing strong emotion.

These obstacles to achieving a client's individual goals are considered resistances to function in a particular way.

When the group presents a shared obstacle to achieving the group goal, group resistance is in effect (Rosenthal, 1985). In this case, if the group began to giggle when a member presented a difficulty in achieving some aspect of performance, the group would be resisting having difficult feelings in relation to the member's presentation. If all group members arrived late to each session, investigation of this resistance would likely reveal avoidance of negative feelings that could not be expressed in the group.

Resistances are barriers to cooperative function that do not get expressed in words by the individual or group.

Monopolizing

Sometimes resistances are not dealt with, and the integrity of the group is affected. Monopolizing is a destructive resistance found in groups because it denies others their treatment time (Rosenthal, 1994). When left unresolved, this resistance can have a deleterious effect on the group.

Case Scenario

In a high-functioning music group at a senior center with a goal to achieve emotional wellness, a group member named Sam needed to be the favorite of Marcy, the occupational therapy leader. To gain Marcy's attention, he would come early to speak with her, struggle with technique problems that would require her lengthy attention during the music activity, and talk to the group during any opportunity about his knowledge of composers. This group member's insistence on monopolizing the leader and the group created tension and disharmony among the members, which was communicated by facial expressions. Marcy was uncomfortable with her own feelings and the disinterest she was beginning to experience from the group. Ultimately, the group resistance, in this case, unexpressed hostility toward a monopolizing group member, was enacted. The rest of the group began ignoring Sam and lost interest in the project, and Marcy withdrew emotionally.

Marcy's counterresistance was acted on in a way that demonstrated that she was not comfortable with using her own feelings to help the group work cooperatively within the context of the activity. She did not realize that she was angry with the group, and working in a community setting as a consultant occupational therapy practitioner, she had no supervisor with whom to discuss the dynamics of her group. Unwittingly, she felt pressured to try a new musical activity that would curtail Sam's monopolizing. Marcy selected two other group members for a duet, leaving out Sam. Although the two members selected were delighted, Sam experienced a feeling of rejection and dropped out of the group without any notice. With his exit, the rest of the group felt abandoned and, at the same time, guilty for regaining their opportunity to interact freely. They no longer wanted to work together, and the group soon fell apart. How would you have intervened in this circumstance?

The individual and group resistances that occurred in this activity group were wonderful opportunities to explore the emotions that interfered with cooperative group function. When practitioners understand their own reactions in response to group members, they can intervene with appropriate activities that will free people to express their thoughts and feelings in a way that will be maturational for themselves and the group. In this case, Marcy could have considered including some psychodrama activities, such as sculpting. Sculpting is a living picture of a family or group in which the main character and other role players are used (Dayton, 1994). This type of activity may have helped the group to learn about their own past roles in the family and in the present when confronted with a monopolizer.

Rivalry

Another powerful group resistance is rivalry (Rosenthal, 1985). Rivalry in groups can reject new group members. Once a group has become cohesive and is working well on individual and group goals, a sense of boundary and bonding has developed. The practitioner, however, keeps the group alive with enough members. If members drop out because of illness, moving away, or anger, the practitioner must bring in new members (Yalom, 1985). The entrance of a new group member can raise a multitude of feelings in the group, with a desire to eject him or her as soon as possible. The group's behavior to "get rid of the new baby" can be identified as resistance when the group excludes the new member, tells the group member horrible stories about group members who have since left, attacks the new member, or demands that the new member reveal personal details in the first two meetings. Very often, the group is really angry at the practitioner for bringing in a new member and displaces the anger onto the new member rather than risk jeopardizing the relationship with the practitioner. The intensity of this reaction may be tempered by adequate preparation of the group for the new member's entrance.

Group members learn that the practitioner and each client can handle thoughts and feelings. When this situation is handled properly by embracing the resistances of the group members, the group, depending on its level of understanding, will talk in some way about fears of loss and desire for dominance in the face of a new member. For many group members, conflicts they experienced within their early family life will be remembered. With the occupational therapy practitioner's help, they can be empowered to appreciate this history and how it interferes with their own effectiveness in achieving their personal goals. A practitioner should carefully select an activity that highlights the group members' reactions to changes in the group. A historical time line activity can provide the opportunity for the group members to identify patterns of responses and adaptations to changes. A mural art project using collage (e.g., pattern, torn paper, cut paper, texture, paint) can offer group members an opportunity for an emotional, sensory, and symbolic representation of their experiences, with time for processing this aspect of their experience (Silberstein-Sorfer & Jones, 1982; Thomson, 1997).

Sabotage

Sabotage—uncooperative behavior—is another form of resistance that interferes with goal achievement if it is not understood. Sabotage of the treatment goals can occur when an individual or the group believes that there needs to be a change and cannot find or is unable to communicate this need in an appropriate way. When the purpose of the sabotage is brought to attention, the practitioner has the opportunity to evaluate, in collaboration with clients, what goals need to be changed.

Case Scenario

In working with school-age children in a private office, occupational therapy practitioners have the opportunity to set the time, frequency, and fee and to collaborate with the child and family on goal setting. In one case, a mother unwittingly sabotaged the occupational therapy of her son, Lance, by getting him to the sessions more than 20 minutes late each time. This tardiness placed Tina, the occupational therapist, in a difficult position because Lance, who was working on increasing social competency skills, was upset that he was arriving late and was afraid to let his mother know that he wanted to be at the sessions on time. With Lance's permission, Tina invited his mother and twin sister into the sessions. Over the course of several sessions, the family worked together on group art projects, such as making masks and tissue-paper collage lunch boxes, with a group goal to have fun together and verbalize individual needs. Lance confidently began to tell his mother that he wanted to be on time and found it stressful to be late. As his mother listened, she explained that she was stressed and tired. Tired and feeling overwhelmed, it was hard for her to leave early in the morning for the therapy sessions. She herself needed new activities to balance the long hours of working in an office. By selecting a family events calendar, Tina was able to engage the mother and Lance in a discussion of what they could do together to resolve both of their issues.

Had the mother of this child behaved compliantly by getting to the sessions on time, the practitioner would not have explored a hidden problem that was affecting the whole family. Tina needed to address the resistance in a way that empowered Lance with his newly achieved assertiveness, which also helped Lance's mother. Activity group process is an excellent medium for developing new skills, new ways of relating, and empowering a sense of self. When occupational therapy practitioners conduct the activity group in a safe environment with low stimulation, meaning that the practitioner allows the process to unfold and responds to the communications of the members, they establish an optimum setting for goal achievement.

Transferring and Application of Goals to the Community

Occupational therapy clients eventually are ready to leave individual therapy or the activity group. Sometimes, clients leave the treatment setting prematurely because of external circumstances, curtailment of insurance coverage, or closing of a program. Discharge from occupational therapy, whether an agreed-on or a premature termination, means that clients must transfer what they have learned to a new setting or a familiar setting in the community. These settings could be classrooms, job sites, homes, recreational centers, or institutions (e.g., long-term-care facilities, prisons). These settings could be in a different state, county, or country.

Activity-Goal Partners Peer Collaboration

In peer collaboration—pairing one client with another—clients can support each other as they transition back to the community. With a link to a resource support person from a group, the client has the help of a peer who can troubleshoot or serve as a consultant in difficult situations. Peer support gives clients someone to whom they can relate regularly as they adjust to demands of their postdischarge communities. The relationships that often are established support group members for many years as they face new obstacles and challenges to the goals they set for themselves. This structure is used in many self-help groups.

Case Scenario

Female adolescents hospitalized for depression were members in an activity group to promote assertiveness in school, work, family, and friendships. Each member had been working on individual goals, such as speaking up and taking the appropriate share of time in the group, becoming aware of others' needs and offering assistance, controlling urges to withdraw, and resolving to engage in tasks. The group goal was to become cooperative, where members get one's own needs met while helping others get their needs met. Over time, the group became cohesive, with members supporting each other. When it was time for discharge, the group members were presented with the task of how they could support each other once

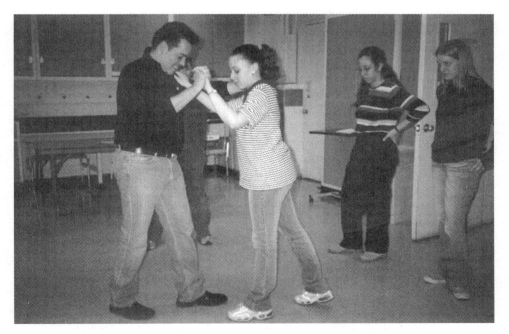

Figure 9.2. Dancing provides an excellent activity for interacting with members of the opposite sex.

back in the community. The members wanted to maintain connections with one another and spent several sessions planning for a support network. Their final plan included pairing members (activity-goal partners) with each other around activities that would occur in their communities. Each pair of activity-goal partners had someone with whom to talk, go to a movie, or have dinner or coffee.

Group-Linking Collaboration

Another method of easing the transition from an institutional group to a community setting is to establish a connection with the support systems within the community. In these situations, occupational therapy practitioners must know about available resources in the community. Additionally, they also must establish relationships with practitioners and other service providers within communities. When group linking, practitioners work with the clients to prepare them for the postdischarge services. During the transition, occupational therapy practitioners serve as consultants to the new group in the community, becoming an important link in the client's rehabilitation.

Case Scenario

Mr. Allen, an elderly gentleman residing in a health care facility, was recovering from a mild stroke that left him with some weakness on the dominant side of his body. He was referred to an activity group in occupational therapy to enhance functional skills. After 3 months, Mr. Allen had learned to doff and don a shirt, tie his shoes, and care for all his grooming activities. He was uncertain about cooking and cleaning his apartment and worried about being isolated in the community without any friends. Recently, many of his friends had died. In planning for his discharge, the occupational therapy practitioner and Mr. Allen visited his new residence in the community. As the practitioner assessed the new living quarters, Mr. Allen expressed a need for a support network of activities in the community. The practitioner knew of several senior day programs that offered activity groups. With Mr. Allen's permission, she worked with the team to refer him to an activity group at a program for seniors in the new neighborhood. On discharge, she met with the occupational therapy practitioner at the new setting. Mr. Allen and both practitioners talked about the carryover of his goals to the new group. Although the new practitioner would make her own evaluation, Mr. Allen had the support during this very important transition to a new group in the community.

Ethics in the Goal-Setting Process

The *Occupational Therapy Code of Ethics* guides ethical behaviors that assist practitioners when dealing with the complexities that emerge when collaborating with clients and activity groups in the goal-setting process (AOTA, 2000). Embedded in all phases of the collaborative relationship are issues of beneficence, confidentiality, autonomy, competence, justice, and veracity (Bailey & Schwartzberg, 2003; Hansen, 2000). The interplay between ethical behavior and difficult feelings that erupt in practitioners, clients, and groups during the goal-setting process requires that practitioners take professional responsibility for the therapeutic relationship and obtain supervision as needed (New York State Board for Occupational Therapy, 1998).

Supervision: Competence, Confidentiality, and Feelings

Beginning practitioners, practitioners who are returning to the profession, and experienced practitioners who decide to work with a new population all benefit from a supervisory relationship. All practitioners must be competent in the areas in which they practice. Although a practitioner who is a beginner or working in a new area may have some insecure feelings, competence will develop over time with experience. Ongoing supervision is an essential means of assuring that practitioners meet the ethical demands of a therapeutic relationship. Supervision ensures that competence of practitioners coincides with the progress of the therapy.

Case Scenario

Jane, an occupational therapy practitioner, had been leading an activity group for geriatric residents in a long-term-care facility for several months. As a new practitioner, Jane had weekly supervision to discuss issues and interactions that came up in her group. During supervision, she discussed that she observed patterns of silence emerge in the group when a member, Mrs. Smith, disappeared from the group because of a serious illness. To complicate matters, Jane had information about Mrs. Smith's cardiac problems that Mrs. Smith had shared before her hospitalization. Mrs. Smith did not want anyone to know the nature of her illness and had asked Jane to keep it confidential. Jane realized that without Mrs. Smith, several group members were fragile and had difficulty tolerating painful feelings, and she did not bring up Mrs. Smith. Several weeks later, a group member mentioned that Mrs. Smith had been hospitalized and asked Jane, "What is wrong with Mrs. Smith? Tell us why she had to go to the hospital." Jane faced an ethical dilemma. She had two concerns. First, she was ethically bound to honor the confidence of Mrs. Smith.

During supervision, Jane discussed the fact that some group members had unexpressed feelings and fears about Mrs. Smith leaving the group. She also observed that the group members never dealt with missing Mrs. Smith as a group member. Jane and her supervisor questioned whether it would it be better for the members to help one another to talk about illness, death, and dying or whether it would do harm. Although Jane realized that the group resistance needed to be respected, she also became aware that she, as a therapist, had to assist clients in dealing with these issues. Faced with this conflict and not wanting to do any harm, Jane, with the guidance of her supervisor, began the next session of the group by asking members about information they already had about Mrs. Smith. After two sessions, the group members began to explore their own feelings about loss, they talked about themselves, experiences they had in the hospital, and fears about death. During these sessions, Jane introduced a range of activities, such as designing get-well cards, listening to music, reminiscing and sharing stories, sharing photographs of family traditions, and making a welcome-back collage to encourage Mrs. Smith to return to the group.

Through supervision and guided by the principles to do no harm and to honor Mrs. Smith's right to confidentiality, Jane acted competently by paying attention to her own feelings. Supervision gave her support while she struggled through the ethical dilemma of how to maintain Mrs. Smith's confidentiality. Further, Jane succeeded in her role as an occupational therapist in this situation by choosing activities that were meaningful and life giving to her activity group.

Practitioners must honor the privacy and confidentiality of clients and activity groups. When clients and groups consider what they want to achieve, they may talk about sensitive issues and be empowered to make appropriate choices. Clients need to know that the practitioners are concerned for their well-being and will respect their right of confidentiality. Practitioners must not give in to the pressures of family members who want personal information regarding their child, spouse, partner, or friend who is in therapy.

When working with clients who have a history of acting out violently or sexually, practitioners need to acknowledge their fears to decide whether they can work

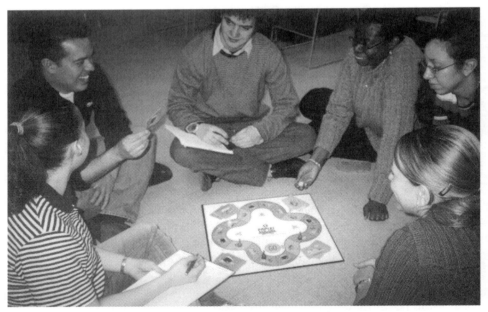

Figure 9.3. Games are important for learning socially appropriate strategies for interacting with others.

with a particular client. Should a practitioner not feel physically safe with a client, the practitioner has the right to request that someone else work with the client. If this is not possible, practitioners should structure the therapy group situation so that they neutralize any potential for aggressive or sexual acting-out behavior. Careful examination of a practitioner's reactions to difficult clients can prevent catastrophic incidents. Difficult clients can induce aggressive and sexual impulses in practitioners, causing them to act impulsively or unethically toward others. Here again, supervision offers practitioners opportunities to reflect on and analyze their areas of difficulty and to create alternative strategies for dealing with these issues. For example, a practitioner who fears a violent client with psychosis on a closed psychiatric unit in a state hospital could be guided to work in a space with low stimulation and with an aide always present. Feelings remain the practitioner's personal source of information needed to understand the dynamics in a therapeutic situation. Reflection and supervision provide the means that practitioners use to reconstruct these feelings to help clients or activity groups meet their goals.

Summary

Activity group work can be stimulating, revealing, gratifying, turbulent, and curative. Just as with any other therapeutic intervention, it can be challenging because it demands our intellectual and social cognitive skill as well as our emotional use of self. It is a complex modality, adding the dimension of activities to group structure and interaction. We hope that readers came to enjoy using activities in groups therapeutically, observing participants' growth as they and you support their rehabilitative efforts. ∎

References

Allen, C. K., Earhart, C. A., & Blue, T. (1992). *Occupational therapy treatment goals for the physically and cognitively disabled.* Rockville, MD: American Occupational Therapy Association.

American Occupational Therapy Association. (2000). Occupational therapy code of ethics (2000). *American Journal of Occupational Therapy, 54,* 614–616.

Bailey, D. M., & Schwartzberg, S. L. (Eds.). (2003). *Ethical and legal dilemmas in occupational therapy* (2nd ed.). Philadelphia: F. A. Davis.

Bair, J. (1998, December). Response to *American Journal of Psychiatry* article. *OT Week, 3,* 10–11.

Barth, T. (1978). *Barth Time Construction.* New York: Health-Related Consulting Services.

Bollas, C. (1987). *The shadow of the object: Psychoanalysis of the unthought known.* New York: Columbia University Press.

Borg, B., & Bruce, M. A. (1997). *Occupational therapy stories: Psychosocial interaction in practice.* Thorofare, NJ: Slack.

Brown, C., & Dunn, W. (2002). *Adolescent/Adult Sensory Profile.* San Antonio, TX: Psychological Corporation.

Bruce, M., & Borg, B. (1993). *Psychosocial occupational therapy: Frames of reference for intervention* (2nd ed.). Thorofare, NJ: Slack.

Bruce, M., & Borg, B. (2002). *Psychosocial frames of reference: Core for occupation-based practice* (3rd ed.). Thorofare, NJ: Slack.

Cole, M. (1998). *Group dynamics in occupational therapy: The theoretical basis and practice application of group treatment* (2nd ed.). Thorofare, NJ: Slack.

Corey, M. S., & Corey, G. (2002). *Groups: Process and practice* (6th ed.). Pacific Grove, CA: Brooks/Cole-Thomson Learning.

Dayton, T. (1994). *The drama within: Psychodrama and experiential therapy.* Deerfield Beach, FL: Health Communications.

Donohue, M. V. (2003). Group profile studies with children's groups: Validity measurements and item analysis. *Occupational Therapy in Mental Health, 19*(1), 1–23.

Duncombe, L. W., & Howe, M. C. (1985). Group work in occupational therapy: A survey of practice. *American Journal of Occupational Therapy, 39,* 163–170.

Early, M. B. (1993). *Mental health concepts and techniques for the occupational therapy assistant* (2nd ed.). New York: Raven.

Freud, S. (1912). The dynamics of the transference. *Standard Edition, 12,* 97–108.

Hansen, R. A. (2000). Guidelines to the *Occupational Therapy Code of Ethics* (2000). In P. Kyler (Ed.), *Reference guide to the Occupational Therapy Code of Ethics* (pp. 14–18). Bethesda, MD: American Occupational Therapy Association.

Howe, M. C., & Schwartzberg, S. L. (1995). *A functional approach to group work in occupational therapy* (2nd ed.). Philadelphia: Lippincott.

Irwin, R. L. (1995). *A circle of empowerment: Women, education and leadership.* Albany: University of New York.

Kaplan, K. L. (1988). *Directive group therapy: Innovative mental health treatment.* Thorofare, NJ: Slack.

Kielhofner, G. (2002). *A model of human occupation: Theory and application* (3rd ed.). Baltimore: Lippincott, Williams & Wilkins.

King, L. J. (1974). A sensory integrative approach to schizophrenia. *American Journal of Occupational Therapy, 28,* 529–536.

Laquercia, T. (1990). Family involvement in the treatment of psychosis. *Modern Psychoanalysis, 7,* 7–28.

Locke, D. C. (1992). *Increasing multicultural understanding: A comprehensive model.* Newbury Park, CA: Sage.

Mosey, A. C. (1986). *Psychosocial components of occupational therapy.* New York: Raven.

Mosey, A. C. (1996). *Applied scientific inquiry in the health professions: An epistemological orientation* (2nd ed.). Bethesda, MD: American Occupational Therapy Association.

New York State Board for Occupational Therapy. (1998, August). Guidelines for supervision. *News From the Office of the State Board for Occupational Therapy,* 1–2.

Olson, L. J. (1999). Psychosocial frame of reference. In P. Kramer & J. Hinojosa (Eds.), *Frames of reference for pediatric occupational therapy* (2nd ed., pp. 323–375). Philadelphia: Lippincott, Williams & Wilkins.

Parten, M. B. (1932). Social participation among pre-school children. *Journal of Abnormal and Social Psychology, 27,* 243–269.

Posthuma, B. W. (2002). *Small groups in counseling and therapy: Process and leadership* (4th ed.). Boston: Allyn & Bacon.

Riley, S. (2001). *Group process made visible: Group art therapy.* Philadelphia: Brunner-Routledge.

Rosenthal, L. (1985). A modern analytic approach to group resistances. *Modern Psychoanalysis, 10*, 165–181.

Rosenthal, L. (1994). *Resolving resistance in group psychotherapy.* Northvale, NJ: Jason Aronson.

Ross, M. (1997). *Interactive group therapy: Mobilizing coping abilities with the five-stage group.* Bethesda, MD: American Occupational Therapy Association.

Sandler, J., Dare, C., & Holder, A. (1995). *The patient and the analyst: The basis of psychoanalytic process* (2nd ed.). Madison, CT: International Universities Press.

Silberstein-Sorfer, M., & Jones, M. (1982). *Doing art together: The remarkable parent–child workshop of the Metropolitan Museum of Art.* New York: Simon & Schuster.

Spotnitz, H. (1985). *Modern psychoanalysis of the schizophrenic patient: Theory of the technique* (2nd ed.). New York: Human Sciences Press.

Stein, F., & Cutler, S. K. (2002). *Psychosocial occupational therapy: A holistic approach* (2nd ed.). Albany, NY: Delmar/Thomson Learning.

Steward, E. C. (1972). *American cultural patterns.* La Grange Park, IL: Intercultural Network.

Thomson, M. (1997). *On art and therapy: An exploration.* London: Free Association.

Toglia, J. P. (1993). *Contextual memory test.* Tucson, AZ: Therapy SkillBuilders.

Yalom, I. D. (1985). *The theory and practice of group psychotherapy* (3rd ed.). Basic (Basic Books, Inc., Publishers): New York.

Zeitlin, S., Williamson, G. G., & Sczepanski, M. (1988). *Early coping inventory.* Bensenville, IL: Scholastic Testing Service.

10

The Ability–Disability Continuum and Activity Match

Lisa E. Cyzner, PhD, OTR

The totality of the impact of serious physical impairment on conscious thought, as well as its firm implantation in the unconscious mind, gives disability a far stronger purchase on one's sense of who and what he is than do any social roles— even key ones such as age, occupation, and ethnicity. These can be manipulated, neutralized, and suspended, and in this way can become adjusted somewhat to each other. (Murphy, 1990, p. 105)

In his book, *The Body Silent*, Robert Murphy (1990), a retired professor from the department of anthropology at Columbia University in New York City, described his experiences living with a chronic illness as the most challenging journey of his life. Invoking the metaphor of a journey, he takes readers with him as he relates how every aspect of his life was affected after learning that he had a spinal cord tumor that eventually led to quadriplegia. If life is the journey, the body is our vessel through which we experience life. The body is our physical, psychological, philosophical, and sociological connection to the world through which we strive to create meaningful lives.

As occupational therapy practitioners, we also must incorporate this multifaceted approach of considering the physical, psychological, philosophical, and sociological perspectives into our evaluation and intervention using purposeful activities. In a sense, we can embrace Murphy's anthropological perspective as a way to individualize our approach. For each person with a disability, the journey is different. For some, the journey begins at birth; for others, it begins after a traumatic event. Families, friends, and significant others take part of this journey as well. For many, the journey of living with a chronic illness is a lifelong process.

This chapter is divided into two major sections. The first discusses the four life perspectives that we, as occupational therapy practitioners, should explore during both the evaluation and intervention processes. In the latter half of this section, a graphic representation of the four continua integrating these perspectives is presented. The second includes a framework of explanations on how we can help clients to construct and reconstruct their lifestyles using purposeful activities, believing that the process of reconstructing lifestyles for many is an evolving, ever-changing process. This section is followed by a work sheet (see Appendix 10.A) developed from this framework that can be used in daily practice.

An Exploration and Integration of the Four Perspectives: Physical, Psychological, Philosophical, and Sociological

World Health Organization Model

In efforts to provide a framework for health professionals providing services for people with disabilities, the World Health Organization (WHO) published the *International Classification of Impairments, Disabilities, and Handicaps* (ICIDH) in 1980. Complete with definitions and information regarding the consequences of disease, the WHO (1980) presented a continuum—an illness trajectory—through which health professionals could communicate by using more uniform terminology than had been used in the past (Knussen & Cunningham, 1988; Rogers & Holm, 1994; Wood, 1980). As Wood (1980) described, one can view this continuum as depicted in Figure 10.1.

Impairment, disability, and handicap are all considered to be consequences of disease. Related to the ICIDH published in 1980, Rogers and Holm (1994) cautioned that the WHO defines these concepts in only terms of dysfunction. Neither aspects of remediation nor compensation were presented within these definitions; however, they are useful and lay a groundwork through which we can begin to explore the physical, psychological, and sociological perspectives affected by disability. Furthermore, Coster and Haley (1992) noted that, although the ICIDH is hierarchical in that each of the four components represents "increasingly complex integrated activities" (p. 13), health professionals should not necessarily view this continuum as linear. They explained that even though an individual presents with problems indicative of a certain component or level of the WHO model, one cannot presume that the same individual also has problems indicative of another component along the con-

---

Disease ⇒ Impairment ⇒ Disability ⇒ Handicap

Figure 10.1. The World Health Organization (1980) *International Classification of Impairments, Disabilities, and Handicaps* continuum.

tinuum. Coster and Haley provided the example of a child with a below-elbow ampu-tation resulting from trauma (an impairment) who could perform all activities of daily living independently with his prosthesis. Thus, according to the WHO system, although the child had an impairment, he would not be considered disabled because he was able to perform all of his activities of daily living independently. Therefore, what we as occupational therapy practitioners must think and question ourselves about is What is an individual able to do, and what is an individual not able to do? We also need to take into account what the individual chooses to do and what level of assistance may or may not be needed.

Coster and Haley (1992) continued to explain that other models of disablement have been both suggested and noted to be conceptually more clear than that of the WHO model, such as that proposed by Nagi (1965, 1991). They described that, unlike the WHO model, Nagi links impairment with disability through functional limitations. Functional limitations encompass a person's ability to perform tasks and to carry out those obligations that are part of his or her role(s) or daily activities.

The WHO published the first ICIDH in 1980 for trial purposes. After multi-ple revisions based on field testing and international consultation, the WHO approved the latest version for use on May 22, 2001, which is now known as the *International Classification of Functioning, Disability, and Health* (ICF; WHO, 2001b). The concepts of impairment, disability, and handicap on one continuum were replaced with a two-level, or two-part, system—Part 1, Functioning and Dis-ability, and Part 2, Contextual Factors—each of which have several components. Within this classification and further breakdown of components, the concepts of impairment and disability are still used; however, they are paired and grouped with other concepts related to functioning so that the presentation and relationship of all of these concepts are no longer linear as the original continuum suggested (see Figure 10.2). Most important, the ICF is intended to have application for all people, not just those with disabilities (WHO, 2001b). Essentially, what Coster and Haley (1992) discussed relative to models of disablement are embodied more so in this version of the ICF than they were in the original ICIDH.

The *International Classification of Diseases, 10th Revision* (ICD-10; WHO, 2001a) is used to classify health conditions such as diseases, disorders, and injuries. The ICD-10 and the ICF, therefore, are complementary, as the ICF provides infor-mation on a person's ability to function with his or her given health conditions. Thus, the ICF now is viewed more as a component of health classification rather than being related to consequences of disease. According to the WHO, the ICF is considered to be a multipurpose classification and conceptual framework that can be used in a vari-ety of contexts related to health care, including management of health care systems; prevention and health promotion programs; and research related to such entities as health care evaluations, health care policy, and applied research to meet the changing needs of society (WHO, 2001).

Figure 10.3 provides what the WHO (2001b) deems an "overview of ICF" (p. 14), which outlines the ICF's overall organization and structure so that one can see

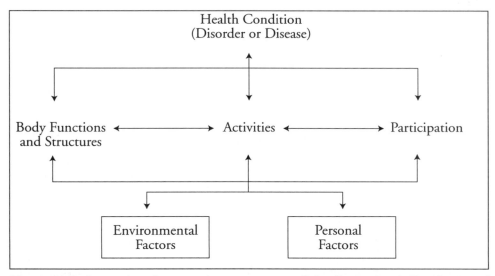

Figure 10.2. Interactions between the components of the *International Classification of Functioning, Disability, and Health* (ICF).

Note. From *ICF: International Classification of Functioning, Disability, and Health. Short version,* by the World Health Organization, 2001, p. 26, Geneva, Switzerland: Author. Copyright © 2001 by the World Health Organization. Reprinted with permission.

that it provides information related to human functioning as well as restrictions to human functioning that can be used by a variety of disciplines. Part 1 of the ICF is related to functioning and disability, which has two components: (a) body functions and structures and (b) activities and participation. What has direct application to occupational therapy is the information related to activities and participation that includes a range of domains covering many aspects of functioning, including looking at functioning from the perspective of both an individual and society. Therefore, the components of Part 1 can be used to indicate a problem, impairment, activity limitation, or participation restriction, all of which can be summarized under the umbrella concept of disability. The components also can be used to indicate aspects of health that are not related to a problem or impairment, and these can be summarized under the concept of functioning (WHO, 2001b). Therefore, as mentioned earlier, it is very important as occupational therapy practitioners that we continue to ask ourselves what an individual both can and cannot do. Also vital for us is to include evaluation and related questioning regarding contextual factors (explained in the next section) and how this also affects an individual's performance of daily life activities. The information gained from this questioning is integral for evaluation, treatment planning, and delivery of the treatment itself.

Part 2 of the ICF is related to components of contextual factors, including (a) environmental factors and (b) personal factors. A person's level of functioning and disability is looked on as an interaction between health conditions, such as a disease,

	Part 1: **Functioning and Disability**		Part 2: **Contextual Factors**	
Components	Body Functions and Structures	Activities and Participation	Environmental Factors	Personal Factors
Domains	Body Functions Body Structures	Life Areas (Tasks, Actions)	External Influences on Functioning and Disability	Internal Influences on Functioning and Disability
Constructs	Change in Body Functions (Physiological) Change in Body Structures (Anatomical)	Capacity Executing Tasks in a Standard Environment Performance Executing Tasks in the Current Environment	Facilitating or Hindering Impact of Features of the Physical, Social, and Attitudinal World	Impact of Attributes of the Person
Positive Aspect	Functional and Structural Integrity	Activities Participation	Facilitators	Not Applicable
		Functioning		
Negative Aspect	Impairment	Activity Limitation Participation Restriction	Barriers/ Hindrances	Not Applicable
		Disability		

Figure 10.3. An overview of *International Classification of Functioning, Disability, and Health.*

Note. From *ICF: International classification of functioning, disability and health. Short version* by the World Health Organization, 2001, p. 14, Geneva, Switzerland: Author. Copyright © 2001 by the World Health Organization. Reprinted with permission.

illness, or injury, and contextual factors, or how the environment affects the person's functioning and disability. Placing value and emphasis on context also is the main focus of the ecology of human performance framework developed by the occupational therapy department faculty of the University of Kansas Medical Center. According to this framework and similar to what the WHO (2001a) described, equal value is given to four constructs that are essential for treatment: person, context, task, and performance. This framework emphasizes the role of context. According to the framework's developers, occupational therapy practitioners as well as programs and professions often neglect context (Dunn, Brown, & McGuigan, 1994; Dunn, Brown, & Youngstrom, 2003). Tham and Kielhofner (2003) agreed and noted that specifically regarding research related to disability, we as a profession lack empirical documentation about how social context affects occupational performance for people with disabilities.

According to the WHO (2001a), environmental factors come from an individual's immediate environment as well as from the surrounding environment, which affects all of the components of functioning and disability. Although personal factors are included and would be considered here, they are not classified in the ICF because there is too much variance related to social and cultural differences to be included in the ICF (WHO, 2001a). Yet to occupational therapy practitioners, information related both to social and to cultural factors is vital because these factors can greatly affect how we work with clients and their families and what our expectations and the families' expectations are relative to treatment. Social and cultural factors also can affect a person and his or her family's view of functioning and disability, which again has a direct impact on choices of treatment, activities integrated into the treatment itself, and modifications to the environment.

As described previously, the sections and components of the ICF particularly related to activities and participation and contextual factors have direct application to occupational therapy practice. I recommend that readers consult the short version of the ICF (WHO, 2001a) for further details on all of the components of the ICF, multiple usages of the classification, and other applications to practice.

To expand on this relationship of the ICF with occupational therapy practice, Lollar (2003) described in his foreword to the text *Perspectives in Human Occupation: Participation in Life,*

> Two major tenets of the new system are that the environment and contextual factors play a crucial role in human function generally and in disability specifically. Second, the outcomes for all people are framed as societal participation. These two components of the new ICF have been the essence of occupation and occupational therapy since their inception: (a) participation and (b) society. This framework allows occupation and occupational therapy to take a leadership role as the field of health and disability move beyond body function to embrace the assessment of classification of health status. The coding system will allow both positive and negative elements of the environment to be included for research, policy development, and program implementation. Evaluation of activity limitations can now be balanced between domains of individuals and their environment. New assessment tools and procedures will grow from this model, and occupational therapists will be at the forefront. (pp. vii–viii)

As noted, many of the components of the ICF appear similar to those areas of human experience in which we as occupational therapy practitioners have expertise. They are reflective of elements of the domain of concern (Mosey, 1996) and of the *Occupational Therapy Practice Framework: Domain and Process* (American Occupational Therapy Association [AOTA], 2002), which officially replaced the third edition of *Uniform Terminology for Occupational Therapy* (UT-III; AOTA, 1994) by a vote of the AOTA's Representative Assembly. The *Framework* includes language to aid occupational therapy practitioners in explaining occupation to their community, particularly how occupation relates to the delivery of occupational therapy intervention. The *Framework* also is more universal, incorporating terminology from the ICF, so that other health professionals can understand it and in turn understand more about the occupational therapy profession, our domain of concern, the client populations with whom we work, and the various settings that we work in on a daily basis (Hinojosa, Kramer, Royeen, & Luebben, 2003; Luebben, 2003; Youngstrom, 2002). (See Figure 10.4 for a comparison of the ICF taxonomy with that of UT-III and the *Framework*.) Thus, considering all the aforementioned, as we as a profession witness the reemphasis and, essentially, a return to our roots of occupation, we also must consider the larger activity performance areas—the occupations—affected by a disability and not just the underlying performance components (Baptiste, 2003; Clark et al., 1997; Coster, 1998; Jackson, Carlson, Mandel, Zemke, & Clark, 1998; Padilla, 2003; Wood, 1998).

Whether the performance of the activity is related to work; play, leisure, recreation, and friendships; family interaction; or activities of daily living, some members of the occupational therapy profession advocate that we should look at these areas first—along with considering context—rather than initially evaluate and subsequently base treatment on problems related to the underlying components affecting the performance. This is better known as a "top-down" approach to evaluation rather than a "bottom-up" approach, which focuses on the underlying components (Coster, 1998; Ideishi, 2003; Trombly, 1993, 1995).

When using a "top-down" approach with a client, an occupational therapy practitioner initially tries to determine the client's ability to perform certain roles and the meaning he or she attaches to these roles. This information is ascertained to determine what activities the client may want to address in occupational therapy sessions. Those roles and related activities that the client engaged in before becoming disabled or coming to occupational therapy (as a result of a recent event or more chronic disability) become the focus of evaluation. If the occupational therapist determines that there is a difference among past, present, and future role performances, then treatment should be implemented. The occupational therapy practitioner explores with the client those role performances and activities that he or she wishes to do and investigates why he or she is unable to do them. This exploration helps the client to understand the need for and what the focus will be in treatment (Trombly, 1993, 1995).

Ideishi (2003) explained that an occupational therapy practitioner can organize his or her practice through implementation of a top-down, bottom-up, or contextual approach. Regardless of the approach chosen, he noted that occupation and the goal of helping clients to engage in meaningful occupations is the commonality among all the approaches. Ideishi stressed,

	Part I: Functioning and Disability	Part II: Contextual Factors
ICF	Activities and Participation — Body Functions and Structures	Personal Factors — Environmental Factors
UT-III	*Performance Areas* — *Performance Components*	*Performance Contexts*
	Activities of Daily Living / Work and Productive Activities / Play or Leisure Activities / * / Sensorimotor / Cognitive / Psychosocial	* / * / Environment / Temporal Aspects
Framework	ADL / IADL / Work / Education / Social Participation / Play / Leisure / Process Skills / Communication/Interaction Skills / Motor Skills / Body Functions / Body Structures / Routines / Habits / Roles / Objects[a] / Physical / Cultural / Social / Spiritual / Temporal / Virtual	
	Areas of Occupation — *Performance Skills* — *Client Factors* — *Performance Patterns* — *Activity Demands* — *Context*	

* Aspects not addressed in UT-III.

a. The aspect, Activity Demands, includes Objects Used and Their Properties, Space Demands, Social Demands, Sequencing and Timing, Required Actions, Required Body Functions, Required and Body Structures.

Figure 10.4. Comparison of three taxonomies: *International Classification of Functioning, Disability, and Health* (WHO, 2001a), *Uniform Terminology for Occupational Therapy—Third Edition* (AOTA, 1994), and the *Occupational Therapy Practice Framework: Domain and Process* (AOTA, 2002).

Note. From "Core Concept of Occupation" by J. Hinojosa, P. Kramer, C. B. Royeen, & A. J. Luebben, 2003, p. 14. In P. Kramer, J. Hinojosa, & C. B. Royeen (Eds.), *Perspectives in human occupation: Participation in life*. Philadelphia: Lippincott, Williams & Wilkins. Copyright © 2003 by Lippincott, Williams & Wilkins. Reprinted with permission.

The challenge for the occupational therapist is to transform and articulate our theoretical concepts into daily practice. If we can articulate what we do and why we do it, our clients, our communities, our colleagues in other disciplines, and the institutions that pay for our services will understand the unique contribution that occupational therapy provides society. (p. 294)

Finally, because ICF is a global taxonomy, it challenges the occupational therapy profession to clarify definitions related to activities and occupation. Occupation is considered to be at the core of our profession as it comprises the daily tasks and purposeful activities, whether mundane or of great importance, that are meaningful to people and are part of who we are as individuals (Hinojosa et al., 2003). Throughout the history of the profession, occupation has been used as both a means during our intervention processes as well as an end that is the goal of our interventions so that our clients can return, or choose new directions regarding their choices, to participation in daily life tasks. Several individuals at the forefront of this debate in our profession and others have contributed valuable discussion to this need to clarify our definitions. Many have suggested that the concept of occupation be defined as a process and activity as the outcome (Hinojosa et al., 2003; Ideishi, 2003; Trombly, 1995).

Whatever an occupational therapy practitioner's view may be, the highest goal of occupational therapy intervention is to help a client to participate in meaningful occupations resulting in participation in life (Ideishi, 2003). Yet, we have little documentation of efficacy regarding occupation, the practice of occupation, and the relationship of occupation to disability (Padilla, 2003). Furthermore, the WHO (2001a) professed through the ICF that we should integrate the medical model of disability with the social model of disability. The WHO defined the medical model of disability as

> a problem of the person, directly caused by disease, trauma, or other health condition, which requires medical care provided in the form of individual treatment by professionals. Management of the disability is aimed at cure or the individual's adjustment and behaviour change. Medical care is viewed as the main issue, and at the political level the principle is that of modifying or reforming health policy. (p. 28)

The WHO defined the social model of disability as

> a socially created problem, and basically as a matter of the full integration of individuals into society. Disability is not an attribute of an individual, but rather a complex collection of conditions, many of which are created by the social environment. Hence the management of the problem requires social action, and it is the collective responsibility of society at large to make the environmental modifications necessary for the full participation of people with disabilities in all areas of social life. (p. 28)

If we as a profession embrace this integration of models, which is also at the core of our philosophical underpinnings, and if we want to align ourselves with the leaders who affect health policy, management, and outcomes, then we must be clear in our definitions and be able to explain our models of intervention to society at large.

A Psychological Continuum: The Disability Process

Much of the psychological literature describing people's reactions to disabilities and the processes they undergo can be found in the area of bereavement and loss as well as in the area of stress and coping (Carroll, 1961; Clegg, 1988; Knussen & Cunningham, 1988; Lazarus & Folkman, 1991; Parkes, 1998; Parkes & Weiss, 1983). Clegg (1988) defined *bereavement* as a state that follows an actual or perceived loss. She described bereavement as including changes in all dimensions of a person's life— physical, psychological, and behavioral—as a result of this loss. Individuals may display their reactions to this actual or perceived loss through their own social, cognitive, physical, and emotional behaviors. Thus again, we are reminded of the integration of the models of disability from both the individual and the societal perspective.

One particular continuum found in the literature was developed specifically from research related to the bereavement process (Parkes & Weiss, 1983). Some of these authors' research focused on participants who had acquired disabilities. The continuum is presented in Figure 10.5.

Clegg (1988) described that in life we tend to live each day on a set of assumptions; these assumptions can be disrupted once we face a loss (also see the next section on philosophical perspectives). She explained that Parkes views the grieving process as part of an individual's letting go of one set of assumptions and adopting another set when coming to terms with such losses as a disability. This is reflected in the continuum, the tasks of grieving. Parkes and Weiss (1983) believed that an individual must go through this grieving process before he or she can truly accept the loss. They stated that an individual facing a recent loss must try to make sense of what has happened in order to begin to answer the omnipresent question, "Why?"

Individuals then move along the continuum toward emotional acceptance when they begin to feel less of a need to avoid reminders of the loss that may evoke other painful feelings and emotional responses, including denial. Some people who receive occupational therapy never will fully come to this level of emotional acceptance. For many, the process may be slow. Each person's experience and ways of dealing with loss will be unique, and we as practitioners must be vigilant about this and sensitive to the client's "place" along this continuum. Finally, Parkes and Weiss (1983) described the adoption of a new identity as dichotomous: "maintaining one identity while acting in another" (p. 159). In other words, if we believe that our identity reflects the set of

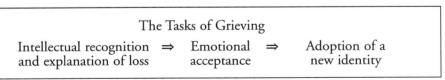

Figure 10.5. The tasks of grieving by Parkes and Weiss (1983).

assumptions or ideas that we have about ourselves, then these are the very same ideas that affect our choices, our activity selections. This emphasis on choice, on engaging in meaningful activity, is central to the occupational therapy profession. Whether using activities in evaluation or treatment to remediate or compensate for a particular disability, the activities chosen must be meaningful to the client. Once again, we are reminded that occupation is the process and activities are the outcome as we help people with disabilities to reenter society and rebuild their lives. Choosing activities for treatment as part of helping a person to reconstruct a lifestyle after a disability is specific to the individual (AOTA, 1993). *There must be an activity match.*

Philosophical Underpinnings: Self, Skills, and Ideas

From philosophy, the concept of figure–ground appears to have direct application to looking at how a disability affects a person's physical and psychological well-being and how he or she learns to cope with the loss (Bateson, 1972, 1979; Idhe, 1991; Popper, 1992). Similar to the ideas presented by Parkes and Weiss (1983), the assumptions on which we operate and carry out our daily activities are part of our "ground," part of what we do not necessarily consciously think about throughout the course of our day. The ground is our background knowledge; it is what we often take for granted. Even habits can become part of our background knowledge. It is not until we have an event that brings about change—a "rupture"—that we see the "figure" (Idhe, 1991; G. Moglia, personal communication, April 22, 1998). In other words, the figure must be brought out of the background for us to realize all that we do automatically. Thus, when a person becomes disabled—when he or she can no longer perform activities as before— the disability becomes part of the figure. A person may realize what he or she had taken for granted in the past. To try to go back to the ground often is a difficult journey.

Related both to the concept of figure–ground and to the idea that we as human beings tend to live by a certain set of assumptions is that we also tend to attach our ideas and skills—and many of our daily activities—to ourselves (see Figure 10.6). Essentially, we embody ideas. We seem to adhere to the belief that our ideas and our skills define who we are. If we relinquish an idea or a skill, especially if we lose a skill and can no longer perform an activity the way we were accustomed to, then a piece of who we are "dies" (Idhe, 1991; G. Moglia, personal communication, April 22, 1998; Popper, 1992).

Although it is very hard to do, we really cannot begin to criticize our ideas and our skills needed to engage in activities until we are able to view those same ideas and skills outside ourselves. This is what makes the process so difficult: accepting that some of our ideas and skills are fallible and that often we have to make mistakes in order to learn more about ourselves. It is only then that we can improve on our ideas and skills (Popper, 1992). This recognition is analogous to an individual's accepting that he or she may not be able to perform an activity the way he or she used to or learning that the same activity can still be performed but that modifications may have to be made to carry it out independently. Assistance may be needed for a person to

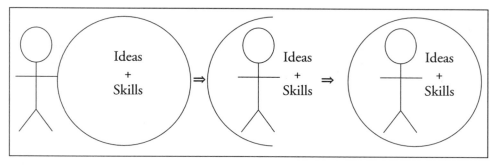

Figure 10.6. We as human beings tend to live by a certain set of assumptions and attach our ideas and skills.

continue to participate in an activity that was part of his or her daily life before becoming disabled. Furthermore, for people living with chronic illness, if symptoms progress, the level to which the person may be able to perform certain activities will change. As the conditions change, so may the need for modifications or assistance.

In the occupational therapy literature, this theme of embodiment of ideas and skills is apparent. Only a few works have been selected for this chapter as examples, yet there are others. For example, Clark (1993) in her Eleanor Clarke Slagle Lecture entitled "Occupation Embedded in a Real Life: Interweaving Occupational Science and Occupational Therapy," told the story of Penny Richardson, a professor from the University of Southern California. She poignantly related the process that Richardson went through to rediscover herself, to realize how she had defined herself before surviving the traumatic event of an aneurysm and what she would have to do to discover a new self. Clark described that, through the use of narrative (telling stories), she was able to help Richardson through the process of recovery and "how rehabilitation can be experienced by the survivor as a rite of passage in which a person is moved to disability status and then abandoned" (p. 1067). Richardson made Clark aware that "occupations were important because they marked the new you versus the old you" (p. 1072). These statements echo not only the information presented in the tasks of grieving as described by Parkes and Weiss (1983) but also the notion that our ideas and our skills—our occupations and the activities that constitute them—define who we are.

Similar to Clark (1993), Price-Lackey and Cashman (1996) presented information gained from life history interviews to describe how Jenny Cashman (the second author of the work and graduate student of library science and archeology) experienced and adapted to becoming disabled after a traumatic brain injury. The authors presented Cashman's use of daily activities that had meaning to her and a narrative construction to help her to regain a sense of identity. Similar to what Murphy (1990) described, Cashman also viewed her recovery process as a challenging journey. The following is an excerpt from Cashman's postscript to her head injury experience, which she wrote and which was included in the article:

The process of healing and redefinition has also been a profound experience, providing new depth and richness to my life. The fact that my life has changed is no longer a source of grief to me, but something I embrace. I am writing again—not in the way I wrote before, but in a new way, and that feels like a gift....I am at this point, working on a book about my experience and my journey. It is somehow fitting that I celebrated my 5-year anniversary of my accident on an archeological dig in Egypt. The joy this gave me makes it clear that I have found my new path, so I have committed to working on the excavation for at least the next five campaigns. Then I'll see what happens next. Life is, after all, an eternal process of being and becoming. (p. 312)

Both Price-Lackey and Cashman (1996) suggested the following to occupational therapy practitioners:

- It is important to understand what daily activities clients engaged in before becoming ill or disabled. This information is important because descriptions of patterns of activities (occupations) may inform about the client's self-identity, and this information is integral to the recovery process.

- Goal setting should be a collaborative effort between the occupational therapy practitioner and the client.

- In treatment, occupational therapy practitioners should take into account both the doing aspects of occupations and the narrative meaning the client expresses regarding his or her daily occupations. Thus, it seems that by doing so, practitioners can truly begin to value the personal meaning that daily, purposeful activities bring to their clients' lives.

In actuality, we do not just have to look to the literature to find examples of the embodiment of ideas and how people attach their ideas to themselves as a way of forming and reforming their own identities. We can see this happening in our everyday practice, and we can see it in ourselves. Until we can understand it in ourselves, it is very hard to recognize the impact of attaching our ideas to ourselves in order to help others.

Related to this, it is important that we as occupational therapy practitioners begin to figure out what type of learner our client may be or what type of learning styles may affect his or her intervention and process of recovery. We must remember that an individual's learning style may evolve as intervention progresses. Thus, we need to create an environment in which clients feel comfortable learning and through which they can learn through trial and error, by making mistakes, by creating their own knowledge as they begin to construct, and by reconstructing their lifestyles with a disability. Perkinson (1984, 1993) described what he labeled an "educative environment," which may be helpful to us as we help others to learn new skills or relearn old ones in different ways. Although Perkinson mainly described the environment created by a teacher for his or her students, his ideas are applicable for occupational therapy practitioners determining what type of treatment environment to set up for clients, whether children or adults. Perkinson (1993) suggested that we create the following when making decisions about the environment needed to help individuals to learn:

- An environment in which the individuals will feel free to "disclose their present knowledge" (p. 34)

- An environment that provides critical feedback regarding individuals' present knowledge (this feedback can come from a variety of sources)

- A supportive environment so that individuals can accept criticism about their present knowledge and begin to eliminate errors.

Thus simultaneously, practitioners also must question whether our clients truly have the idea in their minds of what we have asked them to do. Again, we must question ourselves and ask, "Because my client can perform a certain action while engaging in activity, does he or she really understand the nature of why I have asked him or her to perform this activity in a certain way (based on the understanding that the activity was chosen by the client)?" In other words, "Can we make the assumption that if we set up behavioral objective, 'A,' then we will get 'B'" (Perkinson, 1993)? We must be sure that when a client is performing a certain activity that he or she understands why and for what purpose. The client can then begin to generalize the knowledge learned from these experiences of performing activities during treatment to other activities he or she wishes to do in his or her daily life. Again, there must be an activity match among the activity itself, the underlying reasons for performing it, and the individual.

Sociological Perspective and Personal Transformation

Disability, in many ways, can be described as a culture (Campbell & Oliver, 1996). In a sense, we all probably can think of at least one activity we do that has been defined by our culture, and perhaps by our society, or even an activity that we may actually resist engaging in because it has been deemed unacceptable by our particular culture. Reflecting on the disability movement in Britain and disability movements in general, Campbell and Oliver (1996) described these movements as redefining "the problem of disability as the product of a disabling society rather than individual limitations or loss, despite the fact that the rest of society continues to see disabled people as chance victims of a tragic fate" (p. 105). For a person who has become disabled, these authors explained that part of the redefining is a sociological process that includes redefining oneself and realizing that part of one's personal issues surrounding disability also, in fact, may be political. These issues give rise to social movement. Therefore, when looking at the change process that affects people with disabilities, the change is twofold in that one looks at the changes in oneself and how these changes affect society. Campbell and Oliver described this duality as transforming both a personal and social consciousness, "promoting self-understanding as a platform for change" (p. 145). Certainly, we have seen evidence of this very idea that seems to have influenced American society with the passing of the Americans With Disabilities Act of 1990

(P.L. 101–336) and the reauthorization of the Individuals With Disabilities Education Act of 1997 (P.L. 105–17) (Bailey & Schwartzberg, 1995; Frist, 1995; Johnson, 1996; Murphy, 2003). Much of the lobbying for passage of these laws lies with the power of advocacy groups, which often comprise people with disabilities and their families. This active participation in advocacy groups and other organizations often becomes a highly valued activity for people with disabilities.

Furthermore, when deciding how to describe this change process to others, Campbell and Oliver (1996) mentioned that they resisted separating information and issues surrounding disability, including social theory, political history, action research, individual biography, and personal experience. Each area related to disability influences the other, and this is reflected in what appears to be yet another continuum regarding disability that looks at changes occurring on both a personal and a social level. Thus, two smaller continua represent the sociological perspective regarding disability and the change process associated with it. For the purposes of this chapter, I concentrate on what seems to be a personal transformation continuum that eventually affects the social transformation process as well (see Figure 10.7).

For personal transformation, Campbell and Oliver (1996) suggested that the following occurs. First, individuals may deny that a problem exists. Their initial response may be to assimilate with the rest of society and view being disabled as part of their identity. Next, individuals must be grateful and reasonable. By this, Campbell and Oliver meant that people with disabilities must somehow learn to balance accepting and being grateful to people wanting to help them with being reasonable and more conscious of what they should actually have to accept and even tolerate from society, for example, knowing when to report discriminatory acts.

The next stage is that of bearing witness. This stage begins the bridge between the personal and societal transformations, which is the act of sharing experiences with others, especially those who have encountered similar problems, including those related to societal issues. We can see how such activities may become quite vital for our clients to help establish resources and reestablish connections with their world. Frequently, other people with similar disabilities are the people from whom our clients learn the most, including information such as what type of wheelchair lift to install in a van or what grocery store is the most accessible and accommodating.

Along this continuum, people with disabilities must learn to understand themselves and to differentiate what Campbell and Oliver (1996) believed to be the difference between one's own personal problems and those caused by a disabling society.

Denial ⇒ Be Grateful and Reasonable ⇒ Bearing Witness ⇒
Understanding Ourselves ⇒ Fighting Back

Figure 10.7. The Personal Transformation Continuum adapted from ideas presented by Campbell and Oliver (1996).

Finally, the authors suggested that individuals can arrive at the level of fighting back, especially against the stereotypes depicted by society, by rejecting what one believes is the dominant disabling culture, getting involved in "cultural production" (e.g., the arts) as a way to express what has happened to them and engaging in political practice by getting involved in political organizations and increasing empowerment. Speaking from personal experience, Campbell and Oliver described, like many others, a difficult journey.

When reflecting on the four life perspectives that affect activity performance for people with disabilities, we can begin to see the parallels between them. They overlap in the information presented regarding the change processes that take place in the individual and that these processes seem to happen simultaneously. Changes occur within oneself and within one's environment. Viewed sociologically, disability can be viewed as a "gap between a person's capabilities and the demands of the environment" (Committee on a National Agenda for the Prevention of Disabilities, 1991, p. 1). Thus, to begin to look at how to help clients construct and reconstruct their lifestyles using activities, we must take into account information from all four of these perspectives. This information can be gained in many ways, most often through clinical interviews with the client, family, significant others, and other caregivers. What becomes an overriding theme for our activity reasoning process is that we must continually ask ourselves the question What is an individual able to do, and what is an individual not able to do regarding his or her activity performance? This construct is represented by A in Figure 10.8 (Parts B, C, D, and E represent the physical, psychological, philosophical, and sociological perspectives, respectively). What we also may consider includes, but is not limited to, a client's resources, background knowledge, level of assistance needed, own understanding of what he or she believes he or she is able to do, and his or her level of motivation. As always, for each person, his or her experiences, feelings, and life situations will be unique.

A Framework: Helping People to Construct and Reconstruct Their Lifestyles Using Activities

According to the philosopher Karl Popper, for human beings to learn, we must criticize our ideas and look for errors. Essentially, through the process of trial and error and making mistakes is when we often learn best. What is difficult for us, however, is to criticize our own ideas or to make other guesses about ways in which to solve problems when we are used to addressing problems in a certain manner. Thus, Popper (1992) described one way in which we can learn more (and gain knowledge) about how to address our problems, accepting the idea that we may never come to a true solution. Popper explained that, once we have identified a problem, we should make guesses about how we can address these problems and to criticize each guess. By discovering problems, we advance knowledge. The metaphor of the staircase for Popper's ideas (as described by G. Moglia, personal communication, June 1, 1998) allows us to go through a process of presentation and description of the problem, making a

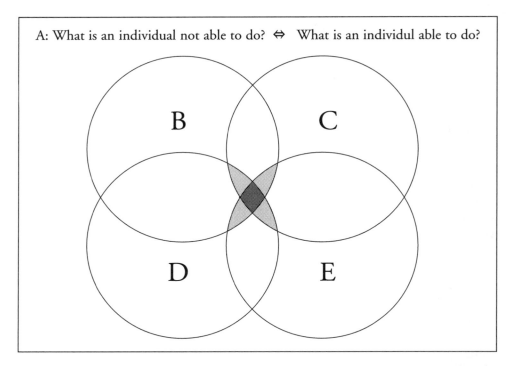

A: What is an individual not able to do? ⇔ What is an individul able to do?

B   C

D   E

Figure 10.8. Integration of the continua from the four life perspectives. A represents the activity reasoning process that requires occupational therapists to continually ask the question: What is an individual able to do, and what is an individual not able to do regarding his or her activity performance? B represents the physical, C the psychological, D the philosophical, and E the sociological perspectives.

guess, criticizing the guess, and making a better guess. This process continues and evolves with each step of the staircase. Thus, while ascending this knowledge staircase, we are able to see our mistakes, and we come to deeper problems and better guesses. A finite end does not exist, only the process to reach better guesses (G. Moglia, personal communication, September 10, 1997; Popper, 1992).

The Occupational Therapy Reflective Staircase, as shown in Figure 10.9, illustrates this process. When we are near the top step of the staircase, we may reach the point in which we must reframe the problem. What we thought was the original problem were deep problems that were either resolved; changed; or, perhaps, underlying the original problem (Schön, 1983). For example, once initiating treatment we begin to realize that a client's depression is affecting physical activity performance more than we had detected in the initial evaluation. Thus, we may need to address the depression first before continuing treatment or concurrently with treatment, or we may need to seek the help of other professionals to assist the client in addressing this problem.

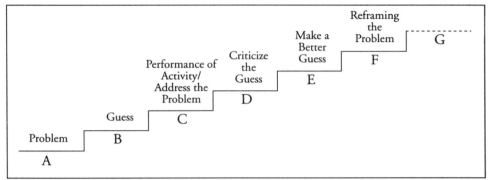

Figure 10.9. The Occupational Therapy Reflective Staircase: Adapting and integrating the ideas of Moglia (1997, 1998), Popper (1992), and Schön (1983) for practice.

For occupational therapy practitioners, this process is similar to our clinical reasoning process. When thinking about how to use activities to help people with disabilities construct and reconstruct their lifestyles, the incorporation of this staircase and the process of analysis (of the problem) and synthesis (making guesses to arrive at possible ways to address the problem) appear applicable and useful.

Using the Staircase in Clinical Practice: The Process

A. Problem

As part of the evaluation process, several questions can be asked regarding the client's current as well as past level of activity performance. The information the occupational therapist seeks through both interview and observation of activity performance is, What is the client able and not able to do? More specifically, what does the client identify as a problem related to activity performance that is interfering with his or her ability to function as independently as possible (based on the activity he or she has chosen), and what does the caregiver identify as a problem related to activity performance? Other questions related to the problem are, What purpose does the activity serve? For example, is the activity part of the client's daily routine; is it a leisure activity, is it an activity that aids the caregiver in assisting the client? We are considering the impact on both performance components, or the underlying problems, and performance areas, while always considering contextual factors. For each client, the focus will be different. It is important to have a clear description and understanding about what the problem is before proceeding with the rest of the process.

Consider the following two case scenarios. Embedded within them are problems that we may choose to address as part of helping these clients to construct and reconstruct their lifestyles using activities. More than likely, we would need more information to develop a complete intervention plan. However, these scenarios may begin to help stimulate your thinking, using the framework presented.

———   ▦   ———

Exercise 10.1—Addressing the Problem

After reading the case scenarios, ask yourself, What is one potential problem related to activity performance that could be addressed in occupational therapy? What other information would I need? Next, describe the problem in your own words. (Also see the work sheet in Appendix 10.A to this chapter for more guidance.)

Case Scenario 1

Mr. Johnson is a 28-year-old man who recently became paraplegic after a motor vehicle accident. Before his accident, he was a manager of a local business supply store. He has been referred by his physiatrist for inpatient occupational therapy now that he has stabilized; thus, it has been determined that Mr. Johnson can participate safely in a rehabilitation program. During an interview, Mr. Johnson relates that he lives alone and plans on returning to his apartment after discharge. His nearest relatives live 400 miles away. On weekends, close friends and family have been visiting him in the hospital. His initial requests during the occupational therapy evaluation are that he wants to be able to dress and bathe himself. At this time, he completely relies on others to carry out these daily living tasks for him. Furthermore, later in the interview, Mr. Johnson describes that he was a member of a men's sports league before his accident and that he has enjoyed competitive sports since childhood.

Case Scenario 2

Karen is a 5-year-old girl who attends public school in a regular education classroom. On initial evaluation, the occupational therapist determines that Karen has sensory defensiveness. (Sensory defensiveness is a defensive reaction to sensations that most people would consider non-noxious [Wilbarger & Wilbarger, 1991, 1997]). She was initially referred to the school occupational therapist by her prekindergarten teacher. Her teacher reports that Karen refuses to participate in most of the daily activities, such as arts and crafts and snack preparation, because she becomes upset (e.g., crying, running around the room attempting to find a place to hide) when she sees that she might have to touch any type of "messy" materials, such as glue or cookie dough. Additionally, Karen fears playing on any moving playground equipment, resulting in her playing alone during recess. She has difficulty making friends. Her mother also relates that Karen is unable to do many self-care activities independently, such as buttoning her shirt. The school therapist also notices that Karen uses a very weak grasp when drawing with crayons, and Karen tells the therapist that, when she grows up, she wants to be an artist.

B. Guess

To begin to make a guess about how to address the problem, the initial question to be asked at this point in the process is, What is constraining activity performance? Similar to using a "top-down" approach as described earlier, after determining the meaning attached to a client's activities and roles, we must explore with the individual (and the caregiver) the possibilities about why he or she is unable to carry out certain activities described as a problem. This exploration helps to focus treatment (Trombly, 1993, 1995). Several guesses or strategies may be used about how to address the problem related to activity performance. For example, we may choose to modify the activity itself, provide adaptive equipment, modify the environment, or provide physical assistance to help a client to perform an activity that he or she identified as part of his or her lifestyle.

Exercise 10.2—Guessing

Considering the two case studies presented, think about what some of your possible guesses may be to address the problems that you have described. Again, you must remember that there is not necessarily one correct guess, as there may be several ways to address the problem. Additionally, when comparing the two scenarios, other issues may affect your thinking, such as Mr. Johnson appears concerned with reconstructing certain activities that were part of his lifestyle before his accident. For a child like Karen, however, the possibility exists that she has never constructed certain lifestyle activities because of her sensory defensiveness. For example, because Karen has avoided touching many objects, the musculature in her hands may not have fully developed, which would affect her fine motor performance and choice of fine motor activities.

C. Performance of Activity/Address the Problem

We must observe clients performing the activity to determine whether our guess regarding the problem was appropriate. Thus, we can *reflect* on the performance to move to the next step of criticizing our guess.

D. Criticize the Guess

This step in the process is crucial in helping a client to construct and reconstruct his or her lifestyle using activities, because this step on the staircase is where the client may see the "figure" (as described earlier in this chapter) of what he or she is still not able to do as a result of the disability. Furthermore, if the client made errors during the performance of the activity, it is important to allow him or her to see the error

(Popper, 1992) and to help the client to gain knowledge from the performance. Occupational therapists also can gain valuable knowledge by looking at our guess, attempting to figure out why it was appropriate or not or why it worked or did not work in addressing the identified problem.

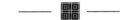

Exercise 10.3—Providing Feedback

Think about how you would provide feedback regarding errors or mistakes to both Mr. Johnson and Karen during their activity performances. For example, if Mr. Johnson attempted to use adaptive equipment during a dressing activity, using it in such a way that he seemed to be expending too much energy, how would you make him aware of this? How could you use the activity as an element of change, helping him to learn energy conservation techniques to be incorporated into his lifestyle? For Karen, if she continues to use a weak or incorrect grasp of her pencil or crayons, how will you make her aware of this? Because she is sensitive to touch, will you physically cue her to place her fingers differently on the shaft of the pencil, or will you need to devise other cuing systems, such as modeling the grasp needed so that she can visually monitor the change needed for more successful activity performance?

E. Make a Better Guess

Several issues can be explored and reflected on here. Perhaps the activity chosen in which a problem was identified was selected appropriately for an initial treatment activity (within the client's capabilities with or without modifications), but the conditions (e.g., amount of time needed for performance of the activity in its entirety) or the context in which it is performed may have to be changed or modified as well. Perhaps a different, related activity would better match the client's or caregiver's current needs. It is only through making these better guesses that we move clients up the staircase so that they can continue to construct and reconstruct their lifestyles.

F. Reframe the Problem

The process described is continuous and evolves over time. But, when guesses still do not seem to be effective, occupational therapists may need to reflect on all that they have done and reframe the problem (Schön, 1983). The original problem we chose to address may in fact not be the one we need to address first to effect change. As professionals, we must ask ourselves questions and reflect on ideas, such as

■ Is the client only physically unable to perform the activity (or elements of a larger activity), or are there other life perspectives that may be affecting performance?

- Considering the previous question, are there underlying reasons why the client cannot perform the activity (e.g., levels of motivation and meaning, difficulty reaching an emotional level of acceptance of his or her disability, difficulty separating ideas from self to learn)?

- Is the underlying problem in the environment or the objects used in the activity and not in the client's physical or psychological capabilities?

- Can the client perform one element of the activity? The problem now becomes the next element, making the activity more complex.

Summary

This chapter takes us on a journey through learning first how we must consider the four life perspectives and how these perspectives can affect people with disabilities and the activity choices they make in their lives. The Occupational Therapy Reflective Staircase, incorporating the process of problem, guess, performance of activity, criticizing the guess, making a better guess, and reframing the problem, can help to guide us as we learn to help clients to construct and reconstruct their lifestyles using activities.

"We can bestow a meaning upon our lives through our work, through our active conduct, through our whole way of life, and through the attitude we adopt toward our friends and our fellow men and towards the world. In this way the quest for the meaning of life turns into an ethical question—the question, 'What tasks can I set myself in order to make my life meaningful?'" (Popper, 1992, pp. 138–139). ■

Appendix 10.A. Constructing and Reconstructing Lifestyles Using Activities: The Occupational Therapy Reflective Staircase Work Sheet

Client's name: ——————————————————————————

Age: ————————————————————————————————

Brief activity history: ——————————————————————

————————————————————————————————————

————————————————————————————————————

————————————————————————————————————

Client's concerns, needs, wants, and priorities that could guide evaluation and treatment related to activity performance: ——————————————

————————————————————————————————————

————————————————————————————————————

————————————————————————————————————

Concerns, needs, wants, and/or priorities of the caregiver or significant other involved that could guide evaluation and treatment related to activity performance:

————————————————————————————————————

————————————————————————————————————

————————————————————————————————————

Additional notes (e.g., medical precautions, disposition plans, contexts in which activities are usually performed, other factors that may affect activity performance):

————————————————————————————————————

————————————————————————————————————

Problem (related to activity chosen together with the client): ——————

————————————————————————————————————

————————————————————————————————————

Guess: ——————————————————————————————

————————————————————————————————————

————————————————————————————————————

Performance of activity/address the problem: _____

_____

_____

Criticize the guess: _____

_____

_____

Make a better guess: _____

_____

_____

Reframe the problem, if needed: _____

_____

_____

References

American Occupational Therapy Association. (1993). Position paper: Purposeful activity. *American Journal of Occupational Therapy, 51,* 864–866.

American Occupational Therapy Association. (1994). Uniform terminology for occupational therapy—Third edition. *American Journal of Occupational Therapy, 48,* 1047–1054.

American Occupational Therapy Association. (2002). Occupational therapy practice framework: Domain and process. *American Journal of Occupational Therapy, 56,* 609–639.

Bailey, D. M., & Schwartzberg, S. L. (1995). Section 504 and Americans With Disabilities Act. In D. M. Bailey & S. L. Schwartzberg (Eds.), *Ethical and legal dilemmas in occupational therapy* (pp. 31–54). Philadelphia: F. A. Davis.

Baptiste, S. E. (2003). Client-centered practice: Implications for our professional approach, behaviors, and lexicon. In P. Kramer, J. Hinojosa, & C. B. Royeen (Eds.), *Perspectives in human occupation: Participation in life* (pp. 264–277). Philadelphia: Lippincott, Williams & Wilkins.

Bateson, G. (1972). *Steps to an ecology of mind.* San Francisco: Chandler.

Bateson, G. (1979). *Mind and nature: A necessary unity.* New York: Dutton.

Campbell, J., & Oliver, M. (1996). *Disability politics: Understanding our past, changing our future.* London: Routledge.

Carroll, T. J. (1961). *Blindness: What it is, what it does, and how to live with it.* Boston: Little, Brown.

Clark, F. (1993). Occupation embedded in a real life: Interweaving occupational science and occupational therapy, 1993 Eleanor Clarke Slagle Lecture. *American Journal of Occupational Therapy, 47,* 1067–1078.

Clark, F., Azen, S. P., Zemke, R., Jackson, J., Carlson, M., Mandel, D., et al. (1997). Occupational therapy for independent-living older adults: A randomized controlled study. *Journal of the American Medical Association, 278,* 1321–1326.

Clegg, F. (1988). Bereavement. In S. Fisher & J. Reason (Eds.), *Handbook of life stress, cognition, and health* (pp. 61–78). Chichester, England: Wiley.

Committee on a National Agenda for the Prevention of Disabilities. (1991). Executive summary. In A. M. Pope & A. R. Tarlov (Eds.), *Disability in America* (pp. 1–31). Washington, DC: National Academy Press.

Coster, W. (1998). Occupation-centered assessment of children. *American Journal of Occupational Therapy, 52,* 337–344.

Coster, W. J., & Haley, S. M. (1992). Conceptualization and measurement of disablement in infants and young children. *Infants and Young Children, 4,* 11–22.

Dunn, W., Brown, C., & McGuigan, A. (1994). The ecology of human performance: A framework for considering the effect of context. *American Journal of Occupational Therapy, 48,* 595–607.

Dunn, W., Brown, C., & Youngstrom, M. J. (2003). Ecological model of occupation. In P. Kramer, J. Hinojosa, & C. B. Royeen (Eds.), *Perspectives in human occupation: Participation in life* (pp. 222–263). Philadelphia: Lippincott, Williams & Wilkins.

Frist, B. (1995). The reauthorization of the IDEA. *Exceptional Parent, 25*(12), 46.

Hinojosa, J., Kramer, P., Royeen, C. B., & Luebben, A. J. (2003). Core concept of occupation. In P. Kramer, J. Hinojosa, & C. B. Royeen (Eds.), *Perspectives in human occupation: Participation in life* (pp. 1–17). Philadelphia: Lippincott, Williams & Wilkins.

Ideishi, R. I. (2003). Influence of occupation on assessment and treatment. In P. Kramer, J. Hinojosa, & C. B. Royeen (Eds.), *Perspectives in human occupation: Participation in life* (pp. 278–296). Philadelphia: Lippincott, Williams & Wilkins.

Idhe, D. (1991). *Instrumental realism: The interface between philosophy of science and philosophy of technology.* Bloomington: Indiana University Press.

Jackson, J., Carlson, M., Mandel, D., Zemke, R., & Clark, F. (1998). Occupation in lifestyle redesign: The well elderly study occupational therapy program. *American Journal of Occupational Therapy, 52,* 326–336.

Johnson, J. (1996). School-based occupational therapy. In J. Case-Smith, A. S. Allen, & P. N. Pratt (Eds.), *Occupational therapy for children* (3rd ed., pp. 693–716). St. Louis, MO: Mosby.

Knussen, C., & Cunningham, C. C. (1988). Stress, disability, and handicap. In S. Fisher & J. Reason (Eds.), *Handbook of life stress, cognition, and health* (pp. 335–350). Chichester, England: Wiley.

Lazarus, R. S., & Folkman, S. (1991). The concept of coping. In A. Monat & R. S. Lazarus (Eds.), *Stress and coping: An anthology* (3rd ed., pp. 189–206). New York: Columbia University Press.

Lollar, D. J. (2003). Foreword. In P. Kramer, J. Hinojosa, & C. B. Royeen (Eds.), *Perspectives in human occupation: Participation in life* (pp. vii–viii). Philadelphia: Lippincott, Williams & Wilkins.

Luebben, A. J. (2003). Ethical concerns: Human occupation. In P. Kramer, J. Hinojosa, & C. B. Royeen (Eds.), *Perspectives in human occupation: Participation in life* (pp. 297–311). Philadelphia: Lippincott, Williams & Wilkins.

Mosey, A. C. (1996). *Applied scientific inquiry in the health professions: An epistemological orientation* (2nd ed.). Bethesda, MD: American Occupational Therapy Association.

Murphy, F. J. (2003). House passes IDEA reauthorization bill. *Exceptional Parent, 33*(6), 28–29.

Murphy, R. F. (1990). *The body silent.* New York: Norton.

Nagi, S. Z. (1965). Some conceptual issues in disability and rehabilitation. In M. B. Sussman (Ed.), *Sociology and rehabilitation* (pp. 104–113). Washington, DC: American Sociological Association.

Nagi, S. Z. (1991). Disability concepts revisited: Implications for prevention. In A. M. Pope & A. R. Tarlov (Eds.), *Disability in America* (pp. 309–327). Washington, DC: National Academy Press.

Padilla, R. (2003). Clara: A phenomenology of disability. *American Journal of Occupational Therapy, 57,* 413–423.

Parkes, C. M. (1998). *Bereavement: Studies of grief in adult life.* Madison, CT: International Universities Press.

Parkes, C. M., & Weiss, R. S. (1983). The recovery process. In C. M. Parkes & R. S. Weiss (Eds.), *Recovery from bereavement* (pp. 155–168). Basic (Basic Books, Inc., Publishers): New York.

Perkinson, H. J. (1984). *Learning from our mistakes: A reinterpretation of twentieth century educational theory.* Westport, CT: Greenwood Press.

Perkinson, H. J. (1993). *Teachers without goals, students without purposes.* New York: McGraw-Hill.

Popper, K. R. (1992). Emancipation through knowledge. In L. J. Bennett (Trans.), *In search of a better world: Lectures and essays from thirty years* (pp. 137–150). London: Routledge.

Price-Lackey, P., & Cashman, J. (1996). Jenny's story: Reinventing oneself through occupation and narrative configuration. *American Journal of Occupational Therapy, 50,* 306–314.

Rogers, J. C., & Holm, M. B. (1994). Nationally speaking—Accepting the challenge of outcome research: Examining the effectiveness of occupational therapy practice. *American Journal of Occupational Therapy, 48,* 871–876.

Schön, D. A. (1983). *The reflective practitioner: How professionals think in action.* Basic (Basic Books, Inc., Publishers): New York.

Tham, K., & Kielhofner, G. (2003). Impact of the social environment on occupational experience and performance among persons with unilateral neglect. *American Journal of Occupational Therapy, 57,* 403–412.

Trombly, C. A. (1993). The issue is—Anticipating the future: Assessment of occupational function. *American Journal of Occupational Therapy, 47,* 253–257.

Trombly, C. A. (1995). Occupation: Purposefulness and meaningfulness as therapeutic mechanisms, 1995 Eleanor Clarke Slagle Lecture. *American Journal of Occupational Therapy, 49,* 960–972.

Wilbarger, P., & Wilbarger, J. L. (1991). *Sensory defensiveness in children aged 2–12: An intervention guide for parents and other caretakers.* Santa Barbara, CA: Avanti Educational Programs.

Wilbarger, P., & Wilbarger, J. L. (1997). *Sensory defensiveness and related social/emotional and neurological problems* [course syllabus]. Oak Park Heights, MN: Professional Development Programs. (original copyright 1992)

Wood, P. H. N. (1980). Appreciating the consequences of disease: The international classification of impairments, disabilities, and handicaps. *WHO Chronicle, 34,* 376–380.

Wood, W. (1998). Nationally speaking—It is jump time for occupational therapy. *American Journal of Occupational Therapy, 52,* 403–411.

World Health Organization. (1980). *International classification of impairments, disabilities, and handicaps.* Geneva, Switzerland: Author.

World Health Organization. (2001). *ICF: International classification of functioning, disability, and health, short version.* Geneva, Switzerland: Author.

Youngstrom, M. J. (2002). *Report of the chairperson of the Commission on Practice, III.C. to the Representative Assembly* (RA charge number 2002M29). Bethesda, MD: American Occupational Therapy Association.

11

Using Activities as Challenges to Facilitate Development of Functional Skills

Joyce Shapero Sabari, PhD, OTR, BCN, FAOTA

Previous chapters of this text have discussed how we use activities in occupational therapy as an end goal. Occupational therapists determine which areas of occupation are meaningful to a client that are now difficult to perform. Interventions include development of compensatory strategies, selection and modification of available assistive devices, design and fabrication of unique assistive devices, and focused practice of relevant tasks.

Critical interventions exist to enable clients to improve performance in selected activities. If underlying impairments remain unchanged, however, these improvements are not likely to generalize to performance of other occupations. When a therapist determines that a client demonstrates potential to improve underlying client factors or performance skills, the client deserves the opportunity to work toward restoration of foundational motor, cognitive, or interactive capacities.

Think about the goals you would set for yourself, or a loved one, if faced with limitations in activity performance. Suppose your friend is unable to perform instrumental activities of daily living because his organizational and problem-solving skills have been affected by a traumatic brain injury. If he exhibits potential to improve these underlying cognitive skills, would an occupational therapy program consisting only of specific task practice be sufficient? What if your younger sister demonstrates impairments in hand coordination that limit her ability to learn handwriting skills? You would want occupational therapy to offer her the opportunity to improve her underlying limitations in addition to specific handwriting practice or the provision of adapted writing utensils. Suppose your grandfather has survived a stroke with intact cognition. He demonstrates some movement throughout his paretic left arm but is unable to use the arm for task performance. Would you be satisfied with an occupational therapy program that is limited to teaching one-handed self-care techniques?

Previous chapters have discussed the *ICF: International Classification of Functioning, Disability, and Health* (World Health Organization, 2001). Occupational therapy practitioners provide interventions that improve performance in areas of occupation through balanced interventions that (a) maximize the client's potential to improve client factors and performance skills (factors internal to the client) and (b) minimize activity limitation through compensatory approaches (factors external to the client). Figure 11.1 illustrates that occupational therapy practitioners balance these internally and externally directed interventions to promote performance of occupations that will enhance participation in family and community situations.

Improvements in internal factors are critical to the occupational therapy process because they enable clients to perform an infinite number of tasks in a variety of situations. Such improvements empower them to create and discover unanticipated occupations and roles.

This chapter describes the use of "occupation as means" (Trombly, 2002) or "enabling activities" (Pedretti & Early, 2001) where occupational therapy practitioners design activities to provide structured challenges to reduce specific impairments and improve specific skills. Practitioners use activities in three major ways to promote improvements in internal factors:

1.   Present an activity to provide the interest level that enables clients to exert more effort, complete more repetitions of a desired behavior, or sustain performance for a longer duration.

2.   Manipulate selected activity and environmental conditions to present graded challenges to specific skills.

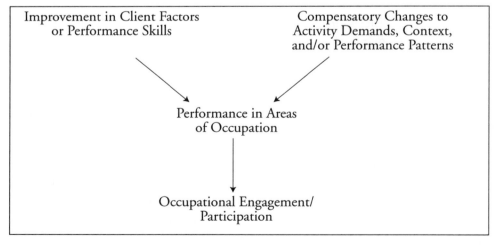

Figure 11.1. Activity-based intervention in occupational therapy is a balance between internally and externally directed interventions to improve performance in areas of occupation and, ultimately, participation in valued roles.

3. Select activities that will provide "problems" that challenge a client to develop effective cognitive or motor strategies that can be generalized to an unlimited variety of future situations.

Although categories overlap somewhat, occupational therapy students must understand when each type of "occupation as means" may be most appropriate and which concepts are most relevant to apply when using occupation as means in each of these three ways.

Using Activities to Elicit Greater Effort, Repetition, or Duration Than Traditional Exercise

Historically, the earliest use of activities in occupational therapy may have been as a medium to facilitate improvement in underlying client factors and performance skills (Taylor, 1929). Research findings (Bloch, Smith, & Nelson, 1989; Kircher, 1984; Steinbeck, 1986) have indicated that healthy adults exert greater cardiovascular and muscular effort, as evidenced by faster heart rate and increased electromyographic activity in selected muscles, when performing activities that they perceive to be fun (e.g., jumping rope) compared to exercises with similar motor components (e.g., jumping in place). Using activities as interventions for this purpose is relevant when treatment goals are to improve cardiopulmonary and specific muscle endurance.

Performance of interesting activity also promotes greater repetition and prolonged duration of physical output than does performance of routine exercise programs (DeKuiper, Nelson, & White, 1993; Hsieh, Nelson, Smith, & Peterson, 1996; Lang, Nelson, & Bush, 1992; Miller & Nelson, 1987; Nelson et al., 1996; Riccio, Nelson, & Bush, 1990; Steinbeck, 1986; Yoder, Nelson, & Smith, 1989). This is well understood in current popular culture, as evidenced by the use of dance routines and embedded games during aerobic exercise and muscle toning sessions at community fitness centers. When muscle endurance or joint flexibility are treatment goals, it is advantageous for the client to produce more repetitions over a longer duration of actions that demand optimal levels of muscle output or soft tissue elongation (Downey & Darling, 1994). When seeking to decrease distal limb edema, repetitive isotonic contractions of muscles in the targeted body segment are a recognized complement to medical and positioning interventions (Burkhardt, 1998; Trombly, 2002).

Research findings provide evidence that people with disabilities exhibit greater range of motion (i.e., perform closer to their maximum potential) when engaged in interesting activities than when performing under conventional exercise conditions. In one study, Van der Weel, van der Meer, and Lee (1991) encouraged children with cerebral palsy who exhibited right hemiparesis to actively perform the forearm movements of pronation and supination. While performing within the experimental condition, the children were instructed to use a drumstick to bang on drums that were positioned to require full forearm range of motion. During the control condition, the same children were instructed to move the drumstick back and forth as far as they could in the frontal plane. Movement range was significantly greater when banging the drums than during the abstract exercise condition.

Sietsema, Nelson, Mulder, Mervau-Scheidel, and White (1993) had similar findings in their study of forward reach in adults with hemiparesis caused by traumatic brain injury. Neurodevelopmental treatment strategies were used to prepare study participants for forward reach from the sitting position. In the exercise condition, participants reached out their hands as far as they could in a rote manner. In the activity condition, they reached forward to control Simon®, a popular computer-controlled game that challenges players to repeat its sequences of flashing lights and sounds by pressing colored panels. Data collected through computerized motion analysis revealed that participants displayed significantly greater mobility when engaged in the activity than when they attempted to reach forward in a purely exercise context.

In pediatric intervention, the use of playful, inviting sensory integration equipment serves, in part, to pique children's interest in and sustain their performance of activities that provide vestibular, tactile, or proprioceptive stimuli they might otherwise avoid. The introduction of imaginative play may engage the child still further and, thus, encourage longer duration of involvement and expenditure of greater effort during treatment sessions.

What makes an activity engaging enough that it will entice a person to continue a performance while repetitively performing a prescribed exercise or practicing a new skill? The answer depends on each person. A person's interest in specific activities is influenced by a complex array of factors, including his or her cultural background, age, and prior experiences. Csikszentmihalyi and Csikszentmihalyi (1988) coined the term *flow* to describe the extremely positive state in which a person is so involved in an activity that nothing else seems to matter. "Flow activities" are those sequences of action that make it easy for people to achieve this optimal experience state. During flow activities, participants reach a state of focused attention and believe that the activity's outcomes are under their own control, and the process becomes as enjoyable as reaching the activity goal.

Understanding the characteristics of flow activities is useful to occupational therapy practitioners when designing activities that will motivate clients to participate in therapeutic interventions. Figure 11.2 illustrates that a state of flow depends on the person's sense of a balance between a task's challenge and his or her own current skill level. When both skill and task challenge are perceived as being low, Csikszentmihalyi and Csikszentmihalyi (1988) predicted that apathy will ensue. A person will be bored (experience boredom) when he or she views his or her skill as far exceeding the task challenge. When task challenges exceed the person's skill, the person is likely to experience anxiety. Only when a task challenge is well balanced with a person's skill is there potential for a sense of flow to occur (see Figure 11.2). Csikszentmihalyi and Csikszentmihalyi described two additional criteria for flow activities: (a) the goals of the activity must be clear to the participant, and (b) the activity itself provides a continuous source of unambiguous feedback about how well the person is doing.

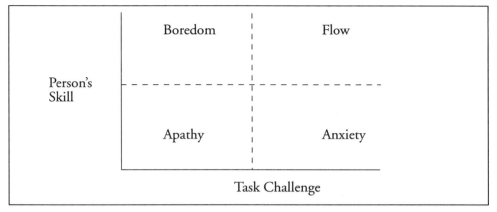

Figure 11.2. A state of flow depends on the person's sense that balance exists between a task's challenge and his or her own current skill level.

Note. From "Introduction to Part IV" by M. Csikszentmihalyi & I. S. Csikszentmihalyi (Eds.), *Optimal experience: Psychological studies of flow in consciousness,* 1988, p. 261, New York: Cambridge University Press. Copyright © 1999 by Cambridge University Press. Reprinted with permission.

In our attempt to create activities that will entice clients to perform repetitive practice of specific movements or skills, occupational therapy practitioners may be tempted to present tasks that are so contrived that they hold little meaning for our clients (Fisher, 1998). If an occupational therapy activity does little to facilitate a flow experience, no advantage exists to choosing activity over exercise as an intervention.

The occupational therapist must learn as much as possible about each client's previous skills, interests, and activity background. This information, combined with our knowledge of the person's current strengths and limitations, is critical to setting feasible treatment goals. Although this information may also be helpful when selecting therapeutic activities, flow activities do not necessarily need to be related to a client's prior repertoire of activity interests. "It does not matter whether one originally wanted to do the activity, whether one expected to enjoy it, or not. Even a frustrating job may suddenly become exciting if one hits upon the right balance" (Csikszentmihalyi & Csikszentmihalyi, 1988, p. 32). For many adults, an enabling activity need not have been a favorite prior pastime. In fact, sometimes a well-meaning practitioner is disappointed to learn that selection of favorite tasks as therapeutic interventions frustrates rather than brings pleasure to a client. The client who worked as an electrician may become disheartened to see that simple wiring tasks are now excessively challenging. The avid puzzle solver may be dismayed to be practicing crossword puzzles designed for children. The match between the intrinsic interest level afforded by an activity and the person's understanding of why the practice is important is key in determining how successful an activity will be in eliciting pleasure during sustained performance. As in all other aspects of occupational therapy, active involvement in the total therapeutic process enhances a client's motivation to participate.

Occupational therapy practitioners must consider a few critical words of caution when using activities to elicit repetitive performance of prescribed movement sequences. First, repetitive movements must be performed only from a position of optimal alignment. The practitioner must avoid activities that are ergonomically unsound while providing appropriate therapeutic positioning and handling to enhance the client's performance and comfort. Second, therapeutic activities are not introduced unless the client demonstrates adequate prerequisite factors and skills. For example, there is no therapeutic value to introducing a task that requires repetitive active reaching unless the client exhibits the necessary joint play and muscle distensibility that will allow adequate passive range of motion at all the joints of the shoulder complex. Finally, practitioners need to remember that repetition must occur naturally within the activity performance. Setting up a checkerboard affords the opportunity for repetitive practice of reach, grasp, and release. The activity component, however, is maintained only if this initial placement of game pieces is followed by an actual game of checkers (with a family member, a volunteer, or another client). In an effort to foster even more repetition, a practitioner may be tempted to ask a client to remove the checkers and begin the task again. Although this contrivance may be effective once or twice, it quickly reduces what may have begun as an interesting activity to a rote exercise that is unlikely to maintain the client's interest over time.

Case Scenario

Jack is a 19-year-old who sustained a spinal cord injury caused by a fracture of the sixth cervical vertebra 4 weeks earlier in a motor vehicle accident. At this time, he demonstrates good strength bilaterally in deltoid, rotator cuff, pectoralis major, biceps, pronator teres, and extensor carpi radialis longus and brevis. One current goal is to develop skill in functionally using a tenodesis grasp pattern (Figure 11.3). This requires repetitive practice picking up lightweight objects by coordinating active wrist extension with the resultant passive tenodesis flexion of his fingers. Wearing an orthosis fabricated by his occupational therapist that maintains his thumb, index, and middle fingers in optimal alignment, Jack tried out his new skill by playing the solitary board game, Think and Jump™ (©Pressman). He finds it pleasurable to try to surpass his record of jumping over and removing pieces from the playing board. For each repetition of the game Jack completes, including setting up the game board, he practices tenodesis grasp and release up to 74 times.

Using Activities to Provide Graded Challenges

Repetition alone will not promote improvements in all client factors and performance skills. When client goals are to enhance muscle strength, range of motion, balance, or coordination, practice sessions must afford opportunities for incremental increases in appropriate demands. The key to effectively using activities to provide graded chal-

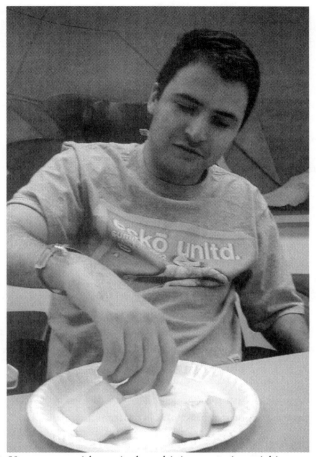

Figure 11.3. Young man with a spinal cord injury practices picking up pieces of apple with a tenodesis grasp.

lenges is the therapist's identification of a specific, relevant continuum on which gradations will be introduced. For example, if the client's goal is to improve active hip and pelvic mobility when sitting, placement of activity objects in relation to the client will represent a relevant continuum. Because the weight or the size of activity objects essentially will be irrelevant to the specific performance of active hip motion, these factors will not be manipulated when making incremental changes to the activity demands. Gentile's (1972, 1987) concept of "regulatory conditions" refers to those environmental features that directly influence a person's choice of strategies for performing a selected task. When designing activities to present graded challenges, practitioners determine which features in the environment and the selected task are "regulatory" to the skills they seek to challenge (Sabari, 1991). Figure 11.4 illustrates the variety of regulatory conditions that can be manipulated to influence the performance requirements for engaging in therapeutic tasks.

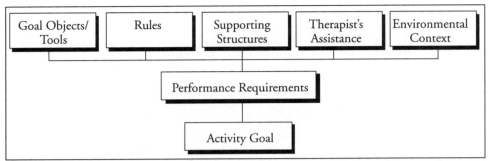

Figure 11.4. Regulatory conditions that can be graded to alter an activity's performance requirements.

Goal Objects and Tools

Goal objects and tools are those items that a person must act on or manipulate within the course of task performance. These objects and tools can be adapted according to size, shape, weight, and texture (American Occupational Therapy Association, 1993; Trombly, 2002). In addition, their position in relation to the person will significantly influence which movements and balance adjustments will be required for task performance. Goal objects also may vary between being static, such as a jar of paint placed next to an easel, or in motion, such as a ball during a game of catch or the action figures in a computer game. When goal objects are moving, their trajectories may be either predictable or unpredictable. Each variation places different demands on the person's requirements to use perceptual–motor skills.

Rules

Rules guide performance of hobbies, crafts, games, and sports. Creative adaptations in rules can tailor an activity to allow for grading along dimensions as varied as turn-taking, cognitive complexity, social interaction, use of imagination, and specific motor skills.

Supporting Structures

Supporting structures can be graded to provide incremental challenges to balance and dynamic motor performance. Whether a supporting structure is a chair, a bolster, a floor surface on which the client stands, or a piece of suspended play equipment, the occupational therapy practitioner can create variations in shape, weight, texture, base of support, and degree of external support. In addition, supporting structures can be graded along a continuum, beginning with stationary support to increasingly unstable or dynamic surfaces.

The Practitioner

The occupational therapy practitioner also may be viewed as a regulatory condition influencing the clients' performance requirements. We can vary the ways in which we provide instructions and feedback as well as the ways in which we provide physical handling to support or assist a client in task performance. Such assistance is graded down incrementally to provide clients with opportunities to develop increasing ability in the skill toward which our intervention is focused.

Environmental Context

Finally, the environmental context introduces a variety of additional regulatory conditions. Competitive noises or visual distractions place higher demands on attentional skills and can be graded through adaptations to the setting in which therapeutic intervention is provided. Physical obstacles, even when they are not central to the actual activity, can be used to pose graded cognitive, perceptual, and motor challenges. Table 11.1 offers examples of selected factors and corresponding "regulatory features" that would be appropriate to adjust when the intervention is designed to present relevant, graded challenges.

The following case scenario provides a clinical example of how one occupational therapist uses activity grading within a group setting to assist clients in achieving specific goals related to trusting others and developing a repertoire of wellness behaviors.

Case Scenario

Cynthia is coordinating a relaxation group for six members who attend an outpatient community mental health day program. All clients are considered to have severe and persistent mental illness. This group is part of a larger wellness program in which participants are learning to manage their psychiatric symptoms and develop healthier lifestyles. Group members exhibit difficulty committing themselves to new styles of behavior and to exposing their vulnerabilities to others. Cynthia will grade the group's activities along a continuum of increasing trust within a group framework and use the clients' strengths and interests in maintaining good health to motivate interest.

At the first session, the group members are required to take off their coats (hanging them on wall hooks that are clearly visible in the same room) and sit in a circle on wooden chairs. Initial activities include practicing deep-breathing strategies and performing active stretching of neck muscles. At subsequent sessions, clients also remove their shoes to practice foot and ankle stretches, then progress to facial exercises with eyeglasses off. Cynthia encourages group members to appreciate the humor in their facial expressions of frowning, grinning, and pouting to enhance their level of trust and comfort in doing awkward and unfamiliar movements. Gradually, larger body movements are added to the

Table 11.1
Regulatory Features of Tasks That Correspond With Grading to Challenge Specific Client Factors or Skills

Factor	*Intervention Strategies*
Figure–ground perception	• Complexity of the visual background or similarity between the visual background and the key foreground object (provided in real-life hide-and-seek games or paper-and-pencil puzzles)
Active range of motion: shoulder flexion	• Height of object placement
Active range of motion: finger flexion	• Size of handles to grasp
Strength of specific muscles	• Placement of objects in relation to gravity (gravity eliminated to lightweight objects to be moved against gravity) • Increased weight (resistance) against gravity • Length of lever arm (short resistance arm to progressively longer resistance arm)
Praxis	• Complexity of a novel motor task
Fine motor coordination and dexterity	• Size and shape of tool (gross to fine grasp) • Size, texture, and shape of objects to be manipulated • Increased demands on speed of performance • Increased demands on manipulation of objects
Standing balance	• Size and stability of base of support (progress from larger, most stable base to smaller, less stable base) • Amount of weight shift required in all planes of motion (achieved through placement of goal objects in relation to the person)
Attention span	• Increased time necessary to complete a task
Social interaction	• The interactive nature of tasks, which may progress from parallel task performance alongside another person, to activities requiring dyadic interaction, to activities requiring increasing amounts of sharing views and feelings with one or more persons

group repertoire. Eventually, Cynthia demonstrates relaxation activities performed supine on a floor mat and encourages group members to try these in private at home as well. An ultimate goal of this grading process is for clients to reach a comfort level in which they are able to sufficiently trust the group to engage in a full repertoire of relaxation exercises considered to be popular and healthful in the larger society and to use these techniques to relieve stress or symptoms.

Similar precautions to those described when using activities to promote repetitive, sustained performance also hold true when practitioners present activities as a series of graded challenges. The practitioner must ensure that in any activity requiring movement, the client is performing from a position of optimal body alignment. Particularly when grading is achieved by altering a support surface or by introducing objects that have been strategically placed at increasingly more challenging locations, the practitioner must pay close attention to the client's general body posture as well as to maintaining appropriate alignment at specific body segments. If the practitioner does not, what he or she planned as a therapeutic intervention may promote inefficient and potentially harmful motor strategies.

Before selecting a treatment sequence that is based on graded activity performance, the therapist must determine whether the client demonstrates potential to benefit from this type of intervention. It is not always the case that simply providing increasingly difficult challenges will result in functional improvements. Occupational therapists must collaborate with other team members to determine what combination of medical, orthotic, physical, and educational measures should precede or accompany graded activity performance.

Occupational therapy practitioners should strive to avoid two common mistakes when using activity grading as a therapeutic intervention. First, activity grading becomes counterproductive when the client perceives it as an unfair "tease." In this situation, a well-meaning but overzealous practitioner constantly upgrades the challenge of therapeutic tasks so that the client never achieves the satisfaction of performing activities more easily. For example, after struggling to achieve improved reach in the context of making a macramé rug, the client deserves an opportunity to work with the materials positioned within reasonable access. The practitioner, however, in an attempt to continually challenge the client's improving abilities, constantly repositions the wall-mounted rug so that it is always just away from comfortable reach. Blanche (1997) has warned practitioners who use toys as lures to motivate young children to reach or ambulate that the practice becomes misguided if the practitioner constantly moves the toy farther and farther away as the child approaches in an attempt to upgrade the child's efforts.

A second problem occurs when a client is participating in an occupational therapy program designed to promote improvements in multiple areas. For example, a child may be working to improve cognitive as well as gross mobility skills. It would be a mistake to grade treatment activities so that cognitive and gross mobility challenges are simultaneously increased. Rather, the practitioner should account for the likelihood that increased demands in one skill domain might have a negative effect on the child's demonstrated skills in other domains. Consider how you might function if you were challenged to your ultimate limits in trying to perform a triple-axel ice skating jump. Would that be the best moment for you to grapple with a difficult mathematics problem? Similarly, a woman who demonstrates dual problems with balance and fine hand coordination may have recently achieved the ability to sit unsupported in a standard chair. When confronted with a challenging task in which she must manipulate objects with both hands, however, her ability to function at her highest level in maintaining sitting balance may be temporarily diminished. In another example, a young woman who has survived a traumatic brain injury may demonstrate problems related to socially appropriate behavior as well as cognitive processing and motor control. When the treatment emphasis is on upgrading demands for social interaction, the intellectual and motoric challenges of a group activity must be kept as simple as possible. The skillful practitioner knows how to alter a task's regulatory conditions so that when grading *up* on one dimension, demands to other domains will be kept at manageable levels. In many cases, the practitioner will structure the activity so that competing demands are temporarily graded *down*.

Using Activities to Promote Development of Effective Strategies for Performance Skills

For many people, the essential occupational therapy goal is to develop performance skills through a process of learning. Teaching and learning as part of occupational therapy intervention are necessary for clients of all ages whose goals are to improve postural control, motor control, cognitive abilities, interpersonal skills, and coping mechanisms. Neither activity repetition nor activity grading may be sufficient interventions when the therapeutic goal is to assist clients in learning and generalizing effective strategies for their performance of daily tasks.

Strategies are organized plans or sets of rules that guide action in a variety of situations (Sabari, 1998). We all have developed a variety of strategies that serve as foundational guidelines for effective participation in daily activities. Many of these strategies have been so well learned that they seem to be automatic. Without them, however, the challenges of performing occupations would be overwhelming.

Motor Strategies

Motor strategies include the vast repertoire of kinematic and kinetic linkages that underlie performance of skilled, efficient movement. For example, when reaching forward to turn on the computer, the strategy of anteriorly tilting the pelvis ensures sufficient mobility of the trunk and scapula. The strategy of abducting and upwardly rotating the scapula enhances the smooth mobility of the arm's trajectory (Neumann, 2002). Specific hand-shaping (Jeannerod, 1990) and visual guidance (Shumway-Cook

& Woollacott, 2001; Wing & Frazer, 1983) strategies enable the index finger to reach the start button with a minimum of effort. Other motor strategies include those automatic plans of action that enable us to maintain our balance throughout infinite varieties of environmental support and challenges to our centers of mass. In addition, we routinely implement strategies that will ensure our "postural readiness" (Abreu, 1998) to perform desired tasks. Think about the task of turning on the computer. What strategies do you use for establishing a base of support and alignment of body segments that ultimately make it easier and more efficient to accomplish your goal?

Cognitive Strategies

Cognitive strategies include the multiple and varied tactics we use to facilitate processing, storing, retrieving, and manipulating information. What cognitive strategies have you found to be useful in negotiating the academic demands of being a college (or graduate) student? Sitting close to a lecturer and jotting down questions to ask after class may be effective strategies that enable one to process information in a large, noninteractive class setting. Reorganizing and rewording class notes regularly aid in storing course information. Categorizing and drawing one's own visual models may be helpful in storing, retrieving, and manipulating information. Cognitive strategies influence our performance of all activities, whether they be simple or complex. Grocery shopping can be achieved more efficiently if one uses the strategies of taking a kitchen inventory, generating a shopping list, organizing the list according to the supermarket layout, and assembling appropriate discount coupons. When basic self-care tasks are challenging to people because of brain injury or developmental disabilities, selection and use of appropriate cognitive strategies make it possible to achieve independence and autonomy.

Interpersonal Strategies

Interpersonal strategies assist us in our social interactions with other people. During child and adolescent development, as well as every time we join a new cultural group, we learn the normative practices of social engagement within a given context. Interpersonal strategies are required for forming and maintaining friendships, for expressing our opinions in various situations, for enlisting assistance by strangers or by family members, and for conducting routine transactions within our communities. Many people requiring occupational therapy intervention can benefit from the opportunity to develop more effective interpersonal strategies.

Coping Strategies

Coping strategies allow people to adapt constructively to stress (Giles, 2003). We experience stress when we perceive that events or factors in our environment exceed our current resources. Effective coping strategies are critical to preventing negative physiological, cognitive, and emotional sequelae to stressful situations. A framework developed by Williamson, Szczepanski, and Zeitlin (1993) postulates that coping strategies are elicited by a sequence of interactions between a person and the environment in a four-step interrelated process. During the first step, the person determines the meaning of a stressful event or situation. A useful strategy at this step would be to logically review the factors that are perceived to be stressful and to analyze the demands of the situation in relation to one's own resources. During this process of "primary appraisal," the person determines whether and how much the perceived stressor is, indeed, harmful or challenging. The strategy of distancing oneself temporarily from the stressful situation may facilitate this appraisal process. The tactic of "cognitive restructuring" (Giles, 2003) may assist a person in identifying cognitive distortions that may lead to inappropriate interpretations of stress.

The second step is to develop an action plan. Effective strategies at this phase include the practice of taking stock of all available options and enlisting appropriate assistance from others. The choice of an action plan that accurately capitalizes on one's own resources and accounts for one's limitations is critical to the effectiveness of the coping process.

Implementing a coping effort based on the action plan is the third step to effectively coping with a stressor. This coping effort produces an outcome that will elicit feedback from the environment. The fourth step, evaluating effectiveness of the coping effort, depends on the person's ability to effectively assess cues from the social and physical environment in relation to his or her own actions. A strategy of identifying and taking pleasure from small achievements is helpful in deriving feelings of success in situations that might otherwise be perceived as overwhelming.

Strategies should be viewed as frameworks rather than as recipes. They provide us with foundational skills that are meant to be adapted to the ever-changing demands of the occupations in which we engage and the infinite variations of multiple environments. Although there never is only one correct strategy, some strategies may have a negative effect on a person's future success or well-being. The practitioner must guide clients toward developing strategies that are likely to have long-term positive implications.

People develop strategies through a process of encountering "problems," implementing solutions, and monitoring the effects of the solutions. "In child development, an experienced adult guides the child through problem-solving activities and structures the child's learning environment by selecting, focusing, and organizing incoming stimuli" (Toglia, 1998, p. 12). "Through transactions in the environment, children try out, practice, and integrate coping strategies into their behavioral repertoire" (Williamson et al., 1993, p. 396).

Strategy development continues throughout our lives. New jobs, new relationships, and new hobbies present us with new sets of problems to be solved. Changes in our physical status, concomitant with normal aging, disease, or disability, create the need for altered strategies when performing familiar tasks.

Sometimes we are lucky enough to get advice or instruction to guide us in the formation of new strategies. Our success in tennis will be enhanced if we learn, early on, some basic rules about postural set, kinematic linkages, and offensive and defensive tactics. Facility at the computer keyboard will be promoted if we practice touch-typing techniques. Ergonomic strategies for positioning of work station materials will have a positive impact on our long-term visual and musculoskeletal health. A coworker's advice about how to interact with a particular administrator will guide us in developing effective on-the-job strategies.

How do practitioners use activities to assist clients in developing useful strategies? We structure tasks within a safe environment that provides clients with opportunities to try out different solutions to actual "problems." The occupational therapy practitioner selects the problems in accordance with the goals for each client. For example, for Trina, who is a preschool child with balance dysfunction, the problem might be to figure out how to stay upright while pushing a doll carriage. Instead of providing solutions, the practitioner offers "suggestions" to Trina through physical handling and artful structuring of the play situation (Pierce, 1997). For Scott, a young adult with schizophrenia, a set of problems might be presented within the context of working as a salesperson in the hospital-run thrift shop. Potential problems could include the challenge of interacting appropriately with customers or the challenge of maintaining interest in the work when business is slow. The practitioner would assist Scott in reflecting on the efficacy of the solutions he has chosen and help him to determine strategies that might guide his future performance in this and other work experiences. The ultimate goal in this type of activity intervention is that the client will develop strategies that perhaps can be generalized to a wide variety of occupations and environments.

Self-awareness and self-monitoring skills are critical prerequisites to a person's ability to generate and apply appropriate strategies. Metacognition (Katz & Hartman-Maier, 1998) is the knowledge and regulation of personal cognitive processes and capacities. It includes an awareness of personal strengths and limitations and the ability to evaluate task difficulty, plan ahead, choose appropriate strategies, and shift strategies in response to environmental cues.

Toglia's (1991, 1998) dynamic interactional model for people with cognitive impairments caused by brain injury emphasizes the importance of metacognition. In this treatment approach, occupational therapy intervention begins by helping clients to develop insight about personal strengths and deficits through a program that challenges them to estimate task difficulty, predict outcomes, and evaluate personal performance. The practitioner then presents tasks that have been synthesized to present selected challenges and that guide the client in selecting appropriate strategies for meeting these challenges. Self-review of one's own performance and guided planning for tackling the challenges of future tasks are key factors in the therapeutic process.

Clients who need to develop improved interpersonal or coping strategies also benefit from therapeutic attention to metacognitive processes. The practitioner plays an important role in guiding the clients' self-reflection on relevant components of task performance.

Self-awareness also is valuable to people with impairments in motor or postural control who wish to learn effective strategies for movement and task performance. Just as assessment of one's cognitive or interpersonal strengths and weaknesses is critical to developing strategies in these areas, the child with cerebral palsy and the woman who has sustained a stroke need to accurately assess when their body segments are optimally aligned or when they are posturally ready to perform particular activities. The practitioner provides effective feedback about kinematic aspects of performance and graded physical guidance to assist these clients in developing effective self-monitoring of their movement strategies (Sabari, 1998).

The use of activities to stimulate strategy development requires extensive knowledge and creativity. Whether the intervention is directed toward developing motor, cognitive, interpersonal, or coping strategies, the practitioner must be an expert about that area of function. A thorough knowledge base, skill in analyzing performance, and the ability to anticipate how environmental and task demands are likely to affect function are required for effective intervention.

A key component is that the activity challenges must be presented in a safe environment that allows for mistakes, self-reflection, and dynamic interaction with the practitioner. Although values exist to provide this type of activity intervention in a naturalistic environment, the practitioner must consider that public spaces may be embarrassing places for clients to be developing basic strategies. For example, a supermarket or public library may not be an appropriate place for trying new motor or cognitive strategies. Occupational therapy interventions should avoid contributing to making clients feel like objects of pity in social or community situations. Rather, the practitioner can simulate challenges in the client's home or in the therapy setting, where it may be emotionally and physically safer to begin the process of strategy development. Once the client has sufficiently mastered the necessary strategies, it is then advisable to provide opportunities to practice in real-world environments.

Case Scenario

Tommy is a 4-year-old boy who has been referred to occupational therapy because his excessive activity level, impulsiveness, and motor incoordination are affecting his ability to function successfully in his preschool classroom. The occupational therapist has determined that Tommy has difficulty identifying environmental cues that are important to successful activity outcomes. Therefore, one occupational therapy goal is to help him to develop strategies to improve his ability to match his motor acts to the requirements of the task.

Because Tommy demonstrates great interest in the "clown" beanbag toss board, the occupational therapist presents a problem. She informs Tommy that the clown has not eaten today and is very hungry. A bucket of beanbags that are chocolate-flavored (and the clown's favorite food) is placed at a distance that the therapist judges to be challenging but still possible for Tommy to be able to throw the "food" through the clown's mouth. The therapist asks Tommy, "What shall we do?" By asking Tommy to tell her what he intends to do before he does it, the therapist ensures that Tommy focuses on the relevant characteristics of distance, size, and position of the clown's mouth and the size and weight of the beanbags. His interest level in the activity will help him to learn to screen out extraneous environmental stimuli. After Tommy throws the "food," he must tell the occupational therapist what happened. To help him learn to assess his own performance, the therapist gives feedback such as, "You threw the food too hard" or "Look at the mouth when you throw." The therapist also can help Tommy to learn to modify his strategies as needed by encouraging him to "try another way" or asking him, "What can you do differently?"

The occupational therapist creates a safe environment with a playful atmosphere where Tommy can feel comfortable experimenting and making mistakes. In this way, Tommy will learn to engage in the following strategies:

- Focus on characteristics that are relevant to the task

- Assess his own behavior and actions about outcome and performance

- Implement changes in his behavior and actions based on the assessment.

In addition, the occupational therapist has collaborated with Tommy's teacher to develop ways of encouraging Tommy to use these strategies during classroom activities.

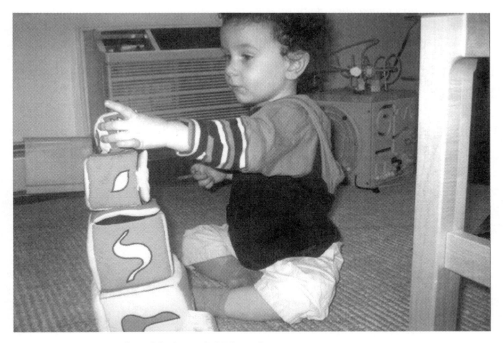

Figure 11.5. Boy stacking blocks with Hebrew letters.

Summary

The use of activities as interventions to improve client factors or develop performance skills is an important component of occupational therapy intervention. Based on a client's goals, the practitioner determines whether the activity program will be structured to (a) elicit repetition or longer duration of a desired behavior, (b) present graded challenges to specific skills, or (c) provide problems that challenge the client to develop appropriate strategies.

Regardless of the treatment setting, client background, or type of activity intervention, several criteria must be met. First, the client must be ready to participate in the selected activity. Prerequisite skills for performance must be assessed and interventions instituted to reduce physical, cognitive, or emotional factors that might constrain performance. Such constraints to performance can render an activity intervention useless or even harmful to a client. Second, the activity must be synthesized for each person. This synthesis is necessary to ensure that the activity will be useful toward developing skills that are specifically relevant for that person and will meet the third criterion, which is that the activity must provide some level of inherent interest to the person. In addition, the client must understand the dual purpose of the activity. Many clients are confused by the occupational therapy process. When an occupational therapy intervention is designed to promote improvements in underlying client factors or performance skills, clients need to be able to differentiate the underlying therapeutic purposes from the activity itself. Finally, occupational therapy intervention to improve client factors or performance skills is never isolated from the projected impact on a client's ability to perform meaningful tasks. The ultimate goal is always to facilitate performance of activities and roles that are meaningful to the person in the context of his or her own life. ∎

Acknowledgments

I wish to acknowledge Suzanne White, MA, OTR, and Margaret Kaplan, PhD, OTR, both clinical assistant professors, SUNY Downstate Medical Center, Brooklyn, New York, for providing the case scenarios about Cynthia and Tommy, respectively.

References

Abreu, B. (1998). The quadraphonic approach: Holistic rehabilitation for brain injury. In N. Katz (Ed.), *Cognition and occupation in rehabilitation: Cognitive models for intervention in occupational therapy* (pp. 51–97). Bethesda, MD: American Occupational Therapy Association.

American Occupational Therapy Association. (1993). Position paper: Purposeful activity. *American Journal of Occupational Therapy, 47,* 1081–1082.

Blanche, E. I. (1997). Doing with—not doing to: Play and the child with cerebral palsy. In L. D. Parham & L. S. Fazio (Eds.), *Play in occupational therapy for children* (pp. 202–218). St. Louis, MO: Mosby.

Bloch, M. W., Smith, D. A., & Nelson, D. L. (1989). Heart rate, activity, duration, and affect in added-purpose versus single-purpose jumping activities. *American Journal of Occupational Therapy, 43,* 25–30.

Burkhardt, A. (1998). Edema control. In G. Gillen & A. Burkhardt (Eds.), *Stroke rehabilitation: A function-based approach* (pp. 152–160). St. Louis, MO: Mosby.

Csikszentmihalyi, M., & Csikszentmihalyi, I. S. (Eds.). (1988). *Optimal experience: Psychological studies of flow in consciousness.* New York: Cambridge University Press.

DeKuiper, W. P., Nelson, D. L., & White, B. E. (1993). Materials-based occupation versus rote exercise: A replication and extension. *Occupational Therapy Journal of Research, 13,* 183–197.

Downey, J., & Darling, R. (Eds.). (1994). *Physiological basis of rehabilitation medicine* (2nd ed.). Boston: Butterworth-Heinemann.

Fisher, A. G. (1998). Uniting practice and theory in an occupational framework, 1998 Eleanor Clarke Slagle Lecture. *American Journal of Occupational Therapy, 52,* 509–519.

Gentile, A. M. (1972). A working model of skill acquisition with application to teaching. *Quest, 17,* 3–23.

Gentile, A. M. (1987). Skill acquisition: Action, movement, and neuromotor processes. In J. H. Carr, R. B. Shepherd, J. Gordon, A. M. Gentile, & J. N. Held (Eds.), *Movement science: Foundations for physical therapy in rehabilitation* (pp. 111–187). Rockville, MD: Aspen.

Giles, G. M. (2003). Interventions to improve person skills and abilities: Stress management. In E. B. Crepeau, E. S. Cohn, & B. A. B. Schell (Eds.), *Willard and Spackman's occupational therapy* (10th ed., pp. 637–642). Philadelphia: Lippincott, Williams & Wilkins.

Hsieh, C. L., Nelson, D. L., Smith, D. A., & Peterson, C. Q. (1996). A comparison of performance in added-purpose occupations and rote exercise for dynamic standing balance in persons with hemiplegia. *American Journal of Occupational Therapy, 50,* 10–16.

Jeannerod, M. (1990). *The neural and behavioral organization of goal-directed movements.* Oxford, England: Clarendon.

Katz, N., & Hartman-Maier, A. (1998). Metacognition: The relationships of awareness and executive functions to occupational performance. In N. Katz (Ed.), *Cognition and occupation in rehabilitation: Cognitive models for intervention in occupational therapy* (pp. 323–342). Bethesda, MD: American Occupational Therapy Association.

Kircher, M. A. (1984). Motivation as a factor of perceived exertion in purposeful versus nonpurposeful activity. *American Journal of Occupational Therapy, 38,* 165–170.

Lang, E. M., Nelson, D. L., & Bush, M. A. (1992). Comparison of performance in materials-based occupation, imagery-based occupation, and rote exercise in nursing home residents. *American Journal of Occupational Therapy, 46,* 607–611.

Miller, L., & Nelson, D. L. (1987). Dual-purpose activity versus single-purpose activity in terms of duration of task, exertion level, and affect. *Occupational Therapy in Mental Health, 7*(1), 55–67.

Nelson, D. L., Konosky, K., Fleharty, K., Webb, R., Newer, K., Hazboun, V. P., et al. (1996). The effects of an occupationally embedded exercise on bilaterally assisted supination in persons with hemiplegia. *American Journal of Occupational Therapy, 50,* 639–646.

Neumann, D. A. (2002). *Kinesiology of the musculoskeletal system: Foundations for physical rehabilitation.* St. Louis, MO: Mosby.

Pedretti, L. W., & Early, M. B. (2001). *Occupational therapy practice skills for physical dysfunction* (5th ed.). St. Louis, MO: Mosby.

Pierce, D. (1997). The power of object play for infants and toddlers at risk for developmental delays. In L. D. Parham & L. S. Fazio (Eds.), *Play in occupational therapy for children* (pp. 86–111). St. Louis, MO: Mosby.

Riccio, C. M., Nelson, D. L., & Bush, M. A. (1990). Adding purpose to the repetitive exercise of elderly women through imagery. *American Journal of Occupational Therapy, 44,* 714–719.

Sabari, J. (1991). Motor learning concepts applied to activity-based intervention with adults with hemiplegia. *American Journal of Occupational Therapy, 45,* 523–530.

Sabari, J. (1998). Application of learning and environmental strategies to activity-based treatment. In G. Gillen & A. Burkhardt (Eds.), *Stroke rehabilitation: A function-based approach* (pp. 31–46). St. Louis, MO: Mosby.

Shumway-Cook, A., & Woollacott, M. (2001). *Motor control: Theory and practical applications* (2nd ed.). Baltimore: Lippincott, Williams & Wilkins.

Sietsema, J. M., Nelson, D. L., Mulder, R. M., Mervau-Scheidel, D., & White, B. E. (1993). The use of a game to promote arm reach in persons with traumatic brain injury. *American Journal of Occupational Therapy, 47,* 19–24.

Steinbeck, T. M. (1986). Purposeful activity and performance. *American Journal of Occupational Therapy, 40,* 529–534.

Taylor, M. (1929). Occupational therapy in industrial inquiries. *Occupational Therapy and Rehabilitation, 8,* 335–338.

Toglia, J. P. (1991). Generalization of treatment: A multicontext approach to cognitive perceptual impairment in adults with brain injury. *American Journal of Occupational Therapy, 45,* 505–515.

Toglia, J. P. (1998). A dynamic interactional model to cognitive rehabilitation. In N. Katz (Ed.), *Cognition and occupation in rehabilitation: Cognitive models for intervention in occupational therapy* (pp. 5–50). Bethesda, MD: American Occupational Therapy Association.

Trombly, C. A. (2002). Occupation. In C. A. Trombly & M. V. Radomski (Eds.), *Occupational therapy for physical dysfunction* (5th ed., pp. 255–281). Baltimore: Lippincott, Williams & Wilkins.

Van der Weel, F. R., van der Meer, A. L. H., & Lee, D. N. (1991). Effect of task on movement control in cerebral palsy: Implications for assessment and therapy. *Developmental Medicine and Child Neurology, 33,* 419–426.

Williamson, G. G., Szczepanski, M., & Zeitlin, S. (1993). Coping frame of reference. In P. Kramer & J. Hinojosa (Eds.), *Frames of reference for pediatric occupational therapy* (pp. 395–436). Baltimore: Williams & Wilkins.

Wing, A. M., & Frazer, C. (1983). The contribution of the thumb to reaching movements. *Quarterly Journal of Experimental Psychology, 35A,* 297–309.

World Health Organization. (2001). *ICF: International classification of functioning, disability, and health, short version.* Geneva, Switzerland: Author.

Yoder, R. M., Nelson, D. L., & Smith, D. A. (1989). Added-purpose versus rote exercise in female nursing home residents. *American Journal of Occupational Therapy, 43,* 581–586.

12

Moving From Simulation to Real-Life Activity and Human Occupation

Anita Perr, MA, OT, FAOTA
Paulette Bell, MA, OTR

This chapter focuses on the significance of activities as part of the last steps in the habilitation or rehabilitation process and in preparation for real-life human occupation. Whereas many textbooks concentrate on occupational therapy and its use of purposeful activities in controlled environments, such as an occupational therapy clinic or lab or a patient's room or client's home, this chapter addresses the value of client-centered activities as part of the end goal of occupational therapy, which is a client's return to real life. Real life involves a client's participation in activities or occupations outside a controlled therapeutic environment. It often requires that a client engage in activities that he or she commonly performed in specific contexts and settings before his or her illness or injury. Additionally, real life for a person with disabilities often requires that he or she engage in new occupations and perform activities in new ways. These new activities may be needed to address changes in the client's ability to participate in activities of daily living, home care, hobbies, and work.

The occupational therapy practitioner assumes a critical role in the integration of a client into his or her natural contexts. Using the therapeutic value of active participation in purposeful activities, practitioners work in collaboration with the client, caregivers, significant others, and other professionals to match the client's engagement in an activity with therapeutic goals. The process by which a client is reintegrated into his or her environment involves a transition along a continuum from performance of contrived activities in a clinical or controlled environment (e.g., stacking blocks), to performance of simulated activities in clinical environments (e.g., role-playing a job interview with other clients), to performance of simulated activities in real environments (e.g., pretending to brush one's teeth at the bathroom sink), to performance of real activities in simulated environments (e.g., shaving at the sink in the occupational therapy clinic), to performance of real activities in real environments (e.g., taking a bus to school, making a meal at home). This process is depicted in Figure 12.1, which illustrates the client's reintegration into his or her environment. Simulation is a central concept in this transition and is discussed in this chapter.

Participation in Real-Life Activity and Occupation as the Goals of Occupational Therapy Intervention

The ability to participate in real life is the ultimate goal for clients receiving occupational therapy. Through a collaborative process, the client and occupational therapist identify and develop client-centered goals. This means that the occupational therapy goals are developed with the client and his or her significant others to meet the client's needs and address his or her specific environmental factors and personal factors.

Closely aligned with this concept of real life is the idea that real-life functioning assumes that the client is able to function independently. Occupational therapy practitioners often are concerned that the client is being independent and able to complete tasks by him- or herself. This goal, however, is only relevant if it is acceptable and appropriate for the client. The client's culture, support systems, and values should

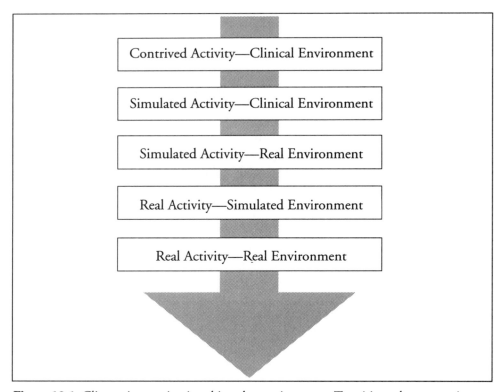

Figure 12.1. Client reintegration into his or her environment. Transitions along a continuum of activities are from contrived simulations to real-life occupations.

be considered when defining optimal participation. The concept of independence is of major importance because many people associate independence with the ability to perform or complete specific tasks, activities, or occupations. For occupational therapy practitioners, the concept of independence is defined from the client's perspective, that is, the ability of the client to direct his or her life. Independence is not necessarily based on the performance of the various tasks; rather, independence is the ability to execute the task in a manner that is acceptable to the client. Thus, independence for one client may be very different from independence for another client. For example, a client who has never cooked a meal and can afford to eat in restaurants may not wish to prepare food but would still be independent in his or her ability to acquire food or to be fed. Another client who needs or wishes to prepare food would need to be able to complete various tasks in order to be considered independent in food preparation. This view of independence becomes complex when one begins to adapt an activity or use assistive devices. Society often judges people with disabilities by a different standard from that used to judge people without disabilities, often viewing people with disabilities as limited in their participation because of the use of an adaptation or assistive device. For example, a client might need to write a list to remember what to do during the day. He or she would be independent related to the organization of daily routines but considered *independent with assistance* because he or she needs to write a daily list.

When independence is a goal, occupational therapy practitioners may modify environmental factors, use assistive technology, or integrate compensatory strategies to facilitate the client's participation in an activity. For instance, one goal for a client who was paralyzed following a cervical spinal cord injury may be to navigate the environment using a manual or power wheelchair. In this instance, independence required the use of a wheelchair (or assistive technology). Ultimately, from an occupational therapy practitioner's point of view, the client would be independent in mobility when the wheelchair is fully integrated into his or her real-life routine and he or she can independently move around in his or her environments. The use of a compensatory strategy, then, does not negate a person's independence; rather, such strategies are simply the means by which the person *is* independent.

Some clients may not be capable of or desire full independence. For a client who does not believe that he or she is capable of full independence in a particular activity, the occupational therapist must first evaluate the client to identify the obstacles. Do cognitive, psychological, or physical impairments limit independence? Is partial independence feasible? The practitioner may intervene by simplifying the activity to match the client's level of function and, thus, encourage the client's participation. In addition, the practitioner may adapt the activity, manipulate the contextual factors, or teach the client the use of assistive devices and compensatory techniques to facilitate task performance. The practitioner also may train the client to instruct others to help meet his or her needs.

In the following example, the occupational therapist and the client determine the client's potential for partial independence and select activities leading to this goal.

Although the client wants to dress independently, she is unable to do so fully because of paralysis in the right-dominant upper extremity, decreased dexterity in the non-dominant left hand, and difficulty sequencing the dressing activity.

The therapist's initial intervention may include a simulated activity in the clinic, such as having the client manipulate various clothing fasteners on a dressing board to improve dexterity in the left hand. Next, the client may learn compensatory one-handed dressing techniques, with the use of assistive devices such as a buttonhook and elastic shoelaces, during dressing at the bedside. In addition, the therapist may set up a contrived or simulated activity in the clinic to improve the client's ability to sequence dressing. The client may then progress to apply sequencing strategies so that she can dress during the morning routine. After the client has maximized the ability to dress, she still may only be partially independent in this area. The client may then need to think about when and how to ask for assistance appropriately.

In another example, a young man (see Figure 12.2) is practicing a sliding transfer with an occupational therapist in an occupational therapy clinic. The eventual goal is for him to transfer independently to and from all surfaces, the hardest of which is the transfer to and from a car. In Figure 12.3, we see another man who has mastered the transfer to and from his car. He is pictured performing this activity in the parking area of his apartment building. As shown, he uses a wheelchair, protective gloves, and a sliding board. When he has these devices, he is independent.

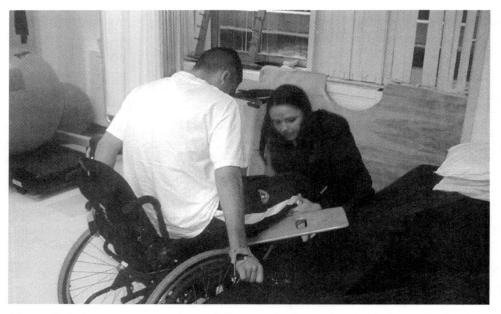

Figure 12.2. A young man practices a sliding transfer from a hospital bed to a wheelchair.

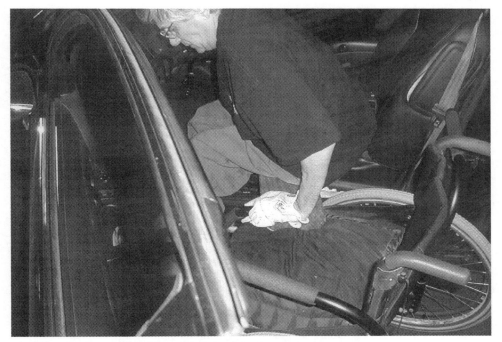

Figure 12.3. A man transfers independently to his car.

A client who does not want to perform all aspects of his or her daily activities personally may still exert control over his or her routine by determining which activities to delegate to others. The practitioner's intervention may include activities that help the client to improve the clarity and manner in which the client gives instructions to caregivers. The practitioner and client may role-play situations to optimize client–caregiver interactions. Activities that begin as simulations (e.g., role-playing) in a controlled environment transition into real life as the client directs the caregiver at home.

The goal of many clients is to become as independent as possible. Let us examine a client who was paralyzed following a spinal cord injury for an example of real-life activities that require assistance. This scenario also illustrates how the client defines independence.

Case Scenario

During the rehabilitation process, the client, Daphne, participates in a seating and wheeled mobility evaluation and eventually receives a power wheelchair and seating system that enable her to negotiate smooth and uneven terrain both indoors and outdoors. She is able to transfer independently to and from her wheelchair. Daphne has not been able to position her wheelchair for charging, to connect her wheelchair to the battery charger in the evening, or to unplug the charger and position the wheelchair for her transfer in the mornings. Daphne lives with a roommate who is able to assist with these activities. Daphne considers herself an independent person and hopes that she will be able to devise a method to charge her wheelchair herself. For now, she is satisfied with her roommate assisting so that she can spend her time with other tasks; this is one aspect of her real life where she uses assistance. Daphne's independence hinges on her ability to instruct others in the appropriate care or assistance that she requires.

This case scenario makes three crucial points. First, Daphne actively participates in some tasks and in delegating others to her roommate. Second, Daphne's delegation does not diminish her sense of independence because she retains control over which tasks she delegates. Third, Daphne continues to strive for even greater independence for the future. Although she requires help in managing the maintenance of her wheelchair, Daphne is independent in managing her routine in this area. She is not, however, independent in performing the task of wheelchair maintenance.

Exercise 12.1—Life as a Student

Consider life as a student away from home and answer the following questions:

■ The context in which you perform activities has changed; the human environment no longer includes your parents. How do you define your new level of independence?

■ Does this independence differ from the independence you had living at home with your family? If so, in what ways?

■ Consider your level of freedom. Who controls or directs your activities and your occupations?

■ Consider the different ways in which people with disabilities may experience independence.

You may consider yourself independent because you have the freedom and the responsibility to make your own decisions, prioritize your activities, and accept the consequences of your decisions. In the same manner, a person with a disability may experience independence by personal performance, by deciding to delegate a time-consuming or difficult task, and by directing others to meet his or her needs.

Dependent or Independent?

Independence is a simple word, and yet, the more one explores it, the more complex it becomes. Try answering the following series of questions. Be open minded and really take the time to think about your answers.

Exercise 12.2—Independent Meal Preparation

Answer the following questions based on your experience:

- What is independent meal preparation?

- Does independent meal preparation require cooking? Using a microwave oven? Using the stove top or range? Following a recipe? Does preparation of a cold meal count?

- Does independent meal preparation include getting packages from cabinets and the refrigerator and opening them, or is it still independent meal preparation if someone else cooks and puts together the meals and you merely put it on the table?

- Does independent meal preparation require independently obtaining the food? Does it require shopping? Making a shopping list? Carrying food home?

- Is it independent meal preparation if you order a meal from a restaurant or from a local delivery service? Does money management matter, or can a personal assistant leave money? Can you run a tab that someone else pays?

Select one of the following clients and answer the same questions for a person who has a disability: a woman who has had a stroke resulting in left hemiparesis, a young man with depression, or a young woman with cerebral palsy resulting in spastic diplegia.

Are the answers different for the client than for you? Why would we hold a person with a disability to a different standard than we do for ourselves? Does this mean that planning for your client to order food in or have someone else prepare meals is an appropriate activity? Absolutely! It means that you have to know your client, his or her family members and support system, and his or her needs and then plan treatment accordingly.

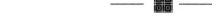

Exercise 12.3—Independent Home Management

Answer the following questions based on your experience:

- What is independent home management? Do you have to be able to mow a lawn?

- What if you live in an apartment and have no lawn? What if you hire someone else to do it?

Do your answers change for a client? The client's neighbor may have a lawn care service, or a child in the neighborhood may do the work. If this arrangement is acceptable for the neighbor, is it acceptable for your client? What if no one else in the neighborhood has this service? Similar questions can be asked for every activity. Why is it acceptable for people without disabilities to hire a maid, but we find it so important for our clients to be able to make a bed or iron a shirt?

What is really important actually depends on the client and his or her own situation. As occupational therapy practitioners, we should not force our values on our clients. Our role is to help our clients to meet their needs as they define them, so if the ability to manage household help is what is important to the client, then *that* is what is important.

Habilitation and Rehabilitation: A Collection of Transitions and Activity Simulations

As was mentioned previously, the process of moving to independence involves many transitions, and practitioners can facilitate these transitions by using various simulations (i.e., performance of contrived activities in a clinical environment and simulated activities in a real environment; see Figure 12.1). When discussing habilitation and rehabilitation, we are concerned with independence and participation in real life. Many changes occur during the transition to real life. Most people like to organize these events in some sort of order. Thinking of the process of habilitation or rehabilitation as a series of transitions may be helpful. The chronology of these transitions generally moves a person from dependence (difficulty or inability to perform life skills) to independence (the ability to perform the life skills without assistance). Each step along the way involves a transition, and at the completion of each transition the individual is closer to independent participation. At each transition, the client actively participates in selecting and performing activities that are specifically chosen to promote the acquisition of skills toward a goal.

The process of habilitation or rehabilitation often does not occur in an orderly, predetermined way. Some clients start the process with total dependence and may require contrived activities in the clinic or other externally structured environment to master initial subskills. Contrived activities can be meaningful to the client if he or she understands their place in the overall treatment plan. The client should understand that these activities are temporary and transitional in nature and provide an opportunity for him or her to learn skills that he or she will later integrate into performance of the real-life occupations.

Case Scenario

Dana gets severe anxiety attacks whenever he takes the elevator to his job on the 15th floor of a high-rise office building. Dana's goal is to become independent in taking the elevator by himself without feeling anxious. Presently, however, he becomes physically ill when simply contemplating the idea. Because of his dependence in this activity, the occupational therapist has decided to initiate intervention by engaging Dana in simple, nonthreatening activities that involve the elevator. Dana and his therapist discuss the activities and, with Dana's input, they make slight modifications. They decide on the following: Dana would watch the elevator doors open and close, watch people get on and off, push the button to summon the elevator, and quickly walk on and off the stationary elevator. During these activities the therapist encourages Dana to discuss his level of comfort or discomfort, and the therapist in turn provides support and encouragement. Although contrived, these activities are meaningful to Dana and actively engage him.

Other clients may start somewhere further along the continuum and focus on learning or relearning actual skills in a simulated environment. Still others start at different points in different performance areas. For example, one client may be dependent in one area (e.g., dressing) and be further along the continuum in another area (e.g., work activities, computer use). In this example, the difference may be because the client has relatively intact fine motor coordination for computer use but has impaired balance and gross motor performance for dressing while sitting on the edge of the bed.

The process, or movement through the transitions, varies among clients and even between the expectations and the actual process for an individual client. No one can say exactly how long a client will stay in any stage of the process or whether he or she will move forward and backward several times during the progression. Some never make the journey all the way to the end. They achieve some level of independence, but they may not achieve total independence or perhaps not the level of independence that they or their family members expected. In addition, a client may choose to receive assistance for a gross motor task that is tiring and time consuming to save energy for another task in which independent performance is a higher priority.

Exercise 12.4—John

John is a bright 6-year-old who, after months of therapy, is now able to maintain good dynamic balance in long sitting. John's goal is to learn to put on his socks and shoes by himself. Where along the continuum would you begin your occupational therapy intervention, and why? Which of these activities would you select? How would you grade the activity you select?

■ Teach John the concepts of "on" and "off" as he places and removes large plastic rings on a pole as he sits on the clinic floor?

■ Teach him how to put the socks and shoes on a rag doll?

■   Teach him how to position himself so that he can put the socks on his own feet?

Occupational therapy should continue by teaching John how to position himself and how to move in order to put on his socks and shoes. He has already mastered the concepts of "on" and "off." Now that his dynamic balance in long sitting is good, he can build on this ability by performing the actual task. Dressing the doll would be an unnecessary detour, as he is moving toward his goal.

Instead of a neat, predictable timetable, the process of habilitation or rehabilitation winds sometimes forward, sometimes backward, and sometimes in a circular pattern. Occupational therapists set goals and expectations in conjunction with their clients on the basis of a wealth of information, including the therapists' previous experiences, the client's current level of functioning, the context, and the therapists' knowledge of the body structures and body functions. The therapist adjusts treatment sessions and revises goals when necessary in response to the winding trail of progress.

Most clients would prefer that the process be more predictable, but this is not possible because of the unpredictable nature of habilitation and rehabilitation. People are not machines, and influences such as attitudes, values, mental functions, and physical geography affect their ability to participate in therapy programs and to perform activities. This unpredictability is sometimes unsettling for occupational therapy students. Clients and family members may have difficulty accepting this as well. Clients and family members often view the repetition of previously learned skills as a step backward. Occupational therapy practitioners must reassure clients, families, and others that the process is complex and somewhat unpredictable and that repetition or movement to a previous step does not signify failure. As new practitioners gain more experience, their expectations may match the actual outcome more closely, but the expected procedure may still require some modification. Practitioners and clients must accept this fact and adjust the program and expectations to meet the clients' current needs and abilities. Occupational therapy otherwise will be less meaningful and less effective.

Although the exact process is unpredictable, some trends are evident in the timing and order of the transitions and stages (see Figure 12.4). At each level of transition, simulation of real-life activity plays a role in occupational therapy. The first transition is one that occurs when a person detects a problem in a body function or structure or a problem with participation. At that instant, the client changes (or transitions) from being a person without a disability to a person with a disability.

After a traumatic injury or illness, the client has a period of medical recovery. During this period, the primary focus for the client is survival. Initiating occupational therapy may be possible at this point. As a result of the client's condition, occupational therapy practitioners often limit sessions to activities that do not closely resemble real life. For example, the practitioner may ask the client to grasp objects of various shapes and sizes, place and release these objects in various planes, and perform certain move-

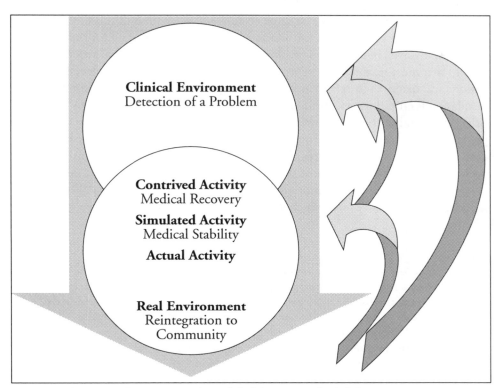

Figure 12.4. Stages of progression through habilitation and rehabilitation.

ment patterns while sitting or lying in bed. These activities, although contrived, are crucial to promote joint range of motion and muscle flexibility throughout the upper extremities. The client may not associate these actions with the accomplishment of an activity (e.g., self-feeding) that he or she will perform in the future. At this stage, the client performs contrived activities in a clinical environment (see Figure 12.1).

As the client becomes more medically stable, he or she may be better able to participate in therapy. During this stage of transition, learning various skills is the focus of occupational therapy. The practitioner may teach the skills individually, and the skills may or may not be related to each other and are sometimes referred to as subskills. After the client masters the subskills to some degree, the practitioner combines the skills in various groupings to simulate various real-life activities. In this case, the client performs simulated activities in a clinical environment (see Figure 12.1).

As therapy progresses, activities more closely resemble real life. Simulation of activities varies greatly and is addressed in greater detail later in this chapter. Initially, a client's treatment session may seem quite different from the expected eventual activity performance. The client sometimes has difficulty identifying the usefulness of a given task in relation to his or her own needs. He or she may perform individual skills out of sequence or in awkward ways or may skip some steps or skills altogether at this point.

The treatment sessions seem to be some abstract representation of real life. When the activity is not representative of real-life activity, it can be frustrating for the client and for others involved in the client's progression. For this reason, the occupational therapy practitioner must reassure the client and family that the simulations reflect real-life situations and that the actual activities will be brought into the clinical environment. The simulation is crucial to treatment, and the simulations become increasingly more realistic. At the end of this phase, the client performs simulations in real environments to prepare for real occupational performance in the real environment. As discussed previously, practitioners may skip steps along this continuum or revisit them until the client achieves maximal performance of the activity in the real environment. The following example demonstrates that individual clients may learn individual skills out of sequence and then later integrate them into a real-life activity or occupation.

Case Scenario

In an outpatient mental health clinic, the client, Mary, has learned, at different times, strategies to control impulsive behavior to foster taking turns, basic money management skills, and appropriate assertiveness. She eagerly participated in the activities to learn these skills and was able to master them individually. Next, Mary and the occupational therapist planned a trip to the local supermarket to shop for the upcoming holiday party. In this situation, she has the opportunity to integrate learned skills into a successful shopping experience.

Simulation

To *simulate* is "to give or assume the appearance of or effect of, often with the intent to deceive," and *simulation* is "the act or process of simulating" (*Webster's Collegiate Dictionary*, 1996, p.1094). Thinking about human performance in terms of using simulation to develop expertise is not unique to habilitation or rehabilitation. Each of us can remember numerous times that we have practiced each component of a skill before putting them together to practice the entire skill in a protected environment. Only then were we able to perform the skill in the real environment. Learning a balance beam routine is one example of this process. A gymnast may begin by practicing each jump and flip on a mat. He or she may also practice walking a straight line marked on a floor. For the gymnast, these subskills only distantly resemble the final routine. Once the gymnast masters the individual skills, he or she then combines the skills. The routine is still not exactly like the form it has in real life, and this is simulation. The gymnast may perform the routine more slowly or on a low or wide beam. Finally, he or she performs the routine in its appropriate context and completes the simulation phase of mastery. For the gymnast, real-life performance of the routine occurs during a competition or exhibition. At any time, however, the gymnast may return to simulation to refine the individual skills.

Simulation is commonplace in other human endeavors, such as in engineering and product design, development, testing, and marketing. These efforts have shown that mechanical simulations or mock-ups, computer-driven simulations, virtual reality, and interactive simulations can provide an accurate representation of the real world. We can analyze product testing, efficiency, and worker and consumer behaviors through simulations. In marketing, the value of testing a concept then building and testing a prototype is that one can measure the viability of ideas long before the product is actually manufactured, thus saving valuable time, effort, and money (Eastlack, 1968). We cannot overstate the value of rigorous testing simulations to determine the durability, effectiveness, and viability of various products and processes.

The Visionary Shopper from Canada Market Research is a computer-driven simulation that uses a virtual reality store to capture shoppers' purchasing behavior (Marney, 1997). Consumers sit at a computer monitor and simulate their purchasing preferences. They can "lift and move" product packages to inspect and read packaging material from different angles. Market researchers are able to determine whether the package design has emotional appeal and provides useful information to encourage purchase.

The SIMUL8 by Visual Thinking International is a computer software visual simulation package designed for use in general engineering. This simulation software allows time-tracking of particular products and assigns fixed and variable costs to simulated activities. It also tracks resource usage, inventory storage, and costs incurred by stocking products (Visual Thinking International, 1998). It allows engineers to explore plant improvements and make recommendations for changes in a timely and cost-effective way.

Physical interactive simulation is a dynamic technique that goes beyond computer simulation or visual interactive simulation to provide a highly accurate representation of the real world (Winarchick & Caldwell, 1997). Through physical interactive simulation, human performance of a task can be simulated and evaluated on a three-dimensional physical model. Delphi Chassis Systems and Sinclair Community College, both of Dayton, Ohio, worked together to establish a workplace prototype lab where analysis of modeling an entire process before pilot production has saved Delphi Chassis Systems millions of dollars. Users of physical interactive simulation are able to interact with models before determining their work-site setups to maximize productivity and to save wasted time and money in development. The models are easy to construct, rearrange, and modify to provide a variety of analyses, including motion economy and ergonomics (Winarchick & Caldwell, 1997).

"The fatigue phenomenon" relates to product durability and has long been a crucial issue not only for the designer and manufacturer of the product (e.g., the automobile, the airplane) but also for the end-user. Automobile manufacturers have produced test programs that simulate road profiles, weather conditions, and the most aggressive maneuvers to ensure that a product meets a desirable target for durability (Weal, Liefooghe, & Dressler, 1997). Impact tests are designed to determine the fatigue strength or crashworthiness of automobiles. Computer-aided engineering models test durability of automobiles and validate design assumptions. Laboratory simulations are efficient and flexible ways of determining durability of products from the design through the manufacturing.

Simulation also plays a major role in the aeronautics industry. One example is the development of airplane engines. Initially, gross drawings are made to design specifications. Next, computer-aided simulations of the designs are made, followed by a critical design review. Solid mock-up parts are made according to specifications of the critical design review team. These parts are assembled in test-cell engines under simulated conditions of aircraft usage. There is a constant flow of information between the designers and those testing the products in simulation (S. Rausch, personal communication, October 15, 1998).

Virtual reality is the ultimate simulation. Through environmental immersion, a person believes that he or she is in an alternative reality. Forms of input of virtual reality include visual, auditory, and tactile. Headsets cover the eyes and ears and allow only input from computer-generated information, thus preventing outside stimuli from affecting the person. The sense of touch (through the field of haptics) is involved, whereby a person feels and manipulates objects in virtual environments, enhancing the realism of virtual worlds. The PHANToM is one example of a haptic device (MIT Artificial Intelligence Laboratory, 1998) that may have applications in occupational therapy. This computer input device allows the user to feel virtual objects. The device exerts an external force on the user's fingertips to provide information about the shape and texture of solid virtual objects. With this haptic interaction with the virtual environment, a user can control a virtual pencil or paintbrush to draw or paint using movements that are free and unimpeded in virtual space.

Many people in the field of driver evaluation and driver (re-)training use virtual reality driving simulators with clients both with and without disabilities as an adjunct to real-life, on-road training. The virtual reality driving simulator technology provides multiple standardized driving environments in which a client can be safely tested or trained without being in a potentially risky on-road situation. Virtual reality driving simulators have been used to train drivers of vehicles such as tractor trailers, trains, fire trucks, passenger cars, and specialized heavy equipment (FAAC Incorporated, 1998).

Occupational therapy practitioners currently use virtual reality alongside more traditional interventions. According to Cunningham (1998), virtual reality provides multisensory input and feedback to clients with stroke who were working on improving their perception, cognition, gross and fine motor coordination, praxis, posture, and safety awareness. Reid (2002) studied how virtual reality may be used to improve the ability of children with cerebral palsy to use their upper extremities.

Simulation in Occupational Therapy

Occupational therapy practitioners use various tools to help clients to achieve their highest level of independence; simulation is one of these important tools. Simulation is an effective tool in various occupational therapy settings, including acute care, rehabilitation, long-term care, home care, and outpatient settings, and is an appropriate tool to use with people who have various cognitive, emotional, physical, and psychological conditions. Simulation is useful regardless of the client's age, ethnic or cultural background, and gender. In almost every scenario, simulation can be used to improve participation.

In psychotherapy, role-playing is an educational tool in which therapists provide people with situations in which they can act out imaginary scenarios. By participating in an imaginary experience, a person may begin to understand problems and improve his or her skills and behaviors. Role-playing provides the participants with simulated examples of how others act in specific situations and how they themselves may act (Corsini, 1966). Role-playing involves the repetition of situations in a therapeutic environment, which allows practice while encouraging exploration and spontaneity. When clients understand that they are participating in an imaginary situation, role-playing is a common part of the simulation process in occupational therapy.

Occupational therapy practitioners plan treatment by designing activities that simulate real life. They identify activities to simulate that are based on client evaluation data. After determining which activities to simulate, the practitioner selects and creates an opportunity to engage in the activities in the clinic, classroom, home, or community setting. While the client is engaged in the activities, the practitioner uses cues and assistance to allow the client to work with only the challenge that is useful and that he or she can tolerate as well as to ensure a positive learning experience. These treatments often involve imagination, and the practitioner asks the client to imagine the circumstances and the context in which he or she will perform occupations.

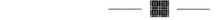

Exercise 12.5—Boy With a Below-Elbow Amputation

You are working with a 14-year-old boy who recently underwent right below-elbow amputation as a result of a traumatic injury. This boy was previously right-hand dominant. As a result of the occupational therapy evaluation, you outline goals with input from both the child and his parents. One long-term goal is for the boy to perform activities of daily living and schoolwork by using the right upper extremity (which has been fitted with a mechanical prosthesis) as an assist. Another goal is to retrain the boy to use his left upper extremity as dominant. Describe one activity that you could use to meet the goal of changing dominance. After you have described the activity, answer the following questions:

■ How have you set up the treatment environment to replicate the real-life setting in which the activity will take place?

■ What are the differences between your simulated environment and the real-life environment?

■ How does the activity itself differ from real life in your simulation?

■   How can you change the demands of the activity and the structure of the context to meet the changing needs of the client as his skills improve?

In this exercise, you were asked to use simulation to target completion of one task that is important to your client. You created the context in which your client played the role of task performer, and you provided the structure that was necessary to match the client's abilities and sufficiently challenging and important to motivate the client to work hard.

Simulation involves the use of some elements of real life and allows the client to explore real-life performance in a protected context. Because the occupational therapy practitioner can control some aspects of the simulation, he or she can design it to meet the clients' needs and abilities at any given time. For example, early in the process, the practitioner may plan the activity so that success is likely. Later, the client can accept more of the responsibility for success. The following is a series of treatment sessions that illustrate this point.

Case Scenario

Brenda is an occupational therapist who works in a community-based center. Her clients are primarily people who live on the street and do not work. Brenda works in a program with social workers, psychologists, and vocational rehabilitation counselors. One goal of the program is to improve the work habits and skills of her clients. Her group meets for 3 months. The members start by talking about what they would like to do in the future and what steps are necessary to reach their goals. After a short period, attendance and participation in the group activities become the "work" of its members.

This scenario of Brenda's community-based program provides a clear example of when a simulation is paramount to the activities. During the group meetings, members discuss work behaviors like grooming, timeliness, and other responsibilities. During some sessions, Brenda encourages group members to role-play specific situations.

The group members then begin to work in the center's gift shop to develop their work skills further. Group members, who are at this point group employees, punch time clocks and meet with their supervisor daily. In addition to working in the gift shop, they continue to meet in their discussion group. During the discussion group, they learn skills to use when interviewing, how to write a résumé, and how to complete a job application. Group members play the roles of the interviewer and the interviewee to practice job interviews. At this point, the group members can apply for specific jobs in the center's shop. For example, some are interested in working in the stockroom, others as cashiers, and others in management.

The clients and the group leaders then work together to answer newspaper advertisements and to work with job placement services. The clients go to their interviews, sometimes with a job coach or assistant, and begin their jobs with the help of a job coach, which is the highest level of simulation. The situation is not quite real life because the job coach influences performance and success by assisting, supervising, and encouraging the client. This job coach continues to work with the client for the required amount of time and then removes him- or herself. At this point, the client is in real life as it relates to working. The client may contact the group leaders anytime, and the group leaders often ask graduates of the group to return to talk to new members about the process and the result.

The ways that occupational therapy practitioners use simulations as part of their interventions are similar in all areas of practice. The process begins with a comprehensive evaluation, development of specific goals, and determination of which performance components need improvement and of which performance skills would benefit from a simulated situation. Of course, the client's motivation, willingness, or preferences are key factors to consider before engaging him or her in a simulated activity. For some clients, simulations are motivating and fun. For others, simulations may have seemingly no value, and they may perceive the simulations to be like child's play. Occupational therapy practitioners should endeavor to provide age-appropriate simulations. Practitioners should clarify or explain the value of the simulated activity in preparing the client for the real-life occupation.

Case Scenario

Belle, a 75-year-old woman who has had a cerebrovascular accident, needs to improve her toileting skills. Initially, Belle participated in tasks and exercises focused on individual steps in the activity. The occupational therapy program included the following activities:

- Sitting to improve balance and the ability to shift weight

- Sitting that encourages weight bearing through the upper and lower extremities

- Forward weight shift and removing weight from the buttocks

- Fine motor and bimanual tasks in preparation for lower-extremity garment management

- Standing to improve balance

- Improving compensation for a visual field cut.

This point during early recovery is when treatment appears the least representative of real life. The simulation is rather abstract. After mastery, or partial mastery, of the individual components of an activity, the client compiles and performs the components in a protected environment. The treatment context is a safe place to practice each individual component and many combinations or collections of components. This context allows clients to make mistakes and to learn from them, to explore alternatives, and to develop strategies for improved performance. Initially, the practitioner sets up the environment to protect the person from distractions and to encourage successful completion of the task.

Case Scenario

At this next stage of intervention for Belle, the occupational therapist uses one or more treatment sessions to bring Belle to a private bathroom where she can practice transfers to and from the commode. During these sessions, the therapist does not address other components of the activity, such as lower-extremity garment management and hygiene after toileting. At some point, the client will perform these simulated activities in a real trial. Initially, with assistance and later with supervision, Belle toilets in the private bathroom. She may practice any task that is difficult for her.

Other occupational therapy sessions focus only on lower-extremity garment management. For example, during part of one treatment session, Belle worked on buttoning and unbuttoning buttons and zipping and unzipping zippers on a dressing board. The therapist designed the activity to begin with large buttons and loose buttonholes and moved on to smaller buttons and tighter buttonholes. Another treatment session began with large zippers on slippery tracks and moved on to smaller zippers with more resistant tracks. Once Belle mastered the task on the dressing board, the next step was to lay a pair of pants smoothly in her lap. The therapist assisted by holding the clothing taut, exposing the zipper or holding the buttonhole steady. As Belle gained the ability to perform this task, the therapist provided less assistance. The next step in this sequence was to have Belle practice the tasks of buttoning, unbuttoning, zipping, and unzipping on her own pants. After she mastered this step, the therapist and Belle worked on removing and replacing the lower-extremity garments in preparation for toileting.

Other interventions focused on the activities of toilet paper management and hygiene. These interventions followed the same procedure of practice and mastery. The therapist used other activities to address other areas in which Belle had difficulty. For example, the therapist used paper-and-pencil tasks, bed making, and computer games to increase her awareness of the visual field cut.

As can be seen from this scenario, practitioners address each component of an activity individually. The client practices and masters the tasks and components of each activity and then groups them together until he or she has addressed the entire occupation (in this case, toileting) sufficiently.

When Belle is able, she completes each activity by herself. This may only be, however, when conditions are optimal, such as when she is already in her wheelchair and wearing sturdy shoes with nonslip soles. In the evenings, when Belle is fatigued, she may continue to require assistance from her husband to perform this task safely. When planning treatment with Belle, the long-term goal is for her to toilet independently regardless of the time of day, the type of clothing she is wearing, or even the layout of the bathroom. When she is able to achieve this goal, Belle will be independent in performing this task in real life. Her occupational therapy sessions will no longer address this goal.

Occupational therapy practitioners frequently use simulation as a key aspect of the intervention plan. The following are a few examples of the way therapists use simulation to ensure that activities are purposeful in occupational therapy.

Work-centered rehabilitation often uses simulation. Work samples such as Valpar Work Samples (Valpar Corporation, 1974) and the Baltimore Therapeutic Equipment Work Simulator (Baltimore Therapeutic Equipment Company) replicate various job skills (see Figure 12.5). Work samples or work simulations can be assessments used to determine a client's abilities and to measure the progress a client makes toward returning to work. Not only are work samples useful for evaluation, but also components of some work samples can be treatment tools. By using these simulation

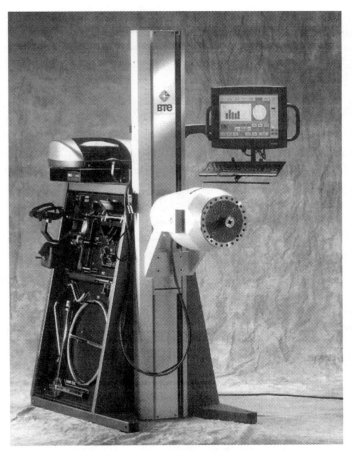

Figure 12.5. Baltimore Therapeutic Equipment Work Simulator.

Note. Baltimore Therapeutic Equipment Company. *Baltimore Therapeutic Equipment Work Simulator.* 7455-L New Ridge Road, Hanover, MD 21076.

tools, practitioners can target specific work skills in an objective, measurable, and repeatable way.

In one Valpar activity, the user must piece together three small metal objects and place them in moving holes on a round track. The rate of movement is adjustable so that the holes move faster as the user's fine motor coordination and speed increase. The practitioner may adjust the time allotted for this activity to meet or challenge a client's endurance. The practitioner counts the number of sets of objects placed in the holes while the client works. The practitioner and client can track progress in several ways: by noting the client's ability as the speed quickens, by noting the amount of time that the client participates in the activity, and by noting the number of sets that the client completes in a fixed or consistent amount of time. This activity that simulates the manipulation of small objects and, in turn, repetitious assembly-line work is useful for several reasons, such as preparing an assembly-line worker for return to work, improving a person's fine motor and bimanual coordination, increasing endurance for fine motor tasks, or even increasing tolerance for repetitious work. This tool may be appropriate for people with various disabling conditions, including traumatic hand injury, medical conditions like diabetes that involve associated sensory impairments, visual impairments in which the purpose of occupational therapy is to improve tactile compensatory strategies, and mental illness that affects a person's concentration and attention span.

Another work-centered simulation involves adults in work rehabilitation who simulate jobs as part of a program (Ellexson, 1989). In a work-hardening program, activities simulate those work skills on which the client must concentrate. Inpatients or outpatients may take contracts from other companies to complete work. For example, a cohort of adults with developmental disabilities may work in a program that has a contract to package plastic knives, forks, and spoons. This job includes counting the utensils, placing them in bags, sealing the bags, labeling the bags, and placing the bags in boxes. This activity demonstrates how simulation allows an occupational therapy practitioner to organize the environment, break down tasks into components, and offer clients purposeful activity as a treatment tool.

Occupational therapy clinics have long included specially built treatment areas that provide treatment to clients in a setting that simulates real life. Examples of specific areas in the occupational therapy department are a kitchen, a bathroom, and a bedroom or living area in which clients practice certain basic activities of daily living skills and instrumental activities of daily living tasks. These treatment locations are useful when the client has improved to the point at which a setting that is more realistic than the occupational therapy clinic or laboratory encourages further progress. A training apartment, for example, may be useful after the client has completed wheelchair transfers in a hospital room and meal preparation in the occupational therapy kitchen area. A client's family members may join him or her in the training apartment so that they can practice the skills of caregiving before discharge. The training apartment offers a transition between the contrived and simulated activities in the clinic and performing activities in real life (in this case, at home).

Occupational therapy practitioners working with children and adolescents often use simulation as part of their interventions. Simulation often is the key to engage young children in a meaningful learning activity. Children develop and explore their environment through the use of their imaginations. Children with disabilities may not be able to use their imaginations or be able to explore their environment as they would without their disabilities. The role of the occupational therapy practitioner is, in part, to create the environment for children to use their imaginations to develop new skills or to become secure or confident with their abilities. Children use play to explore and learn about their environment and to receive the sensory stimulation that they need for development. A child with a disability may be unable to participate in play sufficiently to meet his or her other needs.

Case Scenario

Ricardo is a 5-year-old boy in kindergarten who has a learning disability and attention deficit hyperactivity disorder. He attends regular classes and has occupational therapy, physical therapy, and speech therapy three times weekly. Ricardo switches hand dominance for different activities: he throws a ball with his left hand but writes and uses scissors with his right hand. The occupational therapist, Isadore (Izzy), observed the following problems during writing activities in the classroom: impaired fine motor coordination of both hands, associated reactions in the left hand and arm, squeezing the pencil too hard, pressing too hard on the paper, and difficulty releasing the pencil when finished and repositioning it when writing. He decides that Ricardo needs a fun way to learn to regulate pressure and to learn to grasp and release the pencil appropriately. Izzy decides to play Blockhead™ with Ricardo. Blockhead™ is a game in which the players take turns balancing oddly shaped wood blocks on top of one another until one person causes the tower to topple. The person who causes the tower to topple is the "blockhead." Ricardo does not have the attention span, motor skills, or perceptual skills to play Blockhead™. Izzy adapts the game using its rules but blocks made out of Styrofoam and paper. These materials require Ricardo to regulate his grip pressure and to use larger gross motor skills. Izzy had Ricardo play the game while assuming different positions and with both hands. Sometimes, Ricardo played while seated at a table and other times while standing. Sometimes, Ricardo played while lying in a prone position and resting on his forearms when upper-extremity weight bearing was necessary. Ricardo's mother reported to Izzy that she bought the game and that Ricardo enjoys playing at home with her and his older brother. After playing a simulated Blockhead™ game, Ricardo learned the appropriate rules and developed an attention span adequate to play the real game. Izzy noted that Ricardo's writing skills also improved.

—— ▦ ——

Exercise 12.6—Ricardo

Think about the case scenario about Ricardo and answer the following questions:

■ What real-life activity does this therapeutic intervention address?

■ How did the occupational therapist use simulation to imitate the real-life activity?

■ What modifications did the therapist make to the environment and the demands of the activity?

■ How do the therapist and the family members provide assistance to make the activity possible?

—— ▦ ——

Exercise 12.7—Ricardo: Questions From a Practitioner's Perspective

Take a few minutes to think about more activities that could serve the same purpose for Ricardo. If you were the occupational therapist or the occupational therapy assistant, what would you do? How would you set up the environment? How would you alter the assistance given to meet the changing needs of the child? How would you help the parent and siblings to do this?

Jacobs (1991) discussed the importance of introducing various activities that simulate adult roles in making the transition to becoming an adult worker. She discussed the use of exploratory play and role-playing activities, even in children as young as preschool age. During these role-playing activities, children can explore the physical properties associated with various careers. They also are able to try out different social skills and behaviors necessary for leadership and teamwork. Throughout school, these skills facilitate the development of work behaviors. Behaviors such as punctuality and preparedness are necessary early in a child's schooling, and mastering these skills prepares a child for behaviors that will be necessary later in life at work. Older children may participate in programs in which they develop a mock business and provide some service or product to others.

In the recent past, several rehabilitation departments across North America have begun to use sophisticated, visually appealing, functional simulations of various environments called Easy Street Environments (Habitat, Inc., 1998). The custom environments include more than 30 areas of activity, such as a park, restaurant, bank, supermarket, department store, office, theater, and automobile. Easy Street Environments provide convenient, safe, low-risk, weather-free treatment spaces in which occupational therapy practitioners can effectively treat clients in all age groups who have a wide range of disabilities. With Easy Street Environments, the practitioner and client may address discharge readiness, community reentry, client and family member training, evaluation of possible home adaptations, and assistance needed by the client in the community.

Easy Street Environments are at a level similar to the training apartment discussed earlier. These environments introduce the real world and everyday occupations into the clinical setting and fill the gap between the occupational therapy clinic and real life. After a client demonstrates the ability to perform contrived and simulated activities in an occupational therapy clinic but is not yet ready for community reentry, he or she may practice addressing environmental, community, and work-related obstacles and challenges in the Easy Street Environments. Practitioners who have used these simulated environments claim that their clients' confidence in performing instrumental activities of daily living has increased and that practitioners can use their time more efficiently (Habitat, Inc., 1998). The more realistic the simulation is in the controlled setting, as in Easy Street Environments, the easier or smoother the clients' transition may be when performing these activities in real life.

Occupational therapy practitioners must not make the mistake of thinking that an excellent simulation supersedes real-life training and application. Simulation, by definition is *not* real life. Although the amount of time and the intensity of simulation in occupational therapy may influence the ease of transition to real life, success in simulation does not ensure success in real life.

Simulation is useful in outpatient settings and can provide an even smoother transition to real life. Clients can work on a certain skill during their therapy sessions and practice the skill at home or in another real-life setting. This "homework" is actually an advanced form of simulation because, although still somewhat contrived, it is useful to maximize a client's ability to perform an activity. When clients try techniques at home, they can bring questions back to therapy, and the occupational therapy practitioner can devise simulated activities to use during treatment that target those specific problems. Each time a client masters a skill in the clinic, he or she can perform the skill at home or in the real-life location as a check. As the client performs activities satisfactorily at home, the goals for treatment change. The practitioner can document progress and indicate whether occupational therapy should continue after satisfactory performance of the occupation in the real-life situation.

Real Life

In all of the previous examples, simulations prepare clients for real-life activities and occupations. Transition to real life is the final step in the process we describe in this chapter. The occupational therapy practitioner can foster the transition to real life by keeping the focus on real life foremost in treatment throughout the habilitation or rehabilitation process. The ultimate goal of occupational therapy is for the client to be successful in his or her occupations. Real life is the usual environment in which any given occupation takes place. Real-life environments include the home, workplace, school, places of leisure enjoyment, and private and public transportation. The occupational therapy intervention to prepare a client for real life is limited in scope. Predicting all of the environments in which a client may interact is impossible for the practitioner. It is essential, but not entirely possible, to plan for the unexpected. By addressing occupations in many of the more likely environments in simulation, it is possible to facilitate, but not guarantee, the transition to real life. In occupational therapy, the client learns problem-solving skills and other strategies that will enable him or her to generalize information to various real-life environments and situations.

During therapy, an occupational therapy practitioner must address foundational performance components and purposeful activities that are necessary to engage in real-life occupations. Addressing the psychosocial requirements of an activity is important, including the acceptability of the methods and equipment; embarrassment or pride associated with performance; and support of family members, friends, and others. Real-life performance includes using all of the appropriate activities to engage in an occupation. Real life includes performing activities in the conventional manner, performing activities with alternative techniques and compensatory strategies, and performing activities with assistive technology.

When addressing the real world, occupational therapy practitioners often prescribe and provide adaptive equipment and assistive technology devices. They may focus on simulations with devices and ensure that the client can competently use the device to complete activities in the clinic environment. Everything changes at home, and practitioners must address home issues. In Phillips and Zhao's (1993) study of technology abandonment, they described patterns of abandonment of devices recommended or provided to clients in a physical rehabilitation setting. Four factors were significant in abandoning technology: lack of consideration of user opinion, ease of device procurement, poor device performance, and change in user needs or priorities. The occupational therapy practitioner's role is to address those factors. By ensuring that the device performs as it should, both in the protected therapeutic environment and in the real-life situation, the practitioner can help to provide the best possible solution to clients who require assistive technology. The client's home and other real-life environments should be the focus of treatment, and one should avoid assumptions such as, "If it works in the hospital room, it will work the same at home." In a related study, Bell and Hinojosa (1996) interviewed three participants regarding the effect of assistive devices on their ability to perform their daily routines. They concluded that successful use of these devices in the clinic setting did not necessarily transition to successful use of these devices at home. Follow-up at home, in-home training, or in-home performance is crucial to using the assistive devices or compensatory techniques successfully in the real-life, postdischarge setting.

The human and nonhuman context in which the client performs any activity influences the realism of the simulation. For example, pretending to lift a heavy object in the proper way in an occupational therapy clinic is different from lifting an object of a similar weight on a busy factory floor. In the latter situation, the context includes noise, the space available, the presence of a supervisor and coworkers, and many distractions. These factors make real-life activity performance much more complex than simulated activity. Again, successful performance in a clinic does not necessarily guarantee success in real life.

Summary

As an occupational therapy practitioner becomes more experienced, evaluating the long-term goals of clients becomes easier. In turn, planning and organizing simulated activities to address these needs becomes easier. The visualization of the outcome of occupational therapy may not always be accurate because of the unpredictable nature of human beings, the unpredictability of the setting, and the other demands that influence performance. We believe that as a practitioner gains more experience and builds a repertoire of goal-setting and treatment skills, his or her predictions will be more accurate or will be accurate more often. The practitioner can outline some trends in performance and move from contrived to more purposeful real activities in various environments that range from clinical or simulated to real. The ultimate goal is independent activity performance in a real environment, and occupational therapy practitioners use simulation in this effort. As in industries, simulation in occupational therapy allows clients to test and practice techniques in a safe, controlled environment. Practitioners can address problems, gain insights, and explore solutions before real-life performance. Some practitioners believe that the ultimate setting for providing occupational therapy intervention is at the client's work site or in the client's home or community. In these cases, simulations are already in the real-life setting, which ensures the likelihood of the transition to more optimal real-life performance. ■

References

Bell, P., & Hinojosa, J. (1996). Perception of the impact of assistive devices on daily life of three individuals with quadriplegia. *Assistive Technology, 7*(2), 87–94.

Corsini, R. J. (1966). *Roleplaying in psychotherapy: A manual.* Chicago: Aldine.

Cunningham, D. (1998, April 27). In Alabama, OT is a virtual reality. *Advance for Occupational Therapists, 14,* 19.

Eastlack, J. O. (1968). New products for the seventies. In J. O. Eastlack & J. Tinker (Eds.), *New product development* (pp. 142–148). Chicago: American Marketing Association.

Ellexson, M. T. (1989). Work hardening. In S. Hertfelder & C. Gwin (Eds.), *Work in progress* (pp. 67–126). Rockville, MD: American Occupational Therapy Association.

FAAC Incorporated. (1998). Driving simulators [online]. Retrieved from http://www.faac.com/Driving_Simulators.htm.

Habitat, Inc. (1998). *Easy Street Environments* [product literature]. Tempe, AZ: Author.

Jacobs, K. (1991). *Occupational therapy: Work-related programs and assessments*. Boston: Little, Brown.

Marney, J. (1997). Design testing goes digital. *Marketing, 102*, 10.

MIT Artificial Intelligence Laboratory. (1998). Haptics. [online]. Retrieved from http://www.ai.mit.edu/projects/handarm-haptics.html.

Phillips, B., & Zhao, H. (1993). Predictors of assistive technology abandonment. *Assistive Technology, 5*(1), 36–45.

Reid, D. T. (2002). The use of virtual reality to improve upper-extremity efficiency skills in children with cerebral palsy: A pilot study. *Technology and Disability, 14*(2), 53–61.

Valpar Corporation. (1974). Valpar Work Samples. (Available from Valpar Corporation, 3801 East 34th Street, Suite 105, Tucson, AZ 85713.)

Visual Thinking International. (1998). SIMUL8. [online]. Retrieved from http://www.VTIL.com/simul8.htm.

Weal, P., Liefooghe, C., & Dressler, K. (1997). Product durability engineering: Improving the process. *Sound and Vibration, 31*(1), 68–79.

Webster's collegiate dictionary (10th ed.). (1996). Springfield, MA: Merriam-Webster.

Winarchick, C., & Caldwell, R. (1997). Physical interactive simulation: A hands-on approach to facilities improvements. *IIE Solutions, 29*(5), 34–36.

13

Range of Human Activity: Leisure

Laurette Olson, PhD, OTR
Elizabeth Roarty O'Herron, MS, OTR

Leisure is...freedom from the necessity of labor. (Aristotle)

Leisure is what we do in our spare time and may involve particular activities or a state of mind. Some people define leisure as involvement in any activity that is not work. Others believe that, within the occupation of work, one may find some activities that the person would define as leisure. In this chapter, *leisure* encompasses meaningful activities or occupations that we choose to participate in during our discretionary time. Leisure happens when we engage in an activity that reflects our own true nature (Pieper, 1963). It is a state of mind in which we are available and receptive to the experience of our physical, mental, and social selves. In leisure, we are free to participate or not to participate without consequence. The goals of the activity and the direction the activity takes come from us. Thus, our leisure choices are occupations. Leisure activities or occupations have no external judge of success or failure within them; only the participant decides whether his or her level of participation is adequate for personal enjoyment. Some leisure occupations require new learning that provides a challenge and intellectual stimulation. Others use skills that we have already acquired and may be relaxing, such as reading a novel, knitting, or gardening.

Leisure embodies an extremely broad range of activities that provide entertainment, relaxation, fun and stimulation, or self-development. These activities may be active or passive. Watching television or listening to music are examples of passive activities, whereas traveling or playing a sport are examples of more active activities. During leisure time, people read, play sports, explore nature, dance, paint, tell jokes, do puzzles, help others, worship, engage in religious social activities, watch television, travel, care for pets, drink, gamble, or daydream. Some leisure occupations may resemble adult work, a child's school, or self-care activities. A business person may use leisure time to write a novel or to refinish old furniture; a high school student may explore astronomy; a retired teacher may volunteer a few days a week in a nursing home; a homemaker may design and make clothing in his or her free time.

Leisure provides opportunities to seek out activities that we intrinsically find interesting. When we engage in a leisure occupation, we become so invested in the activity that no other concern or goal matters for the time being (Csikszentmihalyi, 1992). To have a satisfying leisure life, we need to put as much energy into developing a leisure life as we put into work.

Although we frequently associate leisure with adolescence and adulthood, children's play also can be seen as leisure. Leisure play occurs when children participate in an activity for no other reason than because it is interesting to them. During play, children have no overriding desire to please an adult and are allowed to express their true nature in their interactions. Although children may develop motor, cognitive, or social skills in the process, these are not the primary goals for the children. Once children begin to experience the pleasure of mastery of the activity (e.g., jumping rope consecutively, swimming or diving into a pool), nothing else matters for the time being, and other concerns or desires fade to the back of the children's minds.

People of all ages participate in leisure occupations for personal enjoyment and to fulfill personal needs. Throughout life, participation in leisure occupations is a critical safeguard of our mental health. When the external world of school, work, or everyday living does not seem to be offering us affirmation and a sense of mastery, we retreat into leisure to fend off depression and engender optimism in our self and our abilities. We can use these leisure activities as a springboard for redirecting our lives in a more satisfying and productive way.

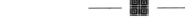

Exercise 13.1—Personal Leisure Activities

Describe your active and passive leisure activities. What activities do you do for relaxation, fun and stimulation, entertainment, and personal development? What are your major leisure occupations?

Needs Met Through Leisure

In modern societies, social control is necessary for humans to maintain order and function every day. As members of a society, people need to fulfill certain roles and put aside their own wishes and impulses for immediate gratification. Sometimes, people must contain their emotions so that work can proceed harmoniously. In modern societies, leisure provides opportunities for people to put their commitments aside and to experience freedom in activities that satisfy their interests. Further, participation in leisure occupations provides opportunities for them to express their desires and express their true range of emotions. This expression of emotions is done with the approval of other people (Neulinger, 1981). For example, an adolescent can write painfully honest poetry about loss and longing and receive praise from others for the beauty and depth of emotion of his or her writing. If the adolescent had shared these feelings at a part-time job, he or she might have made his or her coworkers nervous and cause them to see him or her as a very troubled youth. Another example is the behavior characteristic at a football game; fans cheer and jeer loudly while simultaneously feeling an intense camaraderie. This level of emotion in daily life would be seen as inappropriate or deviant.

Throughout our lives, the activities that have helped us develop, maintain, or strengthen relationships with others are most often leisure occupations. We plan and share special activities or events with family members or friends so that all participants experience pleasure and relaxation. When activities have the desired results, we associate the positive experience with the people with whom we have interacted. This positive interaction cements the relationships, and we will most likely seek out these people when we are looking for companionship in future activities. We may also come to rely on these people when we need assistance in our daily lives, and we are likely to be willing to help them as needed. We are more likely to tolerate and resolve disagreements and frustrations with others when they occur within a relationship that has a history of many pleasurable interactions. We often sustain friendship throughout the life span through shared positive leisure experiences that we associate with these friends.

Literature often emphasizes the relaxing nature of leisure (Kraus, 1994; Neulinger, 1981). Leisure provides us with opportunities to rejuvenate ourselves from the drudgery and stresses of everyday life. For some of us, it is an antidote to work, an opportunity to rest. Some of us seek relief by withdrawing from interactions and reading the newspaper or tending to our gardens. Others revive spirits through having special meals or drinks with others to create a relaxed mood for conversation and interaction.

Leisure occupation provides opportunities to learn more about ourselves, to explore our interests, and to develop skills in activities that bring us pleasure. In our free time, we engage in leisure occupations that are interesting to us without a concern for their usefulness to others (Neulinger, 1981). We may learn to dance, kayak, paint, or play an instrument for no other reason than for the pleasure that it brings us. Developing proficiency in an activity supports our internal sense of mastery and physical sense of control. Traveling may increase our awareness of other cultures, expand our understanding of ourselves and others, and foster an appreciation of activities from other cultures. After a trip through the Middle East, a person may become more interested and invested in religion.

Engaging in leisure occupations also has the power to influence our mood and view of possibilities for everyday living. Success in a leisure activity can be an antidote to a negative experience in another part of our lives. Successful leisure interests and experiences can lead one to have renewed belief in his or her capacity to be effective in all parts of his or her life. Furthermore, leisure activities or experiences can be a

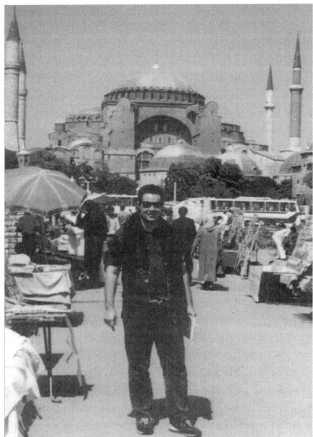

Figure 13.1. Traveling expands one's understanding of the range of human culture.

springboard for making changes in other parts of life. Some people who have become depressed or feel alienated benefit from taking up a new interest (leisure activity) to challenge themselves physically and mentally. The value of a physical challenge that participating in a leisure activity can have has been reported by Gulick (1998) for teenagers with spinal cord injuries who have taken up scuba diving and by Manuele (1998) for adults with disabilities who have learned to ride horses. In these cases, people who may have experienced feeling dependent and less competent than peers without disabilities found that, in spite of their physical limitations they can have adventures; meet the physical challenge of an active sport; and likewise, experience the physical and mental excitement from participation. The impact of their training and participation in these active leisure activities is reported to have had a positive impact on these persons' mental and physical state, thus supporting their everyday functioning in other occupations.

Learning new leisure activities within a structured group can lessen anxiety for learning and promote camaraderie and friendship that foster enthusiasm for living and affirmation of the self. Developing the discipline one needs to master a new activity often is easier when one participates in a group of like-minded and equally skilled individuals. The initial work of mastering a skill or preparing for participation can seem less daunting when we experience the camaraderie of others. When we are "in the same boat," we can share small triumphs and easily give support to each other when we stumble or make mistakes. Joining in with others and working harmoniously foster engagement and continued interest in a challenging activity. In the United States, many nonprofit clubs as well as profit-making companies offer structured group activities. These groups afford various options for us to discover and explore new leisure activities with others.

Independent mastery of a leisure occupation gives us pleasure. When we become overly compliant with external demands and lose our individuality within the needs and desires of others, our individuality disappears, and life becomes meaningless. Within solitary time, we may learn to play a musical instrument, write, read, or participate in a range of other activities for our own individual pleasure idiosyncratically. In an individual leisure occupation, our activity pace is more likely unhurried, and our imaginative and creative abilities can flourish in the presence of only the self. Through this process, we get to know ourselves more deeply and gain an awareness of what moves us beyond being with people that we love. Storr (1988) discussed two opposing human drives: the drive toward closeness to other human beings and the drive toward independence and self-sufficiency. Although love and friendship are important parts of what makes life worthwhile, solitude has great value. When we learn to make good use of solitude, we have the opportunity to focus on our own desires and interests separate from the needs and desires of others.

People also seek leisure for emotional stimulation. Elias and Dunning (1986) stated, "Unless an organism is intermittently flushed and stirred by some exciting experience with the help of strong feelings, overall routinization and restraint...are apt to engender a dryness of emotions, a feeling of monotony" (p. 73). We can potentially experience a full range of human emotion that we avoid in everyday life in leisure activities. Many children love to frighten or be frightened on Halloween; adults pay high ticket prices to become engrossed in the pain and suffering of characters in a play. Sloan (1979) reported studies suggesting that the heartbeat and level of stress in fans at sporting events can be similar to that of the athletes participating. Tension and stress increase, but these feelings are different (and more pleasurable) from tension and stress in everyday life. Aristotle's view that music and tragedy have a cathartic effect and move people's souls the way sports relieve physical tension and energize the body is one that leisure theorists still assert today (Neulinger, 1981).

Leisure, as a social area for loosening nonleisure restraints, is found in all societies and cultures. At a sporting event, a crowd may loudly express very aggressive intentions toward an opposing team that would not be acceptable in a work environment. Roughness and aggression in game play within the confines of the rules of the

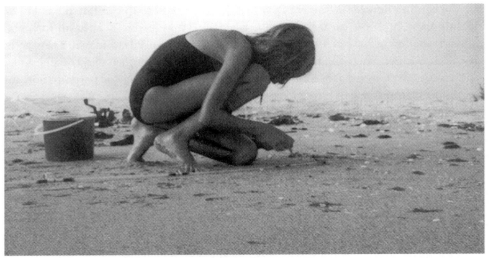

Figure 13.2. Participating in a solitary activity provides opportunity to reflect and collect one's thoughts.

game stimulate enjoyment of watching or playing a game. Aggression assures the participant and the fan a high degree of competitiveness and human drama (Zillman, Sapolsky, & Bryant, 1979). Adolescents can express their sexuality more openly in social dance than they can in other environments. In some cultures, the expression of emotion is more condoned than in others. A difference likewise exists in the openness with which people of different ages show their tension and excitement through bodily movement. Older adults are generally more restrained than teenagers.

Spectator sports can provide a strong emotional bond to a team. Individuals can feel a sense of belonging to a larger meaningful group. When the team wins, fans get to "bask in reflected glory" (Sloan, 1979, p. 235). Although fans cannot attain a sense of achievement as a team player, they can experience a sense of triumph through cheering on their favorite teams. Spectator sports facilitate social interaction with other fans while watching the game or after the event. A shared love of sports can be the basis for days of enjoyable and stimulating conversations together for some sports fans. Without the common focus on sporting events, these individuals may have little to say to each other.

Leisure occupations can provide an outlet or an adaptive way to ease the frustration of daily life. Through joke telling, children and adults alike can share and laugh about the absurdity of some life events that otherwise may produce intense anger or hurt. Adults may tell jokes about incompetent bosses or thoughtless spouses; children tell jokes about teachers and parents. Thinking about the absurdity of the antagonist removes the sting of the interaction.

For many of us, pets are an important part of our leisure time. Pets meet our needs for closeness and love that human interaction in everyday life may not meet. A relationship with a cat or a dog is fraught with fewer complications than relationships with other people. A pet owner can lavish attention on a pet in ways that he or she may not feel comfortable showing other people. An animal depends on its owner for sustenance. The pet's life is centered around its owner. The pet is always present and provides a routine for its owner, companionship, unconditional acceptance, and potentially affection.

We also can fulfill the need to be altruistic through leisure in ways that most work occupations do not meet. Many people use some of their leisure time to help others and, in doing so, feed their own spirits. Altruistic acts often result in the doer feeling invigorated, effective, and in control.

Factors Affecting Leisure Participation

The focus of leisure may be different at different points in our life. In childhood, engaging parents or other children for fun and stimulation is a primary objective. Children need to engage others in order to receive sufficient nurturance, support, and stimulation for healthy development toward adulthood. They also need physical activity for skill development and physical well-being. Leisure often is a means through which children challenge their physical skills and, without conscious effort, develop the coordination and strength necessary for many human occupations.

Adolescents and young adults may focus on activities that are physically exciting and that offer the opportunity to meet new people. Finding a significant other, a satisfying adult life separate from family of origin, may be an outcome of leisure pursuits. Dating relationships that develop into marital ones in Western societies typically grow from sharing many positive leisure experiences before marriage. During young adulthood, participation in selected leisure activities may provide a career direction for later life. Adolescents and children often discover lifelong leisure or work interests through their leisure pursuits. A passion for exploring the outdoors may lead to a career as a naturalist or to lifelong participation in hiking and outdoor activities.

In adulthood, leisure activities provide a means to reconnect emotionally to spouses, children, and other adults; have respite from work; and reaffirm or find a sense of self that may have gotten lost in everyday routine and responsibility. In old age, leisure activities may be a means of making connections to others and defining a sense of identity, purpose, and personal meaning to life.

Personal Traits

Our temperament, the inborn style through which we approach and respond to the environment, influences our leisure pursuits. Our temperament affects our activity level, our approach and withdrawal tendencies in new situations, our adaptability to change, our sensory threshold, the quality and intensity of our mood states, our persistence, and our attention span (Chess & Thomas, 1984). When a person has a low activity level, he or she may seek out more sedentary leisure activities. When a person has a high activity level and a high sensory threshold, he or she may seek out high-intensity pursuits, such as skydiving or hunting.

Likewise, our personality directs the activities in which we choose to participate and the extent to which we participate in them. If we are extroverted, we tend to take advantage of many social opportunities and enjoy a variety of group activities. If we are introverted, we may spend more time in solitary pursuits or in those requiring the participation of only a few people.

Another personal trait that may influence our leisure activity selection is our physical stamina and skills. Some of us are more suited physically to more strenuous physical activities such as skiing, swimming, or tennis. For those of us with less coordination, skill, and stamina, participation in these activities may feel like work.

Finally, our cognitive skill level or interests may determine the leisure activities that we are comfortable participating in. Those of us with highly abstract cognitive abilities may choose to play chess, do crossword puzzles, or play word games. People with different cognitive skills may find these same activities boring, confusing, or too demanding. People with less cognitive skill may find that participation feels like work.

Cultural Factors

Our family values and culture greatly affect our leisure participation. When our culture values productivity and usefulness to our family and our community, leisure activities may revolve around activities related to organized religion or hobbies that produce functional products. In some groups that believe in the centrality of the family, leisure pursuits may be centered in family activities. In these situations, one's free time and creative talents focus on enhancing family life and celebrating family events. In other families who believe in one's self-fulfillment as a person, each member of the family is encouraged to direct his or her time and energy toward exploring individual interests, which may lead to a person spending more time in solitary activity or in activities with like-minded people outside the family.

Cultural beliefs and values also affect how our gender or age may determine our leisure activities. Some cultures delineate appropriate activities by age, gender, or marital status. Some have specific rules about how and when men and women may participate in selected activities. For example, some cultural groups expect married women to spend their leisure time within the family and not in the community at large.

Personal Choice Considerations

How we use time outside of leisure may affect how we view and use leisure time. Some people view their choice of activities relative to what they do in their career or vocation. Neulinger (1981) postulated that people choose leisure activities that are the direct opposite of the daily work routine. Some examples include the following: A person who works at a desk or a computer may spend free time in physically strenuous sport activities (e.g., ride a bike, hike), a mother who spends most of her time attending to the family needs may seek out solitary activities where she can lose herself in an activity (e.g., jogging, painting, dancing), or a person who spends a significant amount of time in solitary work may actively seek group activities within a family or social network. Others seek leisure activities that are related to their chosen career or vocation. Some examples include the following: a person who attends conferences and socializes with members of his or her profession, a high school English teacher who chooses to read books and attend poetry readings, or a young carpenter who builds a boat in his free time.

Environmental Considerations

Our personal access to leisure environments, materials, and equipment strongly influences how we spend our free time and what activities we explore to meet our needs. If we live in a rural environment, we are likely to have the opportunity to explore and develop skill in many outdoor activities. In a city environment, we have a greater opportunity to participate as a spectator in a range of sporting and creative arts events. When we have economic resources, we can buy any materials or equipment that we need to participate in an activity of interest. Thus, personal resources have a significant influence on what leisure activities we choose to pursue.

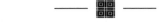

Exercise 13.2—Leisure Pursuits

Think about your leisure pursuits. What factors influence your choice of these leisure activities?

Barriers to Participation in Leisure Activities

Developing healthy leisure pursuits is challenging and threatening. For some of us, work and responsibilities seem to fill up every waking hour. We see leisure activities as frivolous. For others of us, leisure is threatening, frustrating, or a burden. We may be more comfortable having a consistent routine with required activities than to have an expanse of time that we must fill with our own planned activities. To have leisure means to step outside our daily routine. It requires us to challenge ourselves to participate in activities beyond those included in our daily routine. We have the right not to participate in leisure activities and to be passive in our free time. This lack of participation, however, is isolating and may lead to alienation and depression.

In the United States, we have many opportunities to be passive in our leisure time. A major American passive leisure activity is watching television. Television fills time. It sometimes entertains and relaxes us, and it can be a learning tool. Television, however, rarely helps us to understand ourselves more deeply, stretch the range of our intellect or emotions, or engage us with others. Although watching television and participating in other passive activities can help us use our leisure time in a way that makes us feel better than we would if we had nothing to do, it can lead us away from learning to truly experience our leisure time.

When exploring alternative leisure activities, we must recognize that a significant amount of corporate profit in Western society is related to mass consumption of leisure equipment and experiences. Corporations barrage us with advertising about the "perfect" use of leisure time that may interfere with searches for personal definitions of ideal leisure. Relentless advertising attempts to convince us that we want what they are offering. Some of us then begin to value only those leisure activities that are heavily advertised. The "right" pair of running shoes or sports equipment, belonging to the "right" gym, or going on the "right" vacations may become tied to our social status. This may result in our working more hours to afford leisure versus enjoying leisure. We may participate in fewer leisure activities or passive activities because we believe that participation in leisure activities requires a great deal of money.

Quart (2003) addressed the powerful negative influence that marketing targeted at youth has had on adolescents' values and spending habits. She reported that American teens have more than $155 billion in discretionary income. As a cohort, American teens are easy prey for marketers because of their openness to the media, their insecurities, and their desires to be included in their peer groups. The popular marketing strategy (i.e., promoting certain products and services through teen celebrities) has created strong desires among a growing segment of American youth for expensive, name-brand merchandise and physical perfection. More teens are working extra hours to buy the products and services that are heavily advertised; their money and time are being consumed, leaving less for productive adolescent leisure pursuits.

Stereotypes of others can be a barrier for leisure participation, especially for school-age children, teens, and older adults. A group of children may decide that one child is dumb and, therefore, exclude that child from playground activities or in child-initiated clubs. Adolescents identify themselves and one another with crowds who share certain observable behaviors (Brown, 1990). Typical crowd identifications in a high school may include "jocks, brains, or druggies." Certain crowds have more socioeconomic status than others. An adolescent who is associated with an unpopular or negative crowd may experience rejection and discomfort in trying to participate in some leisure activities that are more associated with another crowd. A healthy, elderly person may feel less included in some community activities that are typically associated with younger adults. The person may need to prove competence before experiencing acceptance in some leisure group activities.

Other barriers to access to leisure activities are our personal traits and internal resources, racial background, religious practices, sexual orientation, community resources, and certain select negative habits or behaviors. Some people have personal character issues that interfere with their ability to engage in leisure activities with others. These people may lack the internal resources (i.e., coping skills) or social skills to explore interests or connect with others through personally meaningful and productive activity. Whalen, Jamner, Henker, Delfino, and Lozano (2002) found that adolescents with attention deficit hyperactivity disorder (ADHD) symptoms were more likely to spend their time in passive, entertaining leisure pursuits than in hobbies and structured activities. The participants with ADHD in this study were 10 times more likely to have smoked and 4 times more likely to have consumed alcohol than adolescents without ADHD. Adolescents with ADHD may lack the skills to modulate their attention, which is important for skill development in active and productive leisure activities.

If communities do not have the resources or facilities for creative arts or organized sports, then these leisure activities are not available to people in those communities. In a study of four inner-city middle schools, Shann (2001) found that the children did not participate in after-school activities. The children reported that they participated primarily in unstructured and passive leisure activities, such as watching television and hanging out with their friends. Shann advocated for greater development of after-school and weekend activities programs for inner-city children. For elderly persons, a lack of transportation to attend their local senior citizens' center severely limits their ability to participate in community activities.

Finally, some barriers to participation are related to a person's negative habits or behaviors, such as abuse of drugs or alcohol or participation in gangs. Petty crime or violence may become means of relaxation, excitement, and connecting with others. Even when substance abuse and illegal activities cease, people who had been habitually involved in these activities may lack the skills to find and participate in satisfying leisure activities. Farnworth (2000) found that her sample of probationary adolescent offenders spent 57% of their time in passive leisure activities, such as watching television and listening to music. They reported being bored 42% of the time.

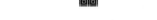

Exercise 13.3—Interests

Think about leisure pursuits that strongly interest you but that you do not participate in. What are the barriers to your participation?

Leisure Experiences Throughout the Life Span

Infancy Through Early Childhood

Leisure for children includes solitary activities and activities with caregivers or peers. Children's first leisure experiences are play. Play is child-initiated activity that an adult has not structured to teach specific skills. The child engages in the activity because he or she wants to and because it is fun. The child is free to participate independently or to negotiate sharing the activity with another. A parent might approach an infant with a busy box, and the infant may bang on it for a few minutes but then crawl away and pick up a pot to bang. The infant is in control of the activity. Thus, this same infant may look toward the parent when he or she wants the parent to join in or move away when he or she wants to play alone. An older child may build with blocks or do a puzzle because he or she finds the activity interesting versus participating in the activity because a parent or teacher instructed the child to complete the activity.

Erikson (1963) said that children's play "is not the equivalent of adult play…it is not recreation. The playing adult steps sideward into another reality, the playing child advances to new stages of mastery" (p. 222). Children's play concerns exploration and discovery in all spheres of human existence. Children's play continuously evolves, and what was once interesting is now boring. Children develop new skills and use them in novel ways during play. Although building skills is not the purpose of play, through play children become more competent in all areas of human functioning. They develop a capacity to cope with their environment and develop ego strength and an investment in life (Cotton, 1984).

Playfulness is an important aspect of children's play. Playfulness exists when a child is intrinsically motivated, internally controlled, and able to suspend reality (Bundy, 1997). Intrinsic motivation means that the child is driven to participate in particular activities because of the innate rewards that the child experiences in the activity. The child does not participate in play activities because he or she is expecting a reward or praise. The child gets involved to have fun. Internal control refers to the child having primary control over what occurs in the activity. When a child suspends reality, he or she uses objects in new ways to discover new uses for everyday things, or he or she makes believe (e.g., imaginary play, games). A child frames an activity by giving cues to others about how they should act toward him or her. For example, a child might cue a playmate that he or she is now going to play house and the other child is going to be the parent. A child who wants to play superheroes and be the "bad guy" may frame the activity so that his or her peers must now fight or run away. This role-playing allows the child to experience life from the perspective of another.

Play begins in infancy when an infant learns to attend to the faces of caregivers. Caregivers smile and make soft sounds at infants and wait for infants to respond in kind. Over time, infants are ready to play peek-a-boo or to imitate facial expressions and sounds that caregivers make. Infants begin to initiate the play, and the child and caregivers receive pleasure from the interaction. This mutual interaction evolves to social play by making a different face or a sound. Through parent–child play experiences in infancy and early childhood, children develop the coping skills necessary for more complex play. The most important variable in a young child's development of coping skills is the mother's leisure experiences with him or her, which is the mother's enjoyment of their play (Murphy & Moriarity, 1976).

Playing and interacting with other children is an important part of the leisure experiences of children from preschool age on up. Children share similar levels of physical activity, exuberance, and open emotional expression, which makes them more attractive to one another than adults are to them. Children share their interests with peers, and enthusiasm for certain activities increases or decreases depending on the reactions that valued peers have to those activities. Children will be more likely to take chances and participate in new activities when other children are participating in those activities. Through leisure play experiences, children learn the joys of friendship and camaraderie and learn to negotiate and compromise in the interest of maintaining peer relationships.

Supportive guidance of caregivers provides young children with confidence that they can successfully participate in an activity and have fun based on past experiences and pleasures. As children grow and enter middle childhood, some leisure activities become recreational ones. These activities have playful elements to them, but they are structured activities that occur as part of a team sport or within a club. Children who enter these activities have begun to accept rules as necessary for group activity. Without defined rules and some accepted order to activities, little pleasurable activity would occur. Children become interested in learning to draw or construct things by following a set plan and in learning new games and sports. This is, of course, important for future leisure participation in adolescence and adulthood.

Leisure for children begins to involve more complex games and group activities. Children master games of chance first, followed by games requiring strategies. In games of chance, children learn first to modulate their intense excitement related to the process of being in the lead or losing a game and accepting the outcome as "just a game" rather than as a statement about their competence. They learn to follow the rules and to inhibit negative emotions that might lead them to quit a game prematurely or to become aggressive when a game does not end in their favor. Depending on children's temperament and innate skills, initially learning games may be challenging to children and their caregivers. Children may be slow to learn or to acclimate to rules. Younger children often change the rules and cheat to win until losing becomes less threatening to them. Once children understand games and begin to accept rules, their animation, physical tension, and excitement in a simple game, such as Old Maid, can bring almost as much enjoyment to caregivers as it does to children.

McHale, Crouter, and Tucker (2001) found that, in making the transition to adolescence, children who participated in structured activities, such as hobbies and sports, were more likely to be well-adjusted adolescents. Children who spent their free time hanging out were more likely to exhibit less adaptive functioning, including poorer school grades and more conduct problems. It is important to balance the findings of this study with the work of Luthar (2003). She studied upper-middle-class suburban youth and found some relationship between overemphasis on achievement along with isolation from parents and the development of adjustment disorders in affluent youth. With two parents with demanding careers, a group of these youths often are left unsupervised or with minimal supervision. They are physically safe in their affluent neighborhoods but have limited resources for emotional support. In addition, these youths often perceive that they must meet or are expected to meet high external standards of performance in their after-school activities. These activities,

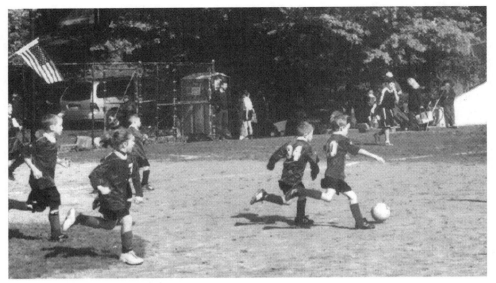

Figure 13.3. In middle childhood, organized sports may become a central leisure activity.

then, are no longer leisure activities where children are free from constraints and able to explore at their own pace and within their own interests.

———   ▦   ———

Exercise 13.4—Childhood

Think about a child whom you know well. What activities does that child participate in that you would consider play or leisure? Why? What underlying skills does the child have that support his or her participation? What needs do you think that the activities meet for the child? What effect, if any, do you think the child's participation will have on his or her overall development?

—————————

Adolescence

Peer groups and peer culture are the central focus of adolescent leisure in the United States (Brown, 1990). Peer friendships are a primary source of activity, influence, and support for most adolescents. Adolescents report enjoying activities with friends more than they do with family members, feeling most understood by friends and that they can be most fully themselves in the company of friends (Savin-Williams & Berndt, 1990). Adolescents tend to see themselves and their peers as fitting into particular groups. Group leisure opportunities increase or decrease depending on where adolescents fit within the culture of their school or community. A football player may be invited to many parties, whereas the president of the chess club may not. Although being a part of a high-status crowd may increase the number of group activities that an adolescent is included in, it may not enhance the adolescent's experience of leisure. Less popular teens may actively pursue individual or small group activities for which they have a passion and, thus, may have deep and satisfying friendships.

American adolescents spend up to 40% of their time in leisure pursuits (Csikszentmihalyi & Larson, 1984). Adolescent moods are the most positive and activity level is the highest when adolescents are engaged in leisure activities as opposed to work or school activities (Fine, Mortimer, & Roberts, 1990). How they use such a large block of leisure time is important to their psychosocial development. Kleiber, Larson, and Csikszentmihalyi (1986) conceptualized adolescent leisure as consisting of two types: relaxed leisure and transitional leisure. Relaxed leisure comprises those activities that are pleasurable but are not challenging, such as listening to music, watching television, or hanging out with friends at a local mall or park. Transitional leisure activities prepare an adolescent for the serious aspects of the adult world. These activities promote concentration and challenge and may include extracurricular school activities and individual hobbies, such as playing a musical instrument or developing high-level painting or dancing skills. This type of activity participation correlates with adult occupational prestige.

When adolescents participate solely in relaxed leisure activities, they are more likely to be less focused and at risk for developing behavior problems that negatively affect their development. Without activities to channel their energies positively, they may be more likely to seek out adventure through drinking, drug experimentation, or early sexual activity. In contrast, adolescents who discover their particular talents and develop habits to cultivate these talents invest a significant amount of time in related activities and develop comfort and the ability to use solitude effectively. As a result, they have a stronger grasp on their developing self-identity, and peers are less likely to influence them negatively. These teens tend to be more open to new experience and exhibit higher levels of concentration than other teens do. Of additional interest, many of these adolescents spend more time with their parents in leisure activities. Parental engagement provides them with a sense of support and consistency, encourages their intensity and self-direction, and enhances their attentional capacities for finding and mastering challenges (Csikszentmihalyi, Rathunde, & Whalen, 1993).

Transitional leisure pursuits can be a sanctuary for adolescents. These activities most often occur in safe and familiar settings that nurture self-expression and exploration. They may involve visiting the science laboratory or an art room of a favorite teacher after school, or may involve participating in a club or extracurricular class. Wilson (as cited in John-Steiner, 1985) studied the experiences of a group of high school students in art. The art room in a public high school was a retreat from the demands of the school environment. Within the room, these adolescents were able to "transcend the limitations of the structure, to engage in acts which are creative or ludic or subversive and to participate in a kind of communitas" (Wilson, as cited in John-Steiner, 1985, p. 94). Sports also are important activities in the socialization of adolescents. Sports are strong foci of adolescent interest. Through sports, adolescents increase their exposure to peers. The adolescent subculture associates athletic participation with adolescent physical fitness, competitiveness, and social status within the adolescent subculture (Savin-Williams & Berndt, 1990). With athletic excellence and physical appearance being so highly valued in the adolescent subculture, some adolescents experiment with anabolic steroids to increase their athletic prowess and muscle mass. Steroids have serious side effects, including increased aggression, irritability, and depression; the long-term risks to physical health include impotency, liver damage, and cancer (Cobb, 2003; Gullotta, Adams, & Markstrom, 2000; Quart, 2003).

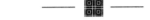

Exercise 13.5—Adolescence

Think back to your adolescent years. Describe your participation in leisure activities at that time. What activities were you regularly involved in that might be described as relaxed leisure activities? What activities were you regularly involved in that might be described as transitional leisure activities? How did these activities influence your experiences as an adolescent and your roles as an adult?

Young Adulthood

As people transition from adolescence into adulthood, shifts in leisure activities occur as individuals continue their education and begin their first real jobs. Many young adults move out of their family homes and enter a different world from that of their childhood and adolescence in which they shared living space with family members. This period becomes one of defining oneself outside one's family of origin. Leisure time may lessen because of work responsibilities or may increase for college students who do not work and who may now live independently with age mates.

When young adults decide to go to college, they pursue courses of study that expand their base of knowledge into new areas. They may develop interests that they were previously unaware of and may come to find that the areas that they were originally interested in are less compelling. The college environment provides numerous new opportunities for leisure activities, with new people to befriend. Many young adults who enter college continue to have a great deal of leisure time. Living independently on a college campus with roommates offers opportunities to explore and experiment. New leisure opportunities may be available at college that were not available in students' communities of origin. Young adults from a large city may find themselves in areas that provided opportunities for outdoor activities such as bike riding, canoeing, hiking, or skiing. Young adults from rural areas may find themselves in a major metropolitan area and discover a love for live music and theater that they never experienced. New friends may come from different backgrounds and expose these young adults to new social opportunities. Additionally, activities that were chores of adolescence may now become valued leisure activities. Preparing a meal in one's own apartment for friends may be a way of expressing one's identity and a way of relaxing. Painting and decorating a dorm room or apartment may be a work of self-expression that a young adult can enjoy for long periods.

This time may also involve the loss of treasured leisure activities secondary to relocation or the responsibilities of being a college student. This transition may be accompanied by difficulty coping with the changes in tasks and activities associated with being a college student in addition to the lack of opportunity to engage in pleasurable and success-assured activities. At this time, many young adults are testing their abilities in pursuit of a future career.

For young adults who enter the workforce, their leisure activities may likewise change. Young adults entering the workforce are entering a new cultural forum in which ethnicity, culture, and gender may be minimized because one is present to perform a job. Pressure may exist to conform to the majority culture, and young adults must learn to adjust their personal values and conduct in the work environment. Leisure is a critical occupational area for workers to explore so that they may find activities that reaffirm their sense of identity, allow them to develop areas of interest and talent, reaffirm a sense of belonging to specific cultural groups, and rejuvenate the soul and spirit. Workers may continue some of the leisure activities of their school years, such as participating in local adult sport leagues; participating in music bands; and attending spectator sports, movies, or live music events. These young adults may remain in the same geographic area and may socialize with the same or similar friends. The major change in their lives is going to work full-time, which results in a notable decrease in their amount of leisure time compared with high school. Their leisure time often is now limited to the weekends or to days off from work.

For all young adults, a considerable amount of leisure time may focus on establishing relationships with a significant other. Sharing leisure activities is a central part of courtship in Western culture. Through these activities, young people socialize in a nonthreatening, neutral environment in which there is a mutually interesting activity, such as dinner, a movie, a sporting event, or a bike ride. Such activities allow a relationship to develop in a relaxed manner. When like-minded people share leisure activities, a bond of friendship may develop. Sharing an activity or adventure with another provides situations in which one learns about him- or herself and the other person.

People may reflect their pleasure in the joint activity by having a positive regard for each other and may develop greater interest in learning more about the other as a person. As a meaningful relationship with a significant other develops, young adults adjust their time commitments to fit the other person's leisure interests. Couples negotiate how much leisure time they will spend together, especially when they have different individual leisure interests and pursuits. Each person in a couple adjusts leisure expectations in the interest of the relationship. One person may give up socializing in a bar or participating in a league sport to please a partner. Another may adjust to a partner's hobby by developing an interest in that hobby to increase shared leisure time. Both partners may take up a new activity together, such as ballroom dancing, to deepen their bond. People may participate individually or with friends in some activities that are particularly rejuvenating, such as spectator sports or physical activities. Couples begin to share holidays and family traditions and events. They begin entertaining friends and family members together. A young woman may accommodate by learning to participate in her husband's traditional Italian family dinner every Sunday.

Young adults with physical disabilities may have limited opportunities for socializing and pursuing leisure activities that interest them. This may severely hinder their ability to pursue a significant relationship. When a person is physically disabled, not only are the activities limited, but also the variety of people involved may be limited. People with disabilities may be limited by the availability of family members for transportation as well as for company as they participate in leisure activities outside their home. Becoming less engaged with family members and more engaged with peers in leisure pursuits may not be possible or may be much more difficult than it is for young adults without disabilities.

In healthy young adulthood, people maintain solitary or group leisure interests that have developed during the life span. Certain activities are part of one's persona, support self-esteem, and rejuvenate. Some people may have a long-standing interest in cars that develops into restoring vintage cars. Sewing, knitting, or jewelry making may be a way of expressing one's artistic side, even though one may work as a store clerk. Others may join adult community sports leagues or coach children's sport activities. Many young adults who enjoyed biking as children and teenagers join biking clubs to maintain physical fitness and rejuvenate their physical beings.

Drinking alcohol as part of social events is often part of the passage from childhood to adulthood in Western culture. The use of substances such as drugs and alcohol may stem from a search for pleasurable feelings that substances can induce (Kraus, 1994). Alcohol can lower one's inhibitions and make socialization easier. When drinking dominates how people spend their leisure time, enjoyment of this activity (as well as other activities) diminishes.

Middle Adulthood

Whether adults choose to marry, remain single, or decide to have children influences how they conceptualize and use leisure time in middle age. People who marry are likely to change how they use some of their leisure time to include their spouses and extended family members. Taking care of children and sharing leisure pursuits with children occupy a large amount of the leisure time of parents.

Single adults continue to seek, establish, and maintain long-term relationships with significant others, but they are likely to pursue and further develop their skills in hobbies and activities in which they have engaged across the life span. Single adults are likely to be settled in their careers and to have adjusted to single adulthood; they have time to devote to enhancing skills in lifelong leisure activities and pursue new interests. In the process, they discover more about themselves as people and their potential to contribute to society in ways other than caring for children. In midlife, some people may become more reflective about community issues or politics and now decide that they have the personal skills and resources to have a positive effect on their community. Others may turn past hobbies into part-time careers; for example, they may write, buy and sell antiques, or design jewelry.

In some ways, single life presents a greater challenge but more opportunity for the development of a rich adult leisure life. Single people confront expanses of unstructured time unencumbered by responsibilities to children or to a spouse. A person may perceive this as freedom or as a burden. They can pursue interests without the restraint of the needs or disapproval of immediate family members. Without an active approach to leisure participation, a single person may experience isolation and discontent. Having solitary leisure interests can be helpful to a single adult because others may not be immediately available for interaction. Finding companions for joint leisure activities is a more active process for single adults than for people with families or spouses. For some, a lack of companionship can present a serious barrier to leisure participation; for others, it is an opportunity to develop new relationships, deepen older relationships, and expand their leisure opportunities through varied companions. Single adults are more likely to participate in group travel or adult leisure organizations than adults with families or spouses. Single adults may be more independent and willing to take risks to participate in activities that interest them. Single women may not experience the retreat from exploration of their own abilities and personal interests that many married women do during their childbearing years.

Women's roles notably change when they become parents. Parenting changes a woman's work life or career to a greater extent than men experience, even if a woman continues to work after childbirth. Although men share in child care and home maintenance activities, most mothers fulfill the role of primary caregiver. Women's former leisure experiences tend to decrease more notably than their husbands' experiences do. Men may share equally in leisure activities with children, but women typically provide more instrumental child care.

Leisure activities of parents who do not work outside the home are usually home centered. Activities may include gardening, sewing, home crafts, cooking, and parent–child play. These parents intersperse these activities among house and child maintenance chores. In families in which both parents work outside the home, family leisure activities often are limited to evenings and weekends. These activities are special because the time together is short. Eating a family meal, reading a book together, and playing a game may be more important than household maintenance activities.

The leisure activities of a family undergo many transitions as children grow. When children are infants, they may greatly curtail parents' leisure activities as parents adjust to parenthood. Leisure may revolve around playful interaction with the infant or sharing parenting experiences with other parents or with older adults who can provide support and guidance to the new parents. Satisfying leisure needs with infants and young children requires effort on the part of the adults. In addition to the home-based leisure activities, parents of young children often visit parks and other public places where other parents and children congregate. They may attend religious functions, parent–child drop-in centers, or gym activities designed to facilitate parent–child interaction and interaction with other families. These community activities provide parents with an opportunity to interact with children in the proximity of other parents, which allows adults to share their parenting joys and frustrations. In these activities, children have the opportunity to meet other adults and children.

Some parents make connections to their children by sharing their leisure passions. Parents may teach their children sports, begin to take them to sporting events, and share the experience of cheering their favorite team. If children show an interest in learning a sport that interests a parent, the sport may provide a means through which the parent and children relate. Positive feelings about the activity become closely associated with positive feelings toward one another, and the sport can bring the two closer together. Parents may return to the leisure activities of their youth as part of their role as parent. A parent may have loved soccer as a child and now coaches his or her child's soccer team.

When children reach adolescence, family-focused leisure time may occur less frequently. Although adolescents may still participate in selected family, religious, or cultural activities, they tend to begin to move beyond their immediate family for leisure pursuits. Parents may feel loss, abandonment, or a new sense of freedom as their adolescent children's leisure increasingly focuses on activities outside the family unit. Parents may experience jealousy as their teenagers' leisure activities become more exciting than their own activities. Activities in adolescence are very different from watching young children participate in the leisure activities of scouting or sports.

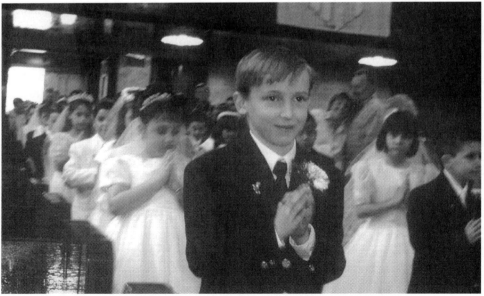

Figure 13.4. Family leisure activities may involve facilitating children's participation in religious rites of passage and activities.

This change may lead parents to question and reevaluate their own leisure activities. The leisure triumphs of an adolescent may facilitate parents' positive moods and interests in activity participation (Steinberg & Steinberg, 1994).

As children grow into adults, parental satisfaction in activities outside their role as parents provides a buffer to the experience of turmoil with the transition. In Steinberg and Steinberg's (1994) qualitative study, parents who were not engaged in satisfying activities beyond that of parenthood were vulnerable to severe distress as their children became adolescents. They interpreted their findings as suggesting that activities such as individual hobbies or community service provide a distraction and support the parents' sense of personal competence and self-worth as the parents adjust to the loss of spending a great deal of time with their children.

When children move on to their own adult lives, middle-aged adults must refocus their leisure pursuits. Although women are more likely to experience psychological turmoil during their offsprings' adolescence before the children leave home, they adjust more easily to the "empty-nest syndrome" than do fathers (Steinberg & Steinberg, 1994). Women are more likely to be engaged in exploring new careers, new interests, or community activities than men. Some believe that change may occur because young women may surrender their own desires in the interest of their husbands and growing family; once their children are grown, women may seek to reclaim their sense of individuality and pursue activities that provide personal satisfaction (Labouvie-Vief, 1994; Niemela & Linto, 1994).

During later middle age, a couple may pursue new joint activities. A parent may reinvest his or her newly acquired time in individual hobbies. Work demands may have lessened so that the time that people focused on career building is now available for leisure pursuits. Leisure travel may become more frequent because the parents' financial situation may be better now that children are independent and parents make fewer demands on their children's time. Middle to older adulthood can be a time to do some of the activities that one has always wanted to do but never did. One begins to see a time limit to one's opportunity to participate in those activities. Some people run their first marathon at 50 years of age. Others use late middle age to challenge themselves intellectually in ways that they wished that they had done as younger adults. Some adults reenter education to finish a high school diploma, pursue a college degree for the sake of knowledge, or pursue another career that they expect may be more fulfilling than their first career. For others, late middle adulthood is an opportunity to connect with other adults in ways that were not possible when they were raising children or focusing on their career. They may develop new or revived passions for activities such as gourmet cooking, golf, bridge, travel, or book clubs.

Middle adulthood is a time when one may have to begin to think about one's physical abilities as awareness grows that minor physical injuries take longer to heal and affect function longer than they did when one was younger. People inevitably experience a decrease in vision acuity and a change in body metabolism, which may result in weight gain or obesity. Some people in middle adulthood may also develop high blood pressure, diabetes, or high cholesterol. These changes and dysfunctions associated with age may interfere with participation in leisure unless people make accommodations in their routines or activities.

Exercise 13.6—Parent Interview

Interview a parent. Discuss the effect of children on his or her participation in leisure activities. What does a parent value in his or her leisure time? How much leisure time does he or she have per day or per week? How does he or she spend it? What leisure activities does he or she participate in alone, with children, with other adults? Compare his or her leisure experiences with that of a single adult you know.

Older Adulthood

Besides successfully avoiding disease and disability, successful aging requires maintenance of physical and cognitive function and engagement in social and productive activities (Hultsch, Hertzog, Small, & Dixon, 1999; Rowe & Kahn, 1997). The importance of establishing or maintaining meaningful occupations in elderly people was demonstrated in a Well Elderly research study (Jackson, Carlson, Mandel, Zemke, & Clark, 1998) that found identification and engagement in meaningful occupations to have an effect on the overall well-being of older adults. Participating in leisure is the most important predictor of well-being among older adults (Zimmer, Hickey, & Searle, 1997).

When older adults retire from paid employment, they have a new opportunity to explore their interests, who they have been during their lifetime, and who they would like to be for the remainder of their lives. If they have maintained some leisure interests throughout their lives, retirement may allow them to expand on those interests and devote more time to the activities that they love. For others, retirement leads to depression or a crisis as they attempt to adjust to a new way of life. When confronted with unstructured time, these older adults may not have the initiative to pursue new or reconnect with old leisure activities. There may be a grieving process related to loss of the previous role. The role of worker is one of the most important roles that one identifies with throughout adult life.

Past participation in leisure activities typically determines the activities that a retiree seeks out. Optimally, people who have neglected developing leisure occupations throughout the earlier part of their lives will begin to explore leisure activities within their community and learn what they really like to do and care about beyond the daily routine of their life's work. Volunteer work in hospitals, schools, or community organizations can provide a structure that organizes daily life in similar ways that paid employment did and may offer older adults an opportunity to find a new life purpose, enhance self-worth, and increase social contact with others (Morrow-Howell, Hinterlong, Rozario, & Tang, 2003; Singleton, 1996).

People's bodies and minds respond differently to the aging process. Although many elderly people may seek out more solitary and sedentary activities, many well elderly people are gregarious and seek out regular exercise. They may swim a few miles every week, in-line skate, enter marathons, take tai chi or yoga classes, or bicycle ride. Others maintain an interest in and regularly participate in outdoor activities. Some older adults actually increase their involvement because they have greater discretionary time. Many people retain solitary interests that have sustained their spirits throughout their lifetimes, including writing, playing an instrument, or painting. As their social obligations lessen, elderly people may become more focused on these activities.

Leisure pursuits may markedly change when adults become grandparents, especially when the grandchildren live nearby. Time spent with family members may now revolve around entertaining and engaging grandchildren. Grandchildren can bring out a more relaxed ability to nurture and play that may not have been possible with one's own children. Grandparents may have increased discretionary time and have the wisdom of experience to be able to enjoy the time they spend with their grandchildren.

Older adults living alone report fluctuations between extremes of involvement with others and projects and periods of isolation (Siegel, 1993). An issue for these adults is how to find a balance in their time and to make the time that they have left to live more valuable and meaningful for themselves. Some people may have difficulty managing this life stage; others seek and find creative aspects of themselves that they have not recognized during earlier years of their lives.

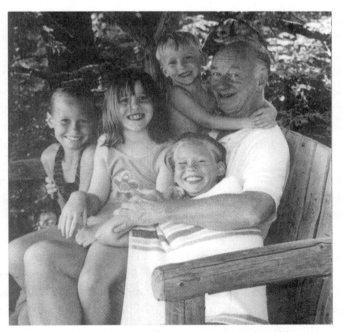

Figure 13.5. Children and grandparents often treasure their shared leisure experiences.

For some mature adults, senior citizens centers become important places of social interaction. Regularly attending meetings and activities may provide the structure and support that some people need to deal with the loss of their jobs and former roles at retirement or with the loss of spouses and friends to death. Activities such as bingo, weekly card games, and day trips with local organizations demonstrate a shift from independent activity to activities that are more interdependent or involve dependence on others. Within the structure of these centers, older adults may find new ways to contribute to their communities; for example, they may make blankets for infants or participate in making products for nonprofit fundraising.

Older adults experience the loss of lifelong partners and close friends, which may result in feelings of isolation and disconnection. Because much of the daily activities of elderly persons is voluntary and is not required work, it is easier to retreat from activity participation. Support groups with adults experiencing similar losses often help these persons in coming to terms with these experiences and in finding ways to reconstruct meaningful lives. In summarizing the experiences of 56 older women who participated in her qualitative study on aging, Siegel (1993) stated,

> With each death of a loved one...we learn something more about who we are within that relationship and who we are without the presence of that person. With each loss, we also learn more about death and dying and about how to cope and survive. (p. 184)

As people near the end of their lives, they are likely to be unable to participate in some past leisure activities because of the infirmities of old age. Some people may cease participation and not seek new activities that interest them, but many older adults replace physically active pursuits with more passive ones in which they can readily participate ("Prevalence of Health-Care Providers Asking Older Adults About Their Physical Activity Levels," 2002; Zimmer et al., 1997). It is not uncommon as one gets older to need to shift from more active occupations to less active occupations; this is not to imply that there is less satisfaction in these occupations (Parker, 1996). Older adults who are likely to feel most in control of their lives will adapt their former interests to their bodies' changes in old age and will work to improve their bodies' functioning for participation through regular exercise, good nutrition, and mental activity (Baltes & Baltes, 1990; Everard, Lach, Fisher, & Baum, 2000).

Frail elderly people may become homebound and gradually lose interest in many leisure activities, including social ones. They may spend more time reflecting on the past and come to depend on adult children or community services for social interaction. In some situations, the adult may require adaptations or assistive devices (e.g., a magnifier to read a book or newspaper, adaptations to a telephone to amplify sound) to participate in leisure activities.

Considering Leisure in Prevention and Occupational Therapy Intervention

The occupation of leisure is a critical aspect of life, and developing the occupation of leisure in clients should be a primary concern for occupational therapy practitioners interested in prevention or working with people with disabilities. As described earlier in this chapter, when people are able to fully participate in the occupation of leisure, the people are more likely to support their mental and physical health.

Leisure skill development as prevention is applicable across the life span but may be particularly important for adolescents, those approaching retirement, and elderly people. The members of these cohorts may have more discretionary time that can potentially enrich their lives, but free time that people do not productively use for activities of interest may be experienced as disorganizing or depressing. Occupational therapy practitioners who are cognizant of the centrality of meaningful occupation for mental health are ideal health providers for assisting these people in developing healthy leisure habits. Those approaching retirement, early retirees, and elderly people may have developed activity limitations or participation restrictions related to arthritis, diabetes, or pulmonary or cardiac dysfunction, and they may need to reconsider their choices of leisure activities, develop new interests, or adapt how they participate in favored activities. It is not uncommon as one gets older to need to shift from more active occupations to less active occupations; this is not to imply that there is less satisfaction in occupations (Parker, 1996).

The Well Elderly Study established occupational therapy as an effective preventive intervention for the well elderly population (Jackson et al., 1998). This study demonstrated that occupational therapy services focused the power of occupation and its ability to enhance health through occupation. The intervention group was provided with education on a variety of topics that are relevant to the engagement in meaningful occupations and opportunities to experience meaningful activities of their choice. Overall, those receiving occupational therapy had more positive gains and fewer declines in function than those who took part in a social activity program.

Limited exposure to the possibilities for leisure engagement within their communities and limited support in developing skills for participation in those activities leave many people with developmental disabilities with a narrow range of interests that may be passive and not supportive of their physical and mental health. For example, studies suggest that adolescents and young adults with Down syndrome typically participate in passive and sedentary recreational activities, such as watching television or listening to music, for as much as 5 hours a day (Heyne, Schleien, & Rynders, 1997). These inactive and passive leisure pursuits are likely to be a contributing factor to obesity and passivity often observed in people with this disorder.

Assessment

Client-centered practice has been defined as "an approach to service which embraces a philosophy of respect for, and partnership with, people receiving services" (Law, Baptiste, & Mills, 1995, p. 253). This approach focuses on the occupational problems identified by the client as he or she relates to his or her ability to carry out role-related occupations. This "top down," occupation-based approach supports the assessing of the occupation of leisure. The Canadian Occupational Measure (Law et al., 1994) is one client-centered assessment used as an individualized measure to detect changes in a person's perception of his or her performance and satisfaction with occupations. Leisure is one of the areas of occupational performance assessed.

In addition, new tools have been developed that not only explore what a person's interests are and how frequently he or she pursued those interests but also facilitate practitioners' exploring what those leisure interests and activities mean to clients. Meaning is central to occupation. For example, Henry (2000) developed the Pediatric Interest Profiles, which are paper-and-pencil surveys of play and leisure for children and adolescents from 6 to 21 years of age. The profiles are simply designed so that children or adolescents can complete them independently or with minimal assistance from an adult in 20 to 30 minutes. A practitioner gains concrete information about a child's or adolescent's interests, actual participation, and view of his or her own participation. These data are meant to be used to facilitate a focused discussion with the child or adolescent about the meaning of their leisure interests, present participation, and desires for further development of their leisure occupations.

The Leisure Activity Profile (Mann & Talty, 1991) is specific to people who are addicted to alcohol. The Leisure Interest Profiles (Henry, 1997a, 1997b) look at the client's interests and participation in play and leisure activities for adults and seniors.

The Barth Time Construction (Barth, 1988), a time chart on which a client pastes colored strips of paper to depict the categories of activities and the amount of time devoted to particular activities over the course of a day and week before a psychiatric hospitalization, is an effective assessment for many clients, especially for clients with substance abuse disorders. The Barth Time Construction provides clients and the occupational therapy practitioner with a graphic picture of time use over the course of a week. Clients with substance abuse disorders frequently are struck by the amount of time that they have devoted to getting, using, and recovering from the effect of alcohol or drugs before seeking treatment. The time chart that clients create can generate a deep discussion about the lack of or minimal amount of meaningful leisure activities in these clients' lives and their individual desires for occupational development for a healthy lifestyle.

Intervention

A client-centered, occupation-based approach to a client should be at the center of occupational therapy intervention. Effective occupational therapy results from our understanding of the client's underlying abilities and needs. Depending on a client's disability, a practitioner may use a variety of frames of reference to assist the client in developing skills or in altering the task or environment for participation in leisure interests. Through applying the sensory integration and motor learning frames of reference, a practitioner may help a child to develop sufficient balance and bilateral coordination for bicycle riding or in-line skating. To assist a client who suffered a hand injury to develop the fine motor strength, endurance, and dexterity to play a musical instrument again, a practitioner may use a biomechanical frame of reference. Adolescents with attention deficit disorder may learn how to modulate their attention and physical states to optimally participate in after-school clubs through working with an occupational therapy practitioner skilled in using an intervention approach that combines concepts of sensory integration with cognitive theory, such as the program developed by Williams and Shellenberger (1994).

Facilitating the development of active and social leisure for people with disabilities may be hindered by the initial resistance to physical activity related to difficulty with fine motor and gross motor skills. When a child has a learning disability or other cognitive disabilities, parents may struggle with interacting with the child in leisure activities. The child may avoid or be unable to attend to learning the typical leisure activities that parents teach and share with the child. The child may stay focused on familiar and repetitive activities or may be emotionally labile or withdrawn when confronted with leisure experiences that are pleasurable to other children. This may result in power struggles between parent and child or a more distant parent–child relationship, with parent and child mutually feeling sad, frustrated, and angry. Occupational therapy practitioners can help parents to guide their children in discovering individual and family leisure activities that are meaningful to both the parents and the child. The therapist may guide parents in learning how to provide support and assistance to their children in confronting new activities or new challenges in old activities. Parents may learn how to modify and adapt activities to foster their children's participation. Parental engagement in helping children in this way facilitates children's development of attentional and coping capacities necessary for future engagement in independent leisure activities. At the same time, satisfying parent–child leisure interaction has positive effects on both the parents' and the children's sense of competence and mood.

Adult clients also may avoid leisure occupations that interest them because of their expectations of failure as a result of pain, being physically unfit or unprepared to undertake the activity, or having limited skills. Assisting clients in adjusting their expectations for their participation, adapting activities or locating adaptive equipment that would allow their participation, and developing the physical skills that they have for participation are important intervention strategies for the occupational therapy practitioner to consider. The practitioner may help a client to make a connection with an organization, such as Tetra Society of North America (www.reachdisability.org/tetra), or may work collaboratively with such a volunteer organization in guiding a person with a disability to participation in leisure occupations of his or her own choosing. Tetra is a volunteer organization developed by a person with tetraplegia who was active in many outdoor sports before his injury. At present, he participates in sailing and many other outdoor activities with adaptations. Tetra is dedicated to finding volunteer engineers and other professionals who work with people with disabilities to design and fabricate assistive devices to make possible participation in particular activities that are important to each person with disability.

Guiding clients to adapt their environments so that they can readily participate in activities is a treatment strategy that an occupational therapy practitioner regularly uses with clients with all levels of disability. A parent may need to simplify game instructions so that a child with a learning disability can play with other children or her family members. Reducing extraneous visual or auditory stimuli in the environment may greatly improve the ability of a person with developmental disabilities to participate in a leisure activity. Other clients may have or may develop sufficient skill during the course of therapy but may lack sufficient external resources for regular participation in activities that interest them. A therapist then may need to evaluate clients' present and required levels of resources necessary for satisfying leisure. A single adult with a physical disability may be interested in travel, or a senior citizen may be interested in finding partners for playing bridge. Helping clients to find community resources or connecting them to another professional or an agency that can find the appropriate external resources for clients are important interventions.

Chronic physical or mental illness in a family may severely weaken marital and parent–child relationships, which reduces the amount and quality of emotional support that children receive from their parents or that spouses receive from each other. Joint leisure activities may be the first activities that the family members sacrifice as stress increases. Playful and relaxed interaction may be minimal or nonexistent. Reexperiencing positive family leisure activities can have a major positive effect on each family member's mood and on the overall emotional atmosphere of the family. Occupational therapy practitioners can help family members to alter their joint leisure activities in response to the effect of the illness and the change in family activities.

Adolescents with disabilities may be isolated from their mainstream peer group and believe that they have few options for activity outside school. Adults with brain injury may lose previous friendships and the ability to participate in some leisure pursuits resulting from reduced cognitive functioning. Life situations related to lack of leisure activities can have a major effect on every area of life functioning; the person may become depressed, passive, and dependent. Participating in a group that focuses on the occupation of leisure may help the person to explore potential leisure interests; develop activity, social, and time management skills for leisure participation; learn how to reduce barriers to leisure participation; and develop a network of similar people who are interested in joint leisure activities. Developing a personally meaningful leisure life is likely to result in a generalized sense of well-being, independence, and personal control.

Whether it is a primary disability or a secondary one related to a physical disability, depression can have devastating effects on the everyday functioning of people.

Developing leisure interests and experiencing successful participation in them may lessen the negative effects of difficult life situations and give people a new perspective on their lives and their ability to exert control over everyday activities. New interests may reduce a sense of alienation and make people more available for interaction with others. Others may need to find leisure outlets to express strong emotions that they cannot express in other everyday activities. Actively participating in sports or games or watching spectator sports may provide a socially acceptable outlet for aggressive impulses. Developing the habit of journal or poetry writing may provide a means for expressing and working through intense feelings for another person.

Adolescents with behavior disorders may have little awareness of their own individual interests and talents and their potential to develop as contributing members of society. They may be solely focused on their role within a negative peer group. Practitioners may engage such adolescents in exploring leisure activities and discovering individual interests and talents. For example, one adolescent may find that he really enjoys the solitary experience of baking; baking may give him time to relax away from peers and to think about his own life issues. Baking may lead to more prosocial individual action on the part of the teen at other times of the day. In addition, he may become aware that he has a talent for baking, be motivated to participate in baking activities regularly, and may begin thinking about education or employment in food services.

Throughout the intervention process, practitioners should be cognizant of clients' innate temperaments. Practitioners' expectations and style of intervention are affected by clients' temperaments. People who are generally positive and easily adapt to changes in their physical status or life circumstances are likely to put practitioners at ease and increase practitioners' expectation for successful interventions. People who tend to have difficulty persevering, have typically negative mood states, and are slow to adapt to changes may be frustrating to practitioners, who may lower expectations of what they and these clients can achieve together. People who are slow to adapt to changes may need more support at any life stage when they attempt to pursue new leisure activities.

The leisure needs of our clients are critical to address despite all of the pressures to first meet the other rehabilitation needs of our clients and the high demands of our health care system. Certainly, we can address some needs simultaneously, but remember that helping clients to develop a rich and personally meaningful leisure life may facilitate their achievement of all other goals of intervention that society values more than leisure.

Summary

Although leisure is a "second thought" that one may consider only after completing required and routine activities of daily life, it can be a powerful buffer for the stresses and negative events of other occupations. Leisure can facilitate relationships and help people to discover their true vocation or life purpose. Through activities that help us express our full emotional range in socially acceptable activities, we maintain emotional equilibrium. One can experience the benefits of leisure only by truly engaging in activities that hold one's interest and possibly one's soul. Leisure is a challenge; it requires as much focused energy as other human occupations. Without active pursuit of a leisure life, free time may be a burden; it may become a time of passivity, boredom, disconnection, unhappiness, confusion, or loneliness.

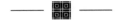

Exercise 13.8—Compare Leisure Values and Experiences

Compare the leisure values and experiences of all of the people of different ages that you talked to or thought about while studying this chapter. What did you learn about leisure across the life span? ■

References

Baltes, P. B., & Baltes, M. M. (1990). Psychological perspectives on successful aging: The model of selective optimization with compensation. In P. B. Baltes & M. M. Baltes (Eds.). *Successful aging: Perspectives from the behavioral sciences* (pp. 1–34). London: Cambridge University Press.

Barth, T. (1988). Barth Time Construction. In B. Hemphill (Ed.), *Mental health assessment in occupational therapy: An integrative approach to the evaluative process* (pp. 115–129). Thorofare, NJ: Slack.

Brown, B. B. (1990). Peer groups and peer culture. In S. S. Feldman & G. R. Elliot (Eds.), *At the threshold: The developing adolescent* (pp. 171–196). Cambridge, MA: Harvard University Press.

Bundy, A. C. (1997). Play and playfulness: What to look for. In L. D. Parham & L. S. Fazio (Eds.), *Play in occupational therapy for children* (pp. 52–66). St. Louis, MO: Mosby.

Chess, S., & Thomas, A. (1984). *Origins and evolutions of behavior disorders: From infancy to early adult life.* New York: Brunner & Mazel.

Cobb, N. (2003). *Adolescence: Continuity, change and diversity* (5th ed.). New York: McGraw-Hill.

Cotton, N. (1984). Childhood play as an analog to adult capacity to work. *Child Psychology and Human Development, 14,* 135–144.

Csikszentmihalyi, M. (1992). A theoretical model for enjoyment. In M. T. Allison (Ed.), *Play, leisure and quality of life: Social scientific perspectives* (pp. 11–23). Dubuque, IA: Kendall/Hunt.

Csikszentmihalyi, M., & Larson, R. (1984). *Being adolescent.* Basic (Basic Books, Inc., Publishers): New York.

Csikszentmihalyi, M., Rathunde, K., & Whalen, S. (1993). *Talented teenagers: The roots of success and failure.* New York: Cambridge University Press.

Elias, N., & Dunning, E. (1986). *Quest for excitement: Sport and leisure in the civilizing process.* New York: Basil Blackwell.

Erikson, E. H. (1963). *Childhood and society* (2nd ed.). New York: Norton.

Everard, K. M., Lach, H. W., Fisher, E. B., & Baum, M. C. (2000). Relationship of activity and social support to the functional health of older adults. *Journal of Gerontology: Psychological Sciences and Social Sciences, 55B*(4), S208–S212.

Farnworth, L. J. (2000). Time use and leisure occupations of young offenders. *American Journal of Occupational Therapy, 54,* 315–325.

Fine, G. A., Mortimer, J. T., & Roberts, D. F. (1990). Leisure, work, and the mass media. In S. S. Feldman & G. R. Elliot (Eds.), *At the threshold: The developing adolescent* (pp. 225–253). Cambridge, MA: Harvard University Press.

Gulick, A. (1998, July/August). Project tide. *Alert Diver,* pp. 39–43.

Gullotta, T. P., Adams, G. R., & Markstrom, C. A. (2000). *The adolescent experience* (4th ed.). San Diego, CA: Academic.

Henry, A. D. (1997a). *Leisure Interest Profile for Adults* (Research version 2.0). Boston: University of Massachusetts Medical Center.

Henry, A. D. (1997b). *Leisure Interest Profile for Seniors* (Research version 2.0). Boston: University of Massachusetts Medical Center.

Henry, A. D. (2000). *Pediatric Interest Profiles: Surveys of play for children and adolescents.* San Antonio, TX: Therapy SkillBuilders.

Heyne, L. A., Schleien, S. J., & Rynders, J. E. (1997). Promoting quality of life through recreation participation. In S. M. Pueschel & M. Sustrova (Eds.), *Adolescents with Down syndrome: Toward a fulfilling life* (pp. 317–340). Baltimore: Brookes.

Hultsch, D. F., Hertzog, C., Small, B. J., & Dixon, R. A. (1999). Use it or lose it: Engaged lifestyle as a buffer of cognitive decline in aging? *Psychology and Aging, 14,* 245–263.

Jackson, J., Carlson, M., Mandel, D., Zemke, R., & Clark, F. (1998). Occupation in lifestyle redesign: The Well Elderly Study Occupational Therapy Program. *American Journal of Occupational Therapy, 52,* 326–336.

John-Steiner, V. (1985). *Notebooks of the mind: Explorations of thinking.* New York: Harper & Row.

Kleiber, D. A., Larson, R., & Csikszentmihalyi, M. (1986). The experience of leisure in adolescence. *Journal of Leisure Research, 18,* 169–176.

Kraus, R. (1994). *Leisure in a changing America: Multicultural perspectives.* New York: Macmillan College.

Labouvie-Vief, G. (1994). Women's creativity and images of gender. In B. F. Turner & L. E. Trol (Eds.), *Women growing older: Psychological perspectives* (pp. 140–165). Thousand Oaks, CA: Sage.

Law, M., Baptiste, S., Carswell, A., McColl, M. A., Polatajko, H., & Pollock, N. (1994). *The Canadian Occupational Performance Measure* (2nd ed.). Toronto, Ontario: Canadian Association of Occupational Therapists, ACE.

Law, M., Baptiste, S., & Mills, J. (1995). Client-centred practice: What does it mean and does it make a difference? *Canadian Journal of Occupational Therapy, 62,* 250–257.

Luthar, S. S. (2003). The culture of affluence: Psychological costs of material wealth. *Child Development, 74,* 1581–1593.

Mann, W. C., & Talty, P. (1991). Leisure activity profile measuring use of leisure time by persons with alcoholism. *Occupational Therapy in Mental Health, 10*(4), 31–41.

Manuele, E. (1998). My rebirth. *NARHA Strides (Spirit Club News Insert), 4,* 2.

McHale, S. M., Crouter, A. C., & Tucker, C. J. (2001). Free-time activities in middle child-hood: Links with adjustment in early adolescence. *Child Development, 72,* 1764–1778.

Morrow-Howell, N., Hinterlong, J., Rozario, P. A., & Tang, F. (2003). Effects of volunteer-ing on the well-being of older adults. *Journal of Gerontology: Psychological and Social Sciences, 58B*(3), S137–S145.

Murphy, L. B., & Moriarity, A. E. (1976). *Vulnerability, coping, and growth: From infancy to adolescence.* New Haven, CT: Yale University Press.

Neulinger, J. (1981). *The psychology of leisure.* Springfield, IL: Charles C. Thomas.

Niemela, P., & Linto, R. (1994). The significance of the 50th birthday for women's individ-uation. In B. F. Turner & L. E. Trol (Eds.), *Women growing older: Psychological perspec-tives* (pp. 117–127). Thousand Oaks, CA: Sage.

Parker, M. D. (1996). The relationship between time spent by older adults in leisure activi-ties and life satisfaction. *Physical and Occupational Therapy in Geriatrics, 14*(3), 61–71.

Pieper, J. (1963). *Leisure: The basis of culture.* New York: Random House.

Prevalence of health-care providers asking older adults about their physical activity levels—United States, 1998. (2002). *Morbidity and Mortality Weekly Report, 51*(19), 412–414.

Quart, A. (2003). *Branded: The buying and selling of teenagers.* Cambridge, MA: Perseus.

Rowe, J. W., & Kahn, R. L. (1997). Successful aging. *The Gerontologist, 37,* 433–440.

Savin-Williams, R. C., & Berndt, T. J. (1990). Friendship and peer relations. In S. S. Feldman & G. R. Elliot (Eds.), *At the threshold: The developing adolescent* (pp. 277–307). Cambridge, MA: Harvard University Press.

Shann, M. H. (2001). Students' use of time outside of school: A case for after school pro-grams for urban middle school youth. *Urban Review, 33,* 339–356.

Siegel, R. J. (1993). Between midlife and old age: Never too old to learn. In N. D. Davis, E. Cole, & E. D. Rothblum (Eds.), *Faces of women and aging* (pp. 173–185). Binghamton, NY: Harrington Park.

Singleton, J. F. (1996). Leisure skills. In C. B. Lewis (Ed.), *Aging: The health care challenge* (3rd ed.; pp. 106–125). Philadelphia: F. A. Davis.

Sloan, L. R. (1979). The function and impact of sports for fans: A review of theory and con-temporary research. In J. H. Goldstein (Ed.), *Sports, games and play: Social and psycho-logical viewpoints* (pp. 219–262). Hillsdale, NJ: Erlbaum.

Steinberg, L., & Steinberg, W. (1994). *Crossing paths: How your child's adolescence can be an opportunity for your own personal growth.* New York: Simon & Schuster.

Storr, A. (1988). *Solitude: A return to the self.* New York: Ballantine.

Whalen, C. K., Jamner, L. D., Henker, B., Delfino, R. J., & Lozano, J. M. (2002). ADHD spectrum and everyday life: Experience sampling of adolescent moods, activities, smok-ing and drinking. *Child Development, 73,* 209–227.

Williams, M. S., & Shellenberger, S. (1994). *How does your engine run?* Albuquerque, NM: TherapyWorks.

Zillman, D., Sapolsky, B. S., & Bryant, J. (1979). The enjoyment of watching sport contests. In J. H. Goldstein (Ed.), *Sports, games, and play: Social and psychological viewpoints* (pp. 297–336). Hillsdale, NJ: Erlbaum.

Zimmer, Z., Hickey, T., & Searle, M. S. (1997). The pattern of change in leisure activity behavior among older adults with arthritis. *The Gerontologist, 37,* 384–392.

14

Range of Human Activity: Work Activities

Jane Miller, MA, OT

All work, even cotton-spinning, is noble; work is alone noble....A life of ease is not for any man, nor for any god. (Thomas Carlyle, as cited by Beck, 1980, p. 474:4)

What Is Work?

Say the word *work*, and many thoughts come to mind. Work conjures up myriad positive and negative thoughts. Throughout the world, people are working: children work during play, at school, and in the home during chores; adults have jobs, homemaking tasks, and hobbies. Whether engaged in job seeking, paid employment, volunteering, or retirement activities, most individuals are working.

A job, an occupation, a vocation, a trade, employment, labor, a business, a calling, or a pursuit: Work and work-related synonyms are very much a part of our lives and vocabulary. Work implies an activity of the body, mind, machine, or nature itself. Usually a sustained physical or cognitive effort, work applies to purposeful activity, especially that of earning one's livelihood.

Work is an area of occupation (American Occupational Therapy Association, 2002) and is a major aspect of occupational therapy's domain of concern. Meaningful or productive occupation is a vital aspect for most people. Work is a part of human occupation. It is both highly valued and defining. The occupational therapy literature is rich with debate surrounding the definition of the term *occupation*. People are occupational beings. Engagement in occupation (doing) is an innate behavior and considered integral with humanness (being) (Wilcock, 2003). Occupations are culturally sanctioned and organize our lives. They enable humans to survive, control, and adapt to our world (Yerxa et al., 1989). Occupation encompasses all human pursuits (cognitive, physical, psychosocial, passive or active, obligatory or elective) or is considered merely a component part (i.e., work as an area of performance).

Briefly, work and productive activities are the purposeful activities of self-development, social contribution, and livelihood. The *International Classification of Functioning, Disability and Health* (ICF; World Health Organization [WHO], 2001) defines work within a broader sphere of major life areas. Major life areas are education, work and employment, and conducting economic transactions. The "tasks and actions required to engage" in these areas are specified. The work and employment section of the ICF (d840–d859) further defines apprenticeship (work preparation); acquiring, keeping, and terminating a job; remunerative employment; and nonremunerative employment.

> d850: Remunerative employment: Engaging in all aspects of work, as an occupation, trade, profession or other form of employment, for payment, as an employee, full- or part-time, or self-employed, such as seeking employment and getting a job, doing the required tasks of the job, attending work on time as required, supervising other workers or being supervised, and performing required tasks alone or in groups. (WHO, 2001, p. 165)

This chapter concentrates on vocational activities. The participation in work-related activities encompasses vocational exploration, job acquisition, work or job performance, retirement planning, and volunteer participation. Vocational exploration is the determination of aptitudes, development of interests and skills, and the selection of appropriate vocational pursuits. Job acquisition consists of the identification and selection of work opportunities and the completion of the application and interview processes. Work or job performance is the timely and effective performance of job tasks and the acquisition and incorporation of work behaviors. Retirement planning involves the determination of aptitudes, development of interests and skills, and the selection of appropriate avocational pursuits. Volunteer participation is the performance of unpaid activities for the benefit of selected people, groups, or causes. These last two areas, retirement planning and volunteer participation, are not explored in this chapter.

Evolutionary Origins and the History of Work

Instinctively and through learned behaviors, animals work to acquire or construct shelter, obtain food, and protect and care for their young. Humans do the same: We gather food (albeit recently through the neighborhood grocery store or from the backyard garden), acquire clothing and housing, defend ourselves from enemies and protect territory, and raise children. Through the ages, from the Stone Age hunters and gatherers until recent times, people have engaged in these activities because the work had to be done. Unless you did the task yourself, either independently or cooperatively with members of your family or community, it was unlikely that you would survive.

Colonial America was a nation of farmers, artisans, and craftsmen. Potters, leather workers, silversmiths, glassblowers, brick makers, and blacksmiths were at the heart of small industries. Work centered on the home and the horse. Along the coast and lakes, maritime activities evolved, including shipbuilding and fishing.

With the emerging factory system, unskilled and semiskilled labor swelled the ranks along with thousands of former agricultural workers. Women, children, and minorities were often exploited. Technological advances introduced during the Industrial Revolution began to make the world of work easier in some respects and more difficult in others. The horse gave way to the automobile; McCormick's reaper performed tasks once completed by hand. The "machine [became] sacrosanct; the worker was [now] expendable" (Fraser, 1992, p. 2). Little attention was paid to the worker's health, safety, or social conditions. The plight of the factory worker, dramatized in the writings of Charles Dickens and others, heightened the public's awareness of dangerous industrial working conditions. One's willingness to perform the task and the apparent lack of any limiting disability were sufficient criteria for evaluating one's fitness for the job.

Sixty percent of the working population was farming in 1850 (Morris, 1976). Agricultural production—farming, ranching, and fishing—still employ approximately 2 million people (*Career Guide to America's Top Industries*, 2002). Air travel, the Internet, and the global market are just a few of the factors influencing today's work in the Information Age. Computerization and robotics have forever changed the way in which we receive, process, and use information; perform tasks; and conduct business. Figure 14.1 projects the number of job openings due to growth and replacement needs.

To further explore the historical development and changes in the United States, I recommend fascinating reading by author Studs Terkel—*My American Century* (1997) and *Working: People Talk About What They Do All Day and How They Feel About What They Do* (1971). Terkel has created an intimate portrait of work, life, and the American people.

> Life grants nothing to us mortals without hard work. (Horace, as cited by Beck, 1980, p. 106:17)

Learning How to Work

In primitive societies, work is clearly visible to children: sowing, threshing, grinding, kneading, dyeing, hunting, kindling, and carrying. Children are taught basic work skills and help in adult tasks as soon as they are able. In developed areas, like the United States, children may not actually see their parents or community engaged in work. They are permitted to spend their time at play and going to school. Childhood games often mimic adult activities. Their experiences may later affect occupational choice and work behaviors (Argyle, 1972).

Basic components of the work personality are established in childhood. The ability to concentrate on a task, being cooperative or competitive with peers, development of appropriate responses to authority, and the meanings and values associated

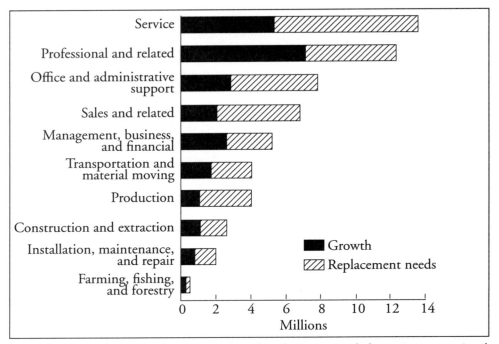

Figure 14.1. Job openings due to growth and replacement needs by major occupational group.

Note. From the online resource of the Bureau of Labor Statistics. Available at www.bls.gov/oco/images/ocotjc11.gif.

with work and achievement prepare the person for future work. During adolescence, teens usually try out various kinds of work through home, school, and neighborhood employment. One difficulty inherent in orienting young people in our modern society is the sheer enormity of occupational choice. A number of studies (e.g., Argyle, 1972; Steele & Morgan, 1991) have shown that teens are attracted to jobs that are viewed as similar to their self-image or require skills that they believe they possess. By the time the person has completed his or her formal education (e.g., high school, vocational program, college, graduate school), he or she is deemed ready to embark on a life's work.

American society tends to look askance at people who are idle and believes that hard work will pay off in the long run. These culturally bound tenets of Judeo–Christian tradition are still evident today. How many times have you heard the expression, "Idle hands are the devil's workshop?" The work ethic is illustrated throughout American history and literature:

> When men are employed, they are best contented for on the days they worked
> they were good-natured and cheerful, and, with the consciousness of having done
> a good day's work, they spent the evening jollily; but on our idle days they were

mutinous and quarrelsome." (Benjamin Franklin, as cited by Beck, 1980, p. 348:21)

Reich (1970) wrote, "Work and function are basic to man. They fulfill him, they establish his identity, they give him his place in the human community" (pp. 367–368).

Bellman's (1996) *Your Signature Path: Gaining New Perspectives on Life and Work* reiterated the theme that work is central to our lives and key to living with meaning. He stated that work feeds our need for growth and accomplishment as well as allows us to demonstrate skill, get attention, exercise discipline, and experience mastery. The benefits of steady employment are psychologically important, along with monetary rewards of a steady income, paid vacations, medical and unemployment insurance, discounts on products, reduced or paid tuition, and other fringe benefits.

> In order that people may be happy in their work, these three things are needed: they must be fit for it; they must not do too much of it; and they must have a sense of success in it. (John Ruskin, as cited by Beck, 1980, p. 572:13)

Trends and Forecasts in Employment

The effect of new technology, economic and political developments, and the job market in various occupational fields is constantly changing. According to the U.S. Department of Labor's Bureau of Labor Statistics (BLS), 150.8 million people (69.3% of the working-age U.S. population 16 years of age and older) worked at some time during 2002 (U.S. Department of Labor, BLS, 2003). Moreover, 66.3% of all employed people worked full time (35 hours or more weekly). Increasing numbers of people are working at home either as wage or salaried workers or are self-employed. Many of these people are in "white collar" occupations, and about 80% use a computer for the work they accomplished at home, which is an increase of almost 20% within the past 5 years.

In December 2001, the BLS issued new 10-year projections for the American workforce from 2000 to 2010. These projections of economic growth, the labor force, and employment by industry are used for developing career information, planning education and training programs, and forecasting employment trends. According to the BLS report, the labor force is projected to increase by 17% (reaching 158 million in 2010). The demographic composition of the cohort of 46- to 64-year-old workers is changing more rapidly as the baby boom generation continues to age. Projected declines in the 25- to 34-year-old age group are caused by decreased birthrates during the late 1960s and early 1970s. Service-producing industries, such as health, business, social, engineering, management, and related services are expected to account for almost half of the growth. Health care practitioners, including technical and health care support occupations, are likely to see a growth of 27.9%. Occupational therapy is projected to have a 33.9% change by 2010 (78,306 employed in 2000 to 104,824 in 2010). The 10 fastest growing occupations are primarily computer related (see Table 14.1).

Table 14.1
Fastest Growing Occupations, 2000–2010
(Numbers in Thousands of Jobs)

Occupation	Employment—Change			
	Year		No.	%
	2000	*2010*		
Computer software engineers, applications	380	760	380	100
Computer support specialists	506	996	490	97
Computer software engineers, systems software	317	601	284	90
Network and computer systems administrators	229	416	187	82
Network systems and data communications analysts	119	211	92	77
Desktop publishers	38	63	25	67
Database administrators	106	176	70	66
Personal and home care aides	414	672	258	62
Computer systems analysts	431	689	258	60
Medical assistants	329	516	187	57

Note. From Bureau of Labor Statistics, www.bls.gov/news.release/ecopro.t06.htm.

Occupations in the American labor market are forever affected by and respond to global, societal, scientific, commercial, and legislative developments. The Balanced Budget Act of 1997 (P.L. 105–33) has dramatically changed the employment outlook for health care providers, such as occupational therapists. The current health care arena is fraught with mergers, downsizing, restructuring, reorganizing, and consolidating. The health services sector, however, hired more workers (270,000) than any other industry in 2002 (McMenamin, Krantz, & Krolik, 2003). The 2.6% growth resulted from increased demand of aging baby boomers, population growth, and technological advances.

> ...the workplace is always in flux, always in transition, always in turmoil—it always has been, and it always will be. (Bolles, 1998, p. 11)

Vocational Exploration

A typical college student will be engaged in approximately 100,000 working hours after graduating (Steele & Morgan, 1991). A person's work influences his or her way of life. Our career choice(s) actually determines who our friends will be, the attitudes and values we develop, the geographic area where we will live, the patterns we will adopt, and how our leisure time will be spent. It shapes and molds our identity. It gives purpose and meaning to our lives. Work confers status in your field of employment; among friends; in your family; and most importantly, to you.

The world of work can be classified in various ways. Some list occupations by their prestige. In this system, judges, physicians, and high-ranking government officials rank at the top, whereas janitors and garbage collectors generally rank at the bottom. Another method of classifying work is by socioeconomic factors or the degree of intelligence, education, and skills required. Holland's (1997) RIASEC theory of careers is the basis for many inventories accepted today. Using a typology of personality and environments, Holland characterized people and their work into six groups:

1. Realistic (concrete and practical activity involving machines, tools, or materials)

2. Investigative (analytical or intellectual activity aimed at problem solving or creation and use of knowledge)

3. Artistic (creative work in the arts or unstructured and intellectual endeavors)

4. Social (working with people in a helpful or facilitative way)

5. Enterprising (working with people in a supervisory or persuasive way to achieve some organizational goal)

6. Conventional (working with things, numbers, or machines in an orderly way to meet regular and predictable needs of the organization or to meet specified standards).

His model provides a framework for what specific personal and environmental characteristics lead to satisfying and stable career decisions.

Just to keep things interesting, the U.S. Employment Service has a different method of classifying work. The *Guide for Occupational Exploration* (GOE; U.S. Department of Labor, Employment Service, 1979) groups work by interests, abilities, and traits required for successful performance. People can identify and explore types of work that closely relate to their own skills and interests. The GOE organizes data into interest areas, work groups, and subgroups. The 14 interest areas correspond to the following broad categories (Farr, Ludden, & Shatkin, 2001):

01 Arts, entertainment, and media (creative expression of feelings or ideas in communicating or performing)

02   Science, math, and engineering (discovering, collecting, and analyzing information about the natural world; manipulating data; and applying technology and scientific research findings to problems in medicine, life sciences, and natural sciences)

03   Plants and animals (activities involving plants and animals, usually in an outdoor setting)

04   Law, law enforcement, and public safety (use of authority to protect people and property)

05   Mechanics, installers, and repairers (applying mechanical and electrical and electronic principles to practical situations, using machines, hand tools, or techniques)

06   Construction, mining, and drilling (assembling components of structures and using mechanical devices to drill or excavate)

07   Transportation (moving people or materials)

08   Industrial production (repetitive, concrete, organized activities in a factory setting)

09   Business detail (organized, clearly defined activities requiring accuracy and attention to detail, primarily in office settings)

10   Sales and marketing (bringing others to a point of view through personal persuasion, using sales and promotion techniques)

11   Recreation, travel, and other personal services (catering to the wishes of others, usually on a one-to-one basis)

12   Education and social services (teaching people or addressing their spiritual, social, physical, or vocational needs)

13   General management and support (making organizations run smoothly)

14   Medical and health services (helping people to be healthy).

Occupational therapists are listed within the work group of medical therapy (14.06.01) under the broader medical and health services area (14).

Exercise 14.1—Selecting a Profession

Think about how you decided to enter the profession of occupational therapy. How did you discover this area of work? Did you have a role model or a personal experience? Where did you go to obtain more information? If you could, how would you do things differently?

Exercise 14.2—Examining Vocational Interests

Read *What Color Is Your Parachute?* (Bolles, 2004). It provides excellent tips and suggestions for analyzing your vocational interests and strengths as well as for obtaining employment. Be sure to visit Bolles's Web site (www.jobhuntersbible.com). The site is designed to supplement his text.

Exercise 14.3—Finding Job Information

Find information related to job seeking on the World Wide Web for special populations. Visit "Job Accommodations" at www.onetcenter.org/links.html or specific conditions at SOAR (Searchable Online Accommodation Resource) at www.jan.wvu.edu.

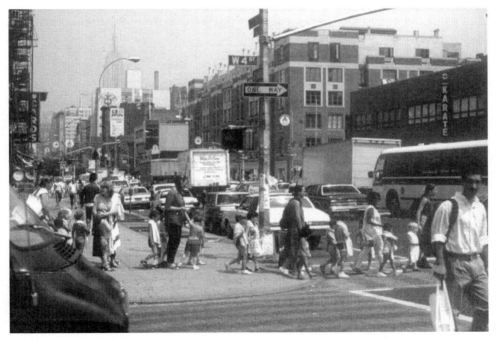

Figure 14.2. Children being guided across a New York City sidewalk. Photograph courtesy of the Public Health Image Library, Centers for Disease Control and Prevention.

The Socratic method of "knowing thyself" consists of asking probing questions, defining terms, and analyzing opinions to reveal their consistency or inconsistency. Career and life planning for each person begins with similar steps. One of the best places to start research and reading is in the *Occupational Outlook Handbook* (U.S. Department of Labor, BLS, 2002), which serves as a guide to career opportunities. It is revised every 2 years, describes approximately 250 occupations, and covers specifically what the worker does on the job, working conditions, education and training needed, and anticipated job prospects and earnings. The Internet version is available at www.bls.gov/oco. Each job title has a unique number. Defined more than 60 years ago by the U.S. Department of Labor, Employment Service (1991), the *Dictionary of Occupational Titles* (DOT) has been replaced with and incorporated into an updated, Internet-based comprehensive database of worker attributes and job characteristics called O*NET—The Occupational Information Network (www.doleta.gov/programs/onet) (U.S. Department of Labor, Employment, and Training Administration, 2003). The eight-digit O*NET code identifies occupations uniquely within the related occupational group and according to worker functions. Now also available in a Spanish version, it can be updated continually with occupational information and labor market research. The direct link to the O*NET database is http://online.onet center.org.

Along with the descriptions of the various job titles and many links to other sites (e.g., America's Job Bank, America's Labor Market Information System, BLS, National Skill Standards Board), this computerized system describes job requirements and worker competencies for approximately 1,100 current occupations. Following are two descriptions of what is included:

- What the worker does; what equipment is used; how closely workers are supervised; how the duties of the worker vary by industry, establishment, and the size of the company; how the responsibilities of entry-level workers differ from those of experienced, supervisory, or self-employed; how technological innovations are affecting what workers do and how they do it; and emerging specialties.

- Typical working and environmental conditions for workers in the occupation; typical hours worked; workplace environment; susceptibility to injury, illness, and job-related stress; necessary protective clothing and safety equipment; basic clothing required; and travel required (see Figure 14.3).

Case Scenario

How is an occupational therapist described in the *Occupational Outlook Handbook* (Department of Labor, BLS, 2002)? Occupational therapy (O*NET 29-1122.00, DOT 076.121-010) is among the fastest-growing occupations. Employment is projected to increase faster than average as a result of a rapidly aging population with increased demand for therapeutic services (Farr, 2003). The book (and Web-based handbook) elaborates on both the pros and cons of

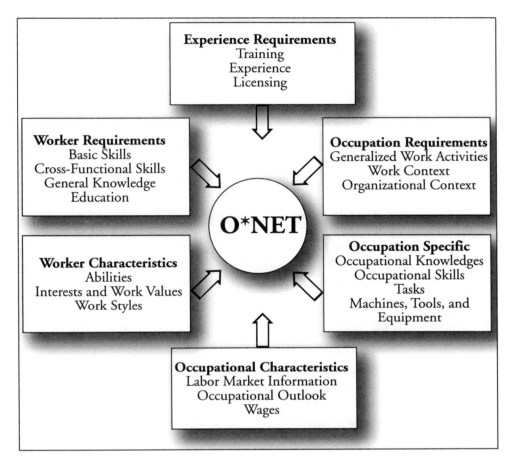

Figure 14.3. The O*NET database.

a particular occupation. For example, the job of the occupational therapist can be tiring because therapists are on their feet much of the time. Those practitioners employed in home health may spend hours driving to and from appointments. Occupational therapists also face job-related hazards, such as back strain from lifting clients and equipment. Some of the qualifications required are patience, strong interpersonal skills to inspire trust and respect, ingenuity, and imagination in adapting activities and environments. Occupational therapists are increasingly taking on supervisory roles; more than one-third work part-time. Read the O*NET description of occupational therapy. You can also use the Skills Search option to see whether your skills and abilities "match" that of the profession.

Role of Occupational Therapy in Work and Work Activities

Historically, work was a modality of treatment rather than the goal of treatment. "Occupational therapy took root in a rich soil of work activities for the mentally ill. In the early 1920's, the first occupational therapists documented steps for a uniform program of curative activity" (Marshall, 1985, p. 297). Today, work and work activities are used as both the treatment approach and the end goal. These applications include, but are not limited to, work-related games for children, welfare-to-work, work-hardening and work-conditioning programs, transition from school to work, supported employment, work readiness, vocational exploration, injury reduction, stress management, tool modification, and job accommodation.

Occupational therapists are uniquely qualified to synthesize the information for the design and implementation of a safe work environment; are able to establish appropriate productivity levels for homebound, sheltered, modified, or competitive work; and are able to implement tool or job-site evaluation and modifications. The therapist develops and guides job-specific programs of graded activity for the worker, performs job task analysis and job station and tool modification, and identifies and remediates behaviors inappropriate to the work environment. The benefits to the worker, employer, and work environment include increased productivity, decreased workers' compensation claims and lost workdays, and prevention and reduction of injury.

Occupational therapists may collaborate with professionals who specialize in ergonomics. *Ergonomics,* the science of work, is the matching of human abilities and capabilities and job requirements within the context of the physical and social work environment. Also known as human factors or human engineering, ergonomics interacts closely with other applied and life sciences, such as engineering, medicine, and psychology, to preserve health, prevent injury, and maximize work efficiency. Its role in rehabilitation is in the redesigning of the external environment to accommodate the worker with disabilities or injuries, thereby enabling each person to contribute fully and independently (Smith, 1989; see Figure 14.4). In disability prevention, ergonomists examine human factors relevant to the job, human capabilities, and the man–machine interaction or interface under given environmental conditions. Ergonomic design is the application of this knowledge to tool, machine, system, job, and environmental design for safe, comfortable, and effective human use. Ergonomists often are engineers (e.g., safety, mechanical) and therapists (e.g., physical, occupational) who have undergone specific educational experiences.

Examining the Workplace and the Worker

Job analysis and worker evaluation is a multiphase process: job description (includes an objective record of job and components, similar to those in the DOT or O*NET), task or job analysis (includes evaluation of selected tasks and activities in terms of human demands, e.g., vision, hearing, cognitive processes, muscle recruitment), and identification of worker capabilities. These phases do not always proceed in a neat and

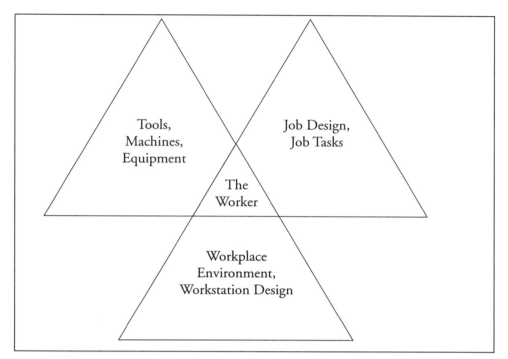

Figure 14.4. Interactions among the workplace, the job, and the worker.

Note. From "Ergonomics and the Occupational Therapist," by E. R. Smith. In S. Hertfelder & C. Gwin (Eds.), *Work in Progress: Occupational Therapy in Work Programs,* 1989, p. 129, Rockville, MD: American Occupational Therapy Association. Copyright © 1989 by the American Occupational Therapy Association. Reprinted with permission.

orderly sequence. Activity analysis is at the core of conducting a job analysis. The process of job analysis will examine the physical demands, cognitive factors, specific tasks, tools and machines used, environment, and the psychological and physical hazards of the work. The following techniques may be used to conduct a job evaluation: interviews with employer and employee(s), questionnaires, photographic documentation (still photos and video recording), anthropometric data collection, and functional and specific work assessments. Identification of potentially hazardous, inadequate work habits, equipment, and environment are noted. After the data analysis, recommendations are offered to (a) reduce risk of work-related injury; (b) provide workers with guidelines for safe, efficient task completion; and (c) suggest possible workstation modifications.

Functional capacity evaluation is a type of procedure used to evaluate a person's level of physical ability to perform basic work tasks. This protocol may be submitted in litigation, pre-employment screens, and return-to-work and work capacity evaluations. Tasks such as lifting, pulling, pushing, and climbing are measured. Numerous standardized and nonstandardized assessments are available.

Case Scenario

Let us examine the work of a typical office worker. According to the U.S. Department of Labor's Employment Service (1991) and BLS (2002), the job title of administrative secretary (O*NET 43-6011.00, DOT 169.167-014) involves the physical demands of sedentary work (maximum lift of 10 pounds) and the abilities to talk, hear, reach, handle, finger, and feel. A limited amount of walking, standing, and carrying of light objects is required. The worker must be able to extend the arms in any direction; seize; hold; grasp; turn; pick; pinch; and perceive size, shape, temperature, or texture of objects. Working conditions are inside (75% or more, with protection from weather conditions but not necessarily from temperature changes).

This job title involves "overseeing and carrying out office operations...and applying clerical skills...including planning own or others' work program, using reasoning, using hands and fingers in typing...and recording data, obtaining and safeguarding confidential information...recognizing and proofing copy to correct errors in spelling, grammar, and punctuation, speaking distinctly...and making decisions involving...policy" (U.S. Department of Labor, Employment, and Training Administration, 2003).

The administrative secretary, a 52-year-old woman with a 2-year employment history with Happy Socks Unlimited, was interviewed by the director of personnel regarding her job tasks and responsibilities and work-related health concerns. She has below-average sick time usage (i.e., less than half of the allotted 12 days per year); absences are usually because of seasonal allergies and sinus headaches. During periods of high keyboarding activity, she reports stiffness in the neck, pain accompanying neck rotation to right, radiating pain down both arms, and nocturnal numbness and tingling in both hands.

The administrative secretary oversees the general functioning of the office and supervises full-time and part-time clerical personnel. The specific job duties and tasks can be categorized as follows:

Cognitive tasks:

- Gathers and develops information

- Stores and retrieves information

- Reads

- Proofreads and edits

- Calculates and analyzes data

- Orders supplies

- Inspects supplies and compares invoices

- Plans and schedules

- Makes decisions.

Social tasks:

- Answers and uses telephone, routes calls
- Confers and meets with people
- Works with other people.

Physical tasks:

- Stores and retrieves documents and files
- Writes with pen, pencil, and marker
- Handles mail
- Collates and sorts
- Photocopies documents
- Types documents from handwritten drafts or typed matter
- Maintains calendar
- Maintains and conducts minor repairs of equipment (e.g., fixes paper jams in photocopier, loads paper, changes printer toner)
- Uses equipment (e.g., pencil, computer, photocopier, printer, telephone).

The physical demands, consistent with the O*NET and DOT description, include the following:

- Standing
- Walking
- Sitting (75% of the time, sedentary work)
- Lifting and carrying (light objects less than 10 kilograms)
- Reaching and grasping
- Handling and fingering
- Stair and step climbing (infrequently)
- Balancing, stooping, and kneeling (infrequently)
- Communicating (talking)
- Hearing
- Vision (near, midrange, far, visual accommodation, color).

Using the guidelines and standards listed in Grandjean (1988), anthropometric measurements were taken with a tape measure. These external body dimensions (e.g., standing height, forward reach, arm span, foot to popliteal length) are compared with group norms. A goniometer was used for measuring range of motion. Hand strength, specifically grasp and pinch, were measured with a dynamometer and pinch gauge. A full upper-extremity evaluation was completed and assessed overall coordination, sensation, and functional abilities. The evaluation confirmed that the worker was within normal limits in all areas (for people of similar age and gender).

Work sampling was conducted. The administrative secretary was seated at her desk in an upright posture. The computer, monitor, and printer were switched on. The task of keyboarding a brief memorandum from a two-page, handwritten draft was analyzed in detail. The steps included the following:

1. Take draft out of "to-do" box on desk or receive draft from originator or courier.

2. Put draft on copy stand.

3. Select word processing icon (software loads).

4. Create document file.

5. Input through typing on keyboard and mouse clicking.

6. Proofread, edit, and spell check document.

7. Click on print icon.

8. Walk to printer location, retrieve paper from storage bin, and load paper, if needed.

9. Walk to printer location and retrieve document.

10. Complete final proofreading.

11. Put finished memorandum in "out" box.

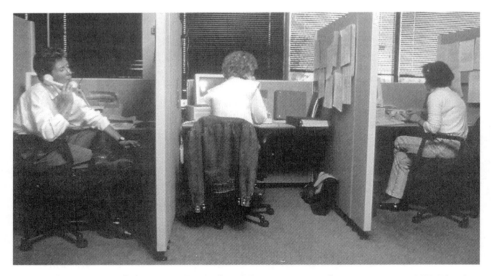

Figure 14.5. Centers for Disease Control and Prevention employees manning AIDS hotline. Photograph courtesy of the Public Health Image Library, Centers for Disease Control and Prevention.

Time studies were conducted to determine approximate hourly keystroke rate. Using a keyboarding assessment, three trials were completed. The documents produced were well formatted; error free; and edited for content, style, spelling, and grammar. The secretary's preferred rate allows for simultaneous conversation with others and does not appear to result in any physical complaints. If the workload warrants, she is able to perform two to three times faster than this rate; however, upper-extremity problems usually result from prolonged exertion.

The work site is housed in a newly renovated facility. The space includes company offices, secretarial areas, reception, and storage. There is a fully equipped lounge with kitchen area (e.g., sink, refrigerator, microwave oven, coffee and hot water system, table, chairs) available for mealtime and snacks. Accessible restrooms are located in the building.

Secretarial workstations contain standard office desks, lateral filing cabinets, shelving, adjustable desk chair, and guest chairs. All enclosed offices are "soundproof" within an acceptable level. Except for the hallways, kitchen, restrooms, and storage areas, all floors are carpeted. The heating ventilation air conditioning (HVAC) system is reportedly a source of irritation: noisy, drafty at certain locations, and not able to regulate the temperature well throughout the office.

The secretary usually sits 24 inches (61 cm) from her monitor and maintains a viewing angle of 18°. Seat height, back angle, elbow angle, keyboard, and screen height are also within acceptable ranges.

Overall, the flexibility inherent in the administrative secretary's job allows her to pace the work. Although the work site is not perfect (e.g., HVAC system) and job demands are more stressful at times, the environment is usually manageable. Her capabilities and task and work requirements are normally balanced. The following suggestions were provided to further enhance performance, reduce work-related injury, and increase worker comfort:

- Modify the workstation by adding task lighting, keyboard wrist rest, angled adjustable footrest (as well as clearing area under desk to allow for more leg room), and chair mat; changing shelf spacing; improving arrangement of work materials; and changing desk, if possible, to a reduced-length, rounded D-shape work surface.

- Reduce repetitive components as much as possible by incorporating varied job tasks, increasing freedom of motion in the workstation area (by ridding area of nonessential storage material), taking frequent "micro breaks" (stretch and exercise periods), and using autosuggestive techniques (such as self-hypnosis) to relax body during activity.

- Avoid excessive extension, flexion, and deviation of the wrist and constrained postures.

- Vary and alternate tasks to reduce the sedentary work.

■   Maintain comfortable environmental temperature and relative humidity and minimize static electricity and drafts.

An Epidemiological Approach

An epidemiological study of a work-related disease is subject to inherent difficulties related to providing evidence of causality (WHO, 1989). Causative factors often have a complex etiology and are influenced by confounding variables such as lifestyle, work habits, and individual capabilities. A disorder requiring a long exposure time or repeated injuries, such as repetitive strain injury (RSI), is more difficult to identify with a specific work activity and onset. The person–environment fit model, based on McGarth's work (Cooper, 1981), depicts the tenuous balance (often an imbalance) between job demands and the abilities of the individual to satisfy those demands (see Table 14.2). The National Institute for Occupational Safety and Health (NIOSH), the federal agency that provides recommendations to prevent work-related illness and injury, agrees that exposure to stressful working conditions can have a direct influence on worker safety and health. Psychological and physiological strain results when demands and abilities are ill matched (U.S. Department of Health and Human Services, NIOSH, 1999; (see Figures 14.6 and 14.7).

Case Scenario

Traditionally, workers in food processing, health services, manufacturing, and craft industries have suffered frequent work-related injuries secondary to repetitive, manual exertions. The rise of the computer in the workplace has introduced another source of work-related concerns. The work of a computer keyboard user may involve rapid, repetitive movements of the upper extremities and static loading (i.e., wrists and shoulders held in same position for extended periods). RSI, also known as cumulative trauma disorder, occupational overuse syndrome, or repetitive motion disorder, is a generic label given to a variety of painful, debilitating, soft tissue conditions believed to be caused by repetitive movements of the hands or arms. Activities such as stooping, sedentary work, and constrained postures and biophysiological factors such as physical size, strength, fitness, range of motion, and work endurance are thought to contribute. Psychological stressors from the job structure (e.g., scheduling, machine pacing), job content (e.g., time pressures and overload, underload, lack of control), and organization (e.g., role ambiguity, competition) can further compound the situation with anxiety, dissatisfaction, psychogenic illness, and absenteeism. A variety of conditions, many ill defined, are involved in RSI. Tenosynovitis, shoulder pain, tension neck, tendinitis, and carpal tunnel injury are but a few of the many musculotendinous conditions included under this disorder. Individuals often list many complaints, such as tenderness, pain, swelling, cramping, and tingling sensations.

Table 14.2
Job Conditions That May Lead to Stress

Condition	Characteristics	Examples
The design of tasks	Heavy workload; infrequent rest breaks; long work hours and shift work; hectic and routine tasks that have little inherent meaning, do not use workers' skills, and provide little sense of control	David works to the point of exhaustion. Theresa is tied to the computer, allowing little room for flexibility, self-initiative, or rest.
Management style	Lack of participation by workers in decision making, poor communication in the organization, lack of family-friendly policies	Theresa needs to get the boss's approval for everything, and the company is insensitive to her family needs.
Interpersonal relationships	Poor social environment and lack of support or help from coworkers and supervisors	Theresa's physical isolation reduces her opportunities to interact with other workers or receive help from them.
Work roles	Conflicting or uncertain job expectations, too much responsibility, too many "hats to wear"	Theresa often is caught in a difficult situation trying to satisfy both the customer's needs and the company's expectations.
Career concerns	Job insecurity and lack of opportunity for growth, advancement, or promotion; rapid changes for which workers are unprepared	Since the reorganization at David's plant, everyone is worried about their future with the company and what will happen next.
Environmental conditions	Unpleasant or dangerous physical conditions, such as crowding, noise, air pollution, or ergonomic problems	David is exposed to constant noise at work.

Note. From *Stress at work* by U.S. Department of Health and Human Services, NIOSH (DHHS Pub. No. 99-101), 1999, p. 9. Cincinnati, OH: Publications Dissemination.

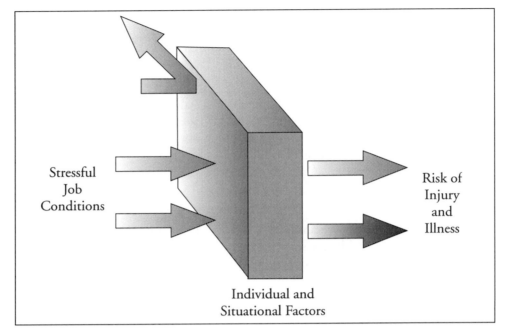

Figure 14.6. National Institute for Occupational Safety and Health model of job stress. *Note.* From *Stress at work* by U.S. Department of Health and Human Services, NIOSH (DHHS) Pub. No. 99-101), 1999, p. 8. Cincinnati, OH: Publications Dissemination.

Health in the Workplace

In the United States, more than 39 million people are hospitalized or receive emergency services for accidental injuries. More than 3 million sustain disabling injuries on the job. Escalating costs from loss of productivity, absenteeism, retraining, and medical and disability insurance have pushed the concern for a healthy worker and a healthy work environment into the spotlight. The switch from a traditional approach of treating illnesses to a health maintenance or preventive medical focus is taking hold. The role of employees' health services has become more comprehensive in many settings. In addition to providing medical care, industrial safety, and compliance with state and federal regulations, the employer may provide the following:

■   Preplacement examinations (baseline medical profiles that protect both the company and the worker)

■   Periodic health and medical surveillance exams (preventive, early detection screens)

■   Return-to-work and disability management (prevent accidents, reinjury, or spread of illness; proper care and rehabilitation to minimize duration of injury) (see Figure 14.7)

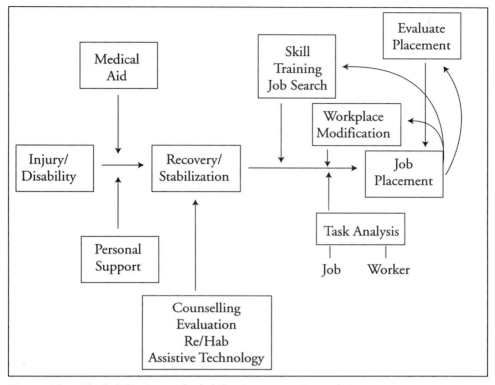

Figure 14.7. The habilitation and rehabilitation process in work injury.

■ Wellness and fitness programs (e.g., promoting fitness, smoking cessation, general nutrition, weight reduction, and stress reduction).

The most important element for control is prevention through environmental protection in the workplace, safety education of workers and managers, the application of appropriate and safe work practices, and the application of basic ergonomic principles (WHO, 1989).

Work injury management and prevention is a multidisciplinary effort (Isernhagen, 1995). Medical, legal, vocational, and insurance professionals, as well as employers and employees, must communicate and cooperate in order to safeguard the worker and prevent job-related injuries. Work evaluation consists of evaluation of the injured worker (or potential worker), the type and method of work performed, and the unique capabilities and interests of the employee. Each professional on the rehabilitation team—occupational therapists, physical therapists, vocational counselor, physician, and psychologist—contributes to the worker's success at the work site. Depending on the situation, occupational health and safety engineers, industrial psychologists, ergonomists, kinesiologists, personnel and human resource staff, attorneys, insurance adjustors, and workers' compensation judges also may be involved in the return-to-work process. It is therefore vital that the resulting documentation be readable, devoid of jargon and highly technical wording, and understandable to a wide audience. To ensure competitiveness in the world market, employers need to maintain a healthy workforce. Providing ongoing safety training and timely rehabilitation of sick and injured workers are sound practices.

Case Scenario

Presenting problem. Immediate employment checking the quality of pecan nuts in a candy factory was being offered to an injured worker. The job is considered light work and thought to be within the worker's capabilities. Subsequent to a back injury sustained while unloading packaging materials from the delivery trucks, the worker had orthopedic surgery in which the L5/S1 vertebrae were fused. The worker was familiar with the job but was not sure whether he would be able to cope with the demands of the work.

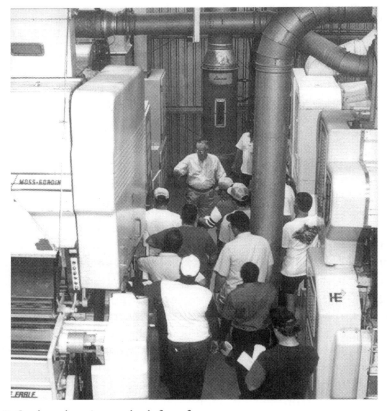

Figure 14.8. Students learning to check for safety.
Photograph courtesy of the Agricultural Research Service, U.S. Department of Agriculture.
Photo by David Nance.

Job description. The employees either sat or stood in front of a slow-moving conveyor belt carrying pecans. Imperfect and broken nuts had to be identified visually, picked out by hand, and placed on another belt (located 10 inches in back of the first belt). Placing the rejected nuts on the second belt required forward reaching. Most workers preferred to stand (as there was little room for their legs) and lean forward over the belt with their forearms resting on the edge of the conveyor. If the employee sat, he or she would need to twist sideways in order to reach the belts.

Conclusion. Both positions available (standing with stooped posture or seated with a rotated spine) would cause considerable load on the lower back. The employee was able to return to work after the candy manufacturer changed the workplace. The modifications included removal of storage bins below conveyor belts, provision of raised stools for sitting, and a foot bar for support while standing. Although these changes required an outlay of capital, they allowed all workers to sit comfortably without rotation. As a secondary benefit to the employer, complaints of neck and low back pain from other workers, absenteeism, and use of sick leave were greatly reduced.

Case Scenario

Presenting problem. An injured tire factory worker had experienced a lumbosacral sprain and right knee sprain and reported ringing in the ears. On inspection, it was noted that the factory had continuous, high-volume background noise and a slight but noticeable floor vibration.

Job description. The job involved identifying and marking defective tires being transported through the area by an overhead carrier. The job was accomplished partly by sight and partly by touch while walking slowly behind the moving tire. Workers also removed surplus rubber left by the molding process with a sharp knife. Rejected tires were removed from the overhead carrier and placed in wheeled carts for reprocessing. The job required standing and walking throughout the work shift. Lifting a tire weighing approximately 30 to 45 pounds occurred once every 4 to 5 minutes.

Conclusion. The lifting requirements were in excess of the worker's capabilities and likely to exacerbate his back condition. Prolonged standing and walking combined with floor vibration also were likely to worsen both his knee and his back pain. Because of a high noise level, communication with coworkers was difficult and a source of stress. It was recommended that the worker be considered for alternate employment. This job and the work site environment has numerous conditions affecting other workers, such as constrained work postures, uneven work rate, and vibration. A thorough ergonomic evaluation was recommended.

Compliance With State and Federal Regulations

The Occupational Safety and Health Act of 1970 (P.L. 91–596) established the Occupational Safety and Health Administration (OSHA) under the Department of Labor to "disseminate and enforce safety and health standards to protect employees at work" (Career Information Center, 1990, p. 55). Places of employment should be free from recognized hazards. A work site with 11 or more employees is mandated to maintain records of work-related injuries and illness and to provide medical surveillance and protective equipment. Specifically, the employer must identify chemical, physical, biological, and ergonomic hazards in the workplace. Medical monitoring for exposure to toxic elements such as asbestos, noise, and lead must be offered along with protective equipment, including safety shoes, helmets, safety glasses, respirators, and hearing protectors.

Hazard communication, or Right-to-Know Compliance, enacted by OSHA in 1983, further requires that all employers notify the workers if they are exposed to or in contact with hazardous materials. All hazardous chemicals must be identified and labeled. Material safety data sheets must be obtained from the manufacturer or supplier. These technical bulletins describe a chemical, its characteristics, health and safety hazards, and precautions. Employees must receive training in the safe handling of the chemical. To learn more about these issues, refer to the Centers for Disease Control and Prevention's Workplace Safety and Health Topics resources at www.cdc.gov/niosh/homepage.html.

The Older Worker

Increasing life expectancy, a low birthrate (which has reduced the numbers of younger replacement workers available), and an aging labor force are changing the age composition of the workplace. The 1986 Amendments to the Age Discrimination in Employment Act of 1967 (ADEA; P.L. 90–202) abolished a mandatory retirement age. The ADEA safeguards the older worker (older than 40 years of age) from age-based distinctions in hiring, salary, promotions, and training. Cost projections for retirement to the individual worker and society are staggering. Legislative actions and policies are being proposed and implemented to extend one's working career. Some programs include the following:

■   Expansion of work opportunities and alternative work schedules through job redesign, phased retirement, job sharing, and part-time jobs

■   Legislation to outlaw age discrimination in employment

■   Training and retraining and second (third, etc.) career opportunities

■   Subsidized employment

■   Pension reform for raising age of eligibility.

There are physical changes that occur with age. As work capabilities vary, every older worker needs to be evaluated individually. Common deficits and limitations are listed briefly:

- Functional capacity, the ability to perform tasks or physiological activities, declines with age. For many people between 30 and 65 years of age, maximum breathing capacity is reduced by 40%, nerve conduction velocity by 20%, and cardiac function by 25%.

- Homeostasis, the body's ability to maintain operation, also is challenged as one ages. Body temperature and glucose regulation may be affected. Older workers exposed to temperature extremes are more easily incapacitated than younger workers.

Cardiovascular changes include a decrease in the mean resting heart rate from 72 beats per minute (bpm) at 25 years of age to 50 bpm by 65 years of age. Maximum heart rate also drops (from 190–200 bpm at 30 to 150–160 bpm at 70). Cardiac output, the volume of blood pumped by the heart with each beat, decreases annually by 1%. Risk of hypertension (secondary to elevated blood pressure), cerebral vascular accident (caused by reduced elasticity of the veins and arteries), and arteriosclerosis (hardening of arterial walls associated with accumulation of fatty deposits) are more frequent in the older worker.

Hearing losses common to older adults include the inability to distinguish low-volume and high-pitched sounds (e.g., consonants *f, g, s, t,* and *z*). Extraneous noises may be filtered out with difficulty. Increased volume of sound may be required to hear.

Other changes in skin (loss of underlying fatty tissue and skin elasticity), gastrointestinal systems, and body composition (reduced muscle mass, loss of calcium in bone) seem less likely to influence work performance but may increase risk of disease and reduce optimal functional capacity. Despite these naturally occurring physiological changes, the older worker is not necessarily an unhealthy or unproductive employee. Age is a poor predictor of the specific person, work capabilities, and performance.

Productivity may not decline with age. Decision-making abilities are enhanced by life experiences. Reaction time slows with age. The older worker tends to be less apt to engage in risk-taking behavior (resulting in lower accident rates). Declines in memory appear to be slight and have little influence on performance. Intellectual functioning does not appear to be altered with age but, rather, by perception, attention, health status, and motivation.

The older worker may be a valuable asset to the workplace. In terms of overall health, the older population displays wide variation. As ill employees tend to leave the workforce voluntarily, the still-employed older worker tends to be physically healthy. Poor work performance, absenteeism, and turnover (often associated with poor health) are less common. Caution must be exercised to fit the right person to the specific job. This caveat, however, concerns all employees, regardless of age.

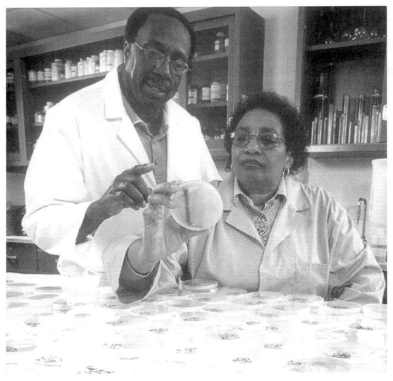

Figure 14.9. Scientists in a lab.
Photograph courtesy of the Agricultural Research Service, U.S. Department of Agriculture.
Photo by Scott Bauer.

The Worker With Disabilities

Work site accessibility is one's ability to overcome barriers to arrive at his or her workstation. A common simplifying assumption is to equate accessibility issues only with wheelchair use. There are many issues that may restrict access, such as reduced endurance for walking, visual impairment, amputation, incontinence, hearing loss, and worker and peer attitudes. A successful job placement depends on surmounting all "barriers" along relevant access routes (see Figure 14.10).

Although I will not discuss specific disabilities, I will list guidelines for optimizing workstations and the general work environment for the worker with disabilities. Application of these principles will enhance work productivity and performance for both the employee with a disability and the employee without a disability. Designing workstations that enhance user capabilities contributes to user comfort, motivation, and productivity. Poor designs result in fatigue, discomfort, and stress.

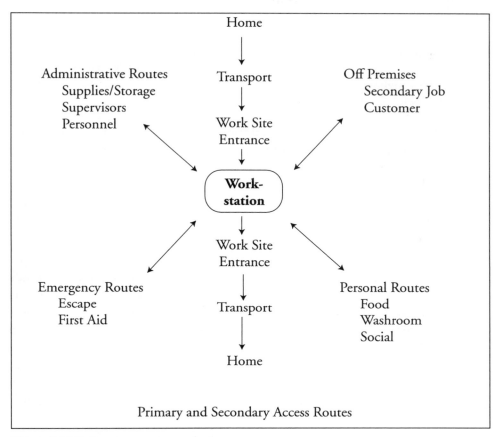

Figure 14.10. Access routes to work site.

Case Scenario

Work site analysis involves identifying jobs and workstations that contain, cause, or pose risk factors for hazards, including identification of symptoms, especially musculoskeletal, and associated risk factors, such as awkward posture, repetitiveness, sustained exertions, extreme temperatures, and vibration.

Case Scenario

Injury and hazard can be prevented through job modification; changing job assignments, tools, or environment to eliminate risk factors through alterations in method or strength required to complete the task; location and position of equipment or tools; speed or frequency; and ambient factors, such as light, noise, and air quality. Common workstation changes include those in layout, seating, and materials handling that promote adjustability for the worker and neutral postures.

Case Scenario

Training and education of employees and management staff in ergonomics principles and safety is an effective means of preventing injury and facilitating a safe working environment.

With increased computer usage and automation equipment in many industries, assistive technology can be applied to increase ease of use. Some of these end-user tools may be as simple as a glare protection screen on a computer monitor to minimize visual fatigue, a large monitor to increase character size in proportion to monitor dimensions, and voice recognition software to eliminate the need for keyboard data entry. Once thought to be costly, impossible dreams, today's computer systems (hardware and software) incorporate many energy-efficient, accessible features.

Computers and robots are now commonplace in routine tasks that are dangerous, boring, or tedious to the human worker. Robotic devices are now capable of skills far beyond simple addition. Sophisticated programming has enabled these aids to imitate the way people solve problems, choose between different courses of action, and make "smart" decisions. The use of robotic aids for people with disabilities has many benefits: cost-effectiveness (lessening dependence on attendant care), improved reliability (always available), and increased environmental control and quality of life. Robotic aids, like a robotic arm, can be used in a workstation. A worker with no or limited arm function can control the robotic arm with switches (e.g., sip-and-puff, chin control, eye gaze).

Accommodation refers to the application of ergonomic principles to maximize the capabilities of all users and thus provide an optimal interface. The Job Accommodation Network (JAN, 2003) is a federally funded operation that assists employers in accommodating workers with disabilities. JAN also provides information about the employability of people with disabilities (www.jan.wvu.edu).

The Americans With Disabilities Act of 1990 (ADA; P.L. 101–336) is perhaps the most far-reaching piece of legislation of our time. The ADA's protection applies primarily, but not exclusively, to people with disabilities: people with a current or prior history of a physical or mental impairment that substantially limits one or more major life activities. Intended to make our society more accessible, the law has five parts: employment (must provide reasonable accommodations, e.g., modifying equipment or restructuring jobs), public services, public accommodations, telecommunications, and a miscellaneous category prohibiting retaliation against people with disabilities. Workers with disabilities also can be accommodated in the workplace through the use of enlarged and raised signage, assistive listening devices, audiotapes, computers, and sign language interpreters.

The sum of wisdom is that the time is never lost that is devoted to work. (Emerson, as cited by Bohle, 1967)

Summary

The performance area of work is a significant aspect of occupational therapy's scope of practice. Work activities include an infinite number of purposeful activities that occupational therapy practitioners use as part of interventions. For many clients, the ultimate goal of occupational therapy intervention is their ability to return to work or to engage in vocational occupations. ∎

References

1986 Amendments to the Age Discrimination in Employment Act. (1967). Pub. L. 90–202, 29 U.S.C. § 621 *et seq.*

American Occupational Therapy Association. (2002). Occupational therapy practice framework: Domain and process. *American Journal of Occupational Therapy, 56,* 609–639.

Americans With Disabilities Act. (1990). Pub. L. 101–336, 42 U.S.C. § 12101.

Argyle, M. (1972). *The social psychology of work.* New York: Taplinger.

Balanced Budget Act. (1997). Pub. L. 105–33, 111 Stat. 251.

Beck, E. M. (Ed.). (1980). *John Bartlett/Bartlett's familiar quotations* (15th ed.). Boston: Little, Brown.

Bellman, G. M. (1996). *Your signature path: Gaining new perspectives on life and work.* San Francisco: Berrett-Koehler.

Bohle, B. (1967). *The home book of American quotations.* New York: Dodd Mead.

Bolles, R. N. (1998). *What color is your parachute? A practical manual for job hunters and career-changers.* Berkeley, CA: Ten Speed Press.

Bolles, R. N. (2004). *What color is your parachute? A practical manual for job hunters and career-changers* (2nd ed.). Berkeley, CA: Ten Speed Press.

Career guide to America's top industries: Essential data on job opportunities in 42 industries (5th ed.). (2002). Indianapolis, IN: JIST Works.

Career Information Center. (1990). *Employment trends and master index* (4th ed.). Mission Hills, CA: Glencoe.

Cooper, C. L. (1981). *The stress check: Coping with the stresses of life and work.* Englewood Cliffs, NJ: Prentice Hall.

Farr, J. M. (2003). *America's fastest growing jobs: Detailed information on the 141 fastest growing jobs in our economy* (7th ed.). Indianapolis, IN: JIST Works.

Farr, J. M., Ludden, L. L., & Shatkin, L. (2001). *Guide for occupational exploration* (3rd ed.). Indianapolis, IN: JIST Works.

Fraser, T. M. (1992). *Fitness for work.* London: Taylor & Francis.

Grandjean, E. (1988). *Fitting the task to the man: An ergonomic approach.* London: Taylor & Francis.

Holland, J. L. (1997). *Making vocational choices: A theory of vocational personalities and work environments* (3rd ed.). Odessa, FL: Psychological Assessment Resources.

Isernhagen, S. J. (Ed.). (1995). *The comprehensive guide to work injury management.* Gaithersburg, MD: Aspen.

Job Accommodation Network. (2003). Retrieved on November 25, 2003, from http://www.jan.wvu.edu.

Marshall, E. (1985). Looking back. *American Journal of Occupational Therapy, 39,* 297–300.

McMenamin, T., Krantz, R., & Krolik, T. J. (2003, February). U.S. labor market in 2002: Continued weakness [Electronic version]. *Monthly Labor Review,* 3–25.

Morris, R. B. (Ed). (1976). *United States Department of Labor bicentennial history of the American worker.* Washington, DC: U.S. Government Printing Office.

Occupational Safety and Health Act. (1970). Pub. L. 91–596, 84 Stat. 1590.

Reich, C. A. (1970). *The greening of America.* New York: Random House.

Smith, E. R. (1989). Ergonomics and the occupational therapist. In S. Hertfelder & C. Gwin (Eds.), *Work in progress: Occupational therapy in work programs* (pp. 127–155). Rockville, MD: American Occupational Therapy Association.

Steele, J. E., & Morgan, M. S. (1991). *Career planning and development for college students and recent graduates.* Lincolnwood, IL: VGM Career Horizons.

Terkel, S. (1971). *Working: People talk about what they do all day and how they feel about what they do.* New York: Pantheon.

Terkel, S. (1997). *My American century.* New York: New Press.

U.S. Department of Health and Human Services, National Institute for Occupational Safety and Health. (1999). *Stress at work* (DHHS Pub. No. 99-101). Cincinnati, OH: Publications Dissemination.

U.S. Department of Labor, Bureau of Labor Statistics. (2002). *Occupational outlook handbook, 2002–2003 edition, bulletin 2540* [online]. Retrieved November 25, 2003, from http://www.bls.gov/oco.

U.S. Department of Labor, Bureau of Labor Statistics. (2003). *News release—Work experience summary* [online]. Retrieved November 25, 2003, from http://www.bls.gov/news.release/work.nr0.htm.

U.S. Department of Labor, Employment and Training Administration. (2003). *O*NET—Beyond information—Intelligence* [online]. Retrieved November 25, 2003, from http://www.doleta.gov/programs/onet.

U.S. Department of Labor, U.S. Employment Service. (1979). *Guide for occupational exploration.* Washington, DC: U.S. Government Printing Office.

U.S. Department of Labor, U.S. Employment Service. (1991). *Dictionary of occupational titles* (4th ed., rev.). Lanham, MD: Bernan.

Wilcock, A. A. (2003). Occupational science: The study of humans as occupational beings. In P. Kramer, J. Hinojosa, & C. B. Royeen (Eds.), *Perspectives in human occupation: Participation in life* (pp. 156–180). Baltimore: Lippincott, Williams & Wilkins.

World Health Organization. (1989). *Epidemiology of work-related diseases and accidents. Tenth report of the Joint ILO/WHO Committee on Occupational Health* (Technical Report Series 777). Geneva, Switzerland: Author.

World Health Organization. (2001). *ICF: International classification of functioning, disability, and health.* Geneva, Switzerland: Author.

Yerxa, E. J., Clark, F., Frank, G., Jackson, J., Parham, D., Pierce, D., et al. (1989). Occupational science: The foundations for new models of practice. *Occupational Therapy in Health Care, 6*(4), 1–7.

15

▦

Range of Human Activity: Self-Care

Anita Perr, MA, OT, ATP, FAOTA

These things we do…no matter the name.

This chapter focuses on the things we do to take care of ourselves. As a group, they are called by many names: *activities of daily living (ADL); daily living skills; basic activities of daily living; instrumental activities of daily living (IADL); self-care skills or activities;* and recently, *occupations of daily living.* The common piece is daily living. The other part, whether you call it *skills, activities,* or occupations, is many *things.* This chapter focuses on a group of *things* (for lack of a better word) that we do frequently. It provides a framework by which one can organize evaluations of a person's self-care and design appropriate interventions for a person who has difficulty with self-care. Finally, this chapter asks you to examine your own thoughts about ADL related to the specific activities and your occupations.

A focus on daily life activities goes back to the beginnings of occupational therapy. Early in the history of occupational therapy there was a focus on the importance of habits and habit training. Eleanor Clarke Slagle developed programs of habit training for people with social and psychiatric conditions. Her focus included self-care and other routine activities.

A focus on ADL goes into and out of vogue in occupational therapy. Often, it is difficult for occupational therapy practitioners who feel the need to defend their profession to focus on such commonplace activities. These commonplace activities, however, make up such a large part of all of our lives. The routines of taking care of oneself are not something most people spend much time thinking about. If, however, any of us were unable to complete these routines, it would come to the forefront of our minds regularly. Focusing on a person's ability to engage in self-care activities is a great service of occupational therapy. Self-care activities are fundamental to human existence and affect our ability to function in society.

Our specific routines differ on the basis of gender, ethnicity, age, and many other factors. These differences, or preferences, need to be addressed in treatment. The way we look at the parts of the routine also should be discussed. As the field of occupational therapy further explores the terms *occupation, activity,* and *task,* it makes sense to think about ADL in these terms as well. At the most basic level, we can look at the category of self-care as the occupation. If occupation can be thought of as a collection of activities, we can think of the various components of self-care as activities. In this organization, the activities are things like combing hair, sexual expression, brushing teeth, toileting, and eating. The way each person puts the activities of self-care together becomes the occupation and is grounded in personal meanings.

Two people, Grace and Jon, will serve as case examples throughout this chapter. Grace and Jon lead very different lives and have different habits, preferences, values, and needs. Their cases will illustrate the various aspects of ADL that occupational therapy practitioners can address. The case scenarios are divided into parts and placed throughout the chapter. Each part is associated with the area of discussion. Although some information is included in each part, a vast amount of information about these two people is not. The information that is included is that which is most relevant to the discussion.

Case Scenario, Part 1: Grace

Grace is a 45-year-old woman who underwent surgery to clip an aneurysm in her brain and bled during the surgery. The result is that she is hemiparetic on the right side. She has flaccid paralysis of the right upper extremity. Grace is right-hand dominant. Although there are some areas of abnormal tone and weakness in the right lower extremity, Grace is able to ambulate for about 10 feet on level surfaces without using an ambulation aid, such as a cane. She also has mild memory impairment and mildly limited executive cognitive functions.

Case Scenario, Part 1: Jon

Jon is a 16-year-old boy who broke his right arm while skateboarding. He has compound fractures of the humerus (mid-shaft) and the ulna and radius. An external fixator is in place at the humerus. Internal fixators, plates, and screws are in place in the forearm. Jon is right-hand dominant.

What Are These Things?

Skills? Activities? Occupations? What do you call them? You may hear *these things* referred to with any of the previous labels. Other labels probably exist that you will hear as well. It is easier to list *these things:* bathing, dressing, grooming, hygiene, toileting, feeding, eating, sexual expression, and communicating. What about home management? Then *these things* also include meal preparation, housekeeping, home finances, shopping, and laundry. Where does one draw the line? Do *these things* include functional mobility? Then *these things* also include bed mobility, transfers, ambulation, and transportation. Where does it end? Eventually, the list of *these things* will include everything that any person does. So now what do we call *these things*? For the purpose of this chapter, I will call all *these things* ADL, and they include everything on the list, and then some. The way that each of us identifies with each of the activities and combines them into our own routine becomes occupation. It is that occupation that fits so easily into the focus of what occupational therapy practitioners do.

Case Scenario, Part 2: Important ADL for Grace

When meeting Grace, her precise dressing and grooming struck me. By her report, it is important that she "look well put-together." She wears her hair in long braids, which she braids herself. She jogs 1 to 3 miles at least three times a week. She showers each morning before leaving for work. An important occupation is cooking, where she attends to nutritional advice and enjoys the challenges of preparing dinner for others. Grace does not drive but uses buses and subways daily, usually for more than just her trip to and from work.

Case Scenario, Part 2: Important ADL for Jon

Jon is a social teenager who spends a great deal of time getting ready to go out with friends. He works at looking well groomed and dressing in the same way as do his friends and their role models, mainly hip-hop rock stars. Jon reports that he has great difficulty putting gel in his hair and getting it to look the way he wants it to since breaking his arm. Jon showers at school after his gym class three times weekly. During his evaluation, Jon revealed that he is uncomfortable dressing and undressing after gym class. He works out about four times a week, primarily lifting weights and working to improve his physique, but he calls himself scrawny. He does not want his classmates to see that he is skinny. He thinks he looks like a little kid and does not understand why he is not bulking up like most of the other teens he is friendly with. Jon has no interest in cooking or preparing meals. His mother prepares meals at home for the whole family. Jon buys lunch in his school cafeteria.

Contextual Factors

Everything takes place within a context. Changing the context changes the activity. Context includes external factors, those that are outside the person, that influence function. When disability is discussed, the impact of the contextual factors may be magnified. Contextual factors need to be identified during the evaluation and included during the intervention. These contextual factors help the therapist to address ADL interventions within appropriate environments and with appropriate foci. By understanding the contextual factors, the therapist is better able to prioritize treatment and determine what is important for each individual client. The context includes both environmental and personal factors.

Environmental Factors

Environmental factors can be further subdivided into physical, social, and attitudinal environments. Environmental factors can be positive and act as facilitators of participation in activity, in this case, ADL. Environmental factors also can be barriers to participation. During the evaluation, the therapist uses environmental facilitators to improve participation in ADL and addresses the environmental barriers to alleviate or lessen their impact. The closet shown in Figure 15.1 was previously an environmental barrier. Initially, only one rod hung in the closet, the higher one. The man in the photo could not reach into the closet from his wheelchair to get his clothes. He installed the second rod and moved the clothing that he wears the most frequently to that rod. Now it is easy to get to the clothing he usually wears. If he needs to retrieve an item from the upper rod, he uses a reacher.

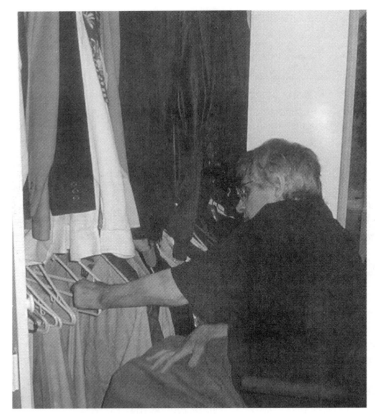

Figure 15.1. A clothes closet with a second rod is no longer an environmental barrier. The rod is actually now an environmental facilitator.

Case Scenario, Part 3: Physical Environment for Grace

Grace lives in a studio apartment in a large east coast city. The apartment is on the second floor, up a flight of 18 steps. There is no elevator in the building. Grace sleeps on a waterbed that is against the wall at the head and left side. She has a small closet in which she keeps the current season's clothing and outerwear. She also has a small dresser for undergarments. Grace's bathroom is very small. The only storage space she has in the bathroom is a small medicine cabinet over the sink. She has a clawfoot bathtub with a shower extension attached to the tub spout.

Case Scenario, Part 3: Physical Environment for Jon

Jon lives in the suburbs, about 2 hours from the same city where Grace lives. He lives in a two-story, four-bedroom house where all of the bedrooms are on the second floor. Jon shares a bedroom with his 14-year-old brother. He sleeps on the bottom bunk. Jon keeps his clothes folded in dresser drawers or hung on hooks or hangers in a closet, but he reports that his room is usually messy, and he usually finds the clothes he wears on the floor or on a chair. The bathroom that Jon usually uses for his morning routine is shared by four children. It has a stall shower. As previously stated, Jon usually showers at school and says this is because if he showers at home there may not be enough hot water.

Case Scenario, Part 4: Social Factors for Grace

Grace is engaged to be married about 6 months from the time of her surgery. She has no immediate or extended family nearby with the exception of her fiancé, Tony. Grace has four or five close friends with whom she speaks or spends time about five times a week. She is very pleasant, although somewhat quiet. She has many acquaintances at work, in her gym, and at church. Grace does not have pets. Before the surgery, Grace never had any medical problems. She sees her physician annually.

Case Scenario, Part 4: Social Factors for Jon

Jon lives with his mother, father, and three brothers. His extended family lives in nearby states and in Taiwan. The family in the area gets together regularly. He has cousins with whom he is very friendly.

Case Scenario, Part 5: Attitudinal Factors for Grace

Grace values her social and economic independence. Although she is very much in love with Tony, both plan to continue to spend time with their own friends pursuing their own interests in addition to building new friendships and developing new pursuits together. She belongs to a church in her neighborhood, attends services regularly, and participates in other church activities. She met Tony during a fund-raising activity that the church sponsored. Graces enjoys yoga and meditation and is learning about eastern religions. She celebrates her African heritage, celebrates Kwanzaa, and plans to "jump the broom" at her wedding.

Case Scenario, Part 5: Attitudinal Factors for Jon

Jon's family is generally conservative in their political views. Jon views his family as too traditional and boring. He says that they are sometimes worried about him because he "tends to be more wild." His family is Catholic, but they do not regularly attend church or actively practice religion. Jon and his friends tend to use curse words when they are with each other, but Jon does not curse when near family members.

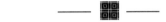

Exercise 15.1—Think About Environmental Factors

In these profiles, what are the physical, social, and attitudinal facilitators and barriers to participation in ADL for Grace and Jon? Think about your own life. What are the environmental facilitators and barriers? How do you use the facilitators? How do you deal with the barriers?

Personal Factors

Personal factors also are contextual. They include age, gender, social status, life experiences, and so on. It is easy to see that the ADL for a 3-year-old differ from those of a teenager, which differ from those of an adult, which further differ from those of an older adult. The young child may be focusing on dressing him- or herself, wearing clothing with elastic waists and shoes with hook-and-loop closures. Most teens have mastered grooming and dressing, and grooming and dressing focus on conforming to some model. Teens may be more focused on other activities like learning to drive or managing their own bank account. Gender-specific and sexual activities are also important activities (occupations) for teenagers. Sex, an often-ignored daily life activity or occupation, is extremely important for adolescents and young and mature adults. Adults may focus on housekeeping. Older adults may have different responsibilities. If they live in a retirement community, they may not have the responsibility for lawn and garden care and may have time to focus on other responsibilities.

Case Scenario, Part 6: Personal Factors for Grace

At 45, Grace cannot believe that she is middle aged, does not like to think about it, and does not want to think about getting older. She is African American and grew up in a small southern town. She has lived on her own since high school. She earned an undergraduate degree and a master of business administration degree from a prestigious New England university. Her fiancé, Tony, is Brazilian and not yet a U.S. citizen. The couple have been involved for 3 years. Grace says that their love life is healthy, that they have sex regularly, and that they both are very caring and compassionate. She says that she likes to experiment a little more than he does. Grace currently works for a small business importing gift items from Africa. She loves to travel.

Case Scenario, Part 6: Personal Factors for Jon

Jon is a 16-year-old Asian American. He attends high school, where his grade-point average is 2.42. He and his male friends often skip school. He has lived his entire life in the same home. He has slept over at friends' houses but not for more than one night consecutively. Jon does not have a girlfriend and is extremely hesitant to talk about close personal relationships. Jon says that he is not sexually active.

Functioning and Disability

All people participate in activities and occupations. The assortment and variety of activities and occupations varies from person to person. As previously established, contextual factors influence our ability to participate. Other factors influence our participation as well. The structural make-up of a person's body provides him or her with a capacity to do something. When an impairment of body structures exists, a person's body functions may be hindered. When body functions are hindered, participation is limited. Using the *International Classification of Functioning, Disability and Health* (ICF; World Health Organization [WHO], 2001) terminology, these difficulties are referred to as *participation restrictions* and *activity limitations*. Body functions and body structures can be compared with the component level of the third edition of the *Uniform Terminology for Occupational Therapy* (American Occupational Therapy Association, 1994).

Case Scenario, Part 7: Body Structure Factors for Grace

Grace suffered a left parietal lobe infarct during the surgery to clip an aneurysm. She presents with muscle imbalance in the trunk and extremely low tone in the right arm. She has spotty decreased strength in her right leg.

Case Scenario, Part 7: Body Structure Factors for Jon

Jon suffered multiple fractures in his right arm and has an external fixator in place for 5 to 7 weeks. He also uses a sling and bolster to support his arm when standing. Jon's arm should also be raised and supported when he is seated, but he says that he is usually not able to do this. Open wounds exist at the pin sites where the external fixator protrudes from his arm.

Case Scenario, Part 8: Body Function Factors for Grace

Since the neurologic insult, Grace has become quieter and now perceives herself as shy. She also complains that she does not know how people will react or whether she will be able to follow the nuances of the conversation. She is somewhat down-hearted about her condition and her impending wedding. Her motivation fluctu-ates from day to day. She tends to be sleepy most of the time and cannot tell whether it is from the new medication because she "just feels crummy." She has mild short-term and long-term memory impairment and mild impairment of high-level cognitive functions. Sensory functions are intact. Grace has a mild balance impairment in standing and mild to moderate impairment in endurance.

Case Scenario, Part 8: Body Function Factors for Jon

Jon's mental and sensory functions are intact and age appropriate.

Evaluation and Intervention

To help a client become more independent in ADL, it is important to complete a thorough evaluation. A comprehensive evaluation identifies the areas of limited par-ticipation and how disability limits participation. The most reliable information is learned by performing the activity in its usual environment, but this is frequently impossible to do. Therapists who work in home-based practice have the advantage of using the client's own environment and materials during the evaluation and the inter-vention. In most situations, however, the evaluation and intervention do not take place in the usual environment. An alternative is to have the person perform the activ-ity using the real tools, such as his or her own clothing or toothbrush, in a simulated setting like a hospital room or an area of an occupational therapy clinic. Care should be taken to bring as much of the usual environment into the evaluation and inter-vention context, including taking into account the client's values and beliefs as well as his or her roles and responsibilities. All of this should be captured in the evaluation.

Some facilities use their own ADL evaluations; some use tools that are com-mercially available. The evaluation the therapist uses should allow him or her to col-lect information about self-care, mobility, IADL, caring for others, and other personal self-management tasks (see Figure 15.2).

The evaluation should include a rating scale that is reliable and valid. Some rat-ing scales use words to describe performance, such as *independent, moderate assistance,* and *dependent.* The ICF uses the qualifiers *no problem, mild problem, moderate prob-lem, severe problem,* and *complete problem* (WHO, 2001). Other ADL evaluations use a numeric scale, such as a scale of 1 to 7 that delineates levels of independence. The preference for the type of rating scale is up to the evaluator as long as the measure is identified and the descriptions make sense for the people who are evaluated and for the environment in which they are evaluated.

The evaluation also should have the capacity to include information that is not actually performed. At times, therapists must rely on reports from the client, his or her family, and others involved in his or her care. This information should be labeled "by report" or similarly, to differentiate it from information gained through observation.

Evaluation Categories

Self-Care Activities
> Sexual expression
> Toileting
> Bathing
> Grooming and hygiene
> Dressing
> Other

Mobility
> Transfers
> Mobility
>> Indoors
>> Home
>> Community
>> Transportation
> Other

Instrumental Activities of Daily Living
> Housekeeping
> Money management
> Other

Caring for Others

Other

Figure 15.2. Evaluation Categories.

Some ADL evaluations are standardized, and others are not. Some are used in many settings, others in very few settings. Table 15.1 lists some commonly used ADL assessments and the areas they cover.

Exercise 15.2—Evaluation

Before moving on to intervention, think about Grace and Jon and perform an imaginary evaluation on them. What areas of ADL are going to be limited? What are the causes for the limitations? Are they body structures? Body functions? Contextual factors?

Table 15.1
Self-Care Assessments

Name	Areas/Domains					
	Communication Emergency Response	Grooming Hygiene	Feeding Eating	Mobility Transfer	Dressing	Other
Arnadottir OT-ADL Neurobehavioral Evaluation (A-ONE; Arnadottir, 1990)	X	X	X	X	X	—
Assessment of Living Skills and Resources (ALSAR; Williams et al., 1991)	Reading Telephone	—	—	X	—	Medication management
OT FACT (Smith, 1990)	X	X	X	X	X	Computer driven
Functional Independence Measure (FIM; Jette et al., 1986)	X	X	X	X	X	Cognitive function
Klein–Bell ADL Scale (Klein & Bell, 1979)	X	X	X	X	X	—
Kohlman Evaluation of Living Skills (KELS; Kohlman-Thompson, 1992)	Telephone	X	—	X	—	Safety, money management
Milwaukee Evaluation of Daily Living Skills (MEDLS; Leonardelli, 1988)	X	X	—	X	X	Money management, medication management
Performance Assessment of Self-Care Skills (PASS, version 3.1; Rogers & Holm, 1994)	—	X	—	X	—	Home management
Routine Task Intervention (RTI; Heinemann, Allen, & Yerxa, 1989)	X	X	—	—	X	Money and time management

x: covered; —: not covered.

Intervention

Occupational therapy practitioners provide intervention to increase a client's ability to participate in activities, in this case, ADL. Areas of disability should be addressed during intervention. Interventions are developed to remedy impairments in body structures and body functions, to maximize facilitating contextual factors, and to eliminate or lessen barriers. The evaluation will help to identify the problem areas. Once the evaluation is completed, the next step is to identify the priorities because it may be impossible to address *everything,* but it is certainly impossible to address everything *first.* Client preferences should strongly influence the priorities for intervention. Safety is even more important than client preference. Although safety often is the client's highest priority, there are instances when the client does not identify problems in judgment and safety awareness. The prevalence of falls in older people may be caused in part by an inability to recognize potential hazards. A client may say to a practitioner that the first thing he or she wants to work on is ironing clothes. The practitioner, however, recognizes that, because of the impairments to body structures, such as the impairments present after a spinal cord injury, the client cannot reach or use the emergency call bell in the hospital room. Everyone should be able to call for help if he or she needs it. This means that the first ADL task addressed for most hospitalized patients is using the call system to call a nurse.

Exercise 15.3—ADL Priorities for Grace and Jon

What are the ADL priorities for Grace and Jon? Are there safety concerns? One ADL task that needs to be addressed with Jon is cleaning the pin sites on his arm. If these sites are not kept clean, infections can develop, slowing his recovery and perhaps leading to further disability. Jon may or may not be mature enough to realize the threat of infection, but one of the first things the therapist should do is discuss this with Jon and his parents. The first ADL priority for Jon may be washing and drying his right arm, caring for the sling and bolster, and addressing issues of positioning in sitting and standing. Did you think of that?

Case Scenario, Part 9: Grace's Priorities

Grace is having a difficult time dealing with the changes that she is undergoing. The stress of her upcoming wedding and the possibility that she may still have residual disabilities at that time sometimes overwhelms her. Through conversation, Grace and the occupational therapist decide that addressing her depression must start immediately and must pervade every other treatment activity. Other priorities are learning to swing her arm when walking and holding objects in both hands. Again, in planning for her wedding, Grace focuses on wanting to be able to carry her bouquet. In addition, she wants to dress, bathe, and groom herself so that she does not have to rely on others to help her. This ADL task is especially important to her because she knows how particular she is in her self-care and thinks that others are bothered by her idiosyncrasies.

Case Scenario, Part 9: Jon's Priorities

Jon identified a priority as being able to gel and set his hair. After addressing the wound sites, the next priority addressed with Jon also was suggested to him—that of toileting independently. Once this was mentioned to Jon, he also identified it as a priority. Toileting often is addressed first. Did you name that as a priority?

What are the limitations that affect Jon's ability to use a bathroom independently? What about Grace's ability to manage toileting by herself? Jon and Grace both may need to work on one-hand techniques and dominance retraining to manage lower-extremity garments and to clean after toileting. Jon's therapist asked about the pants he likes to wear and Jon decided to put away his button-fly jeans until his arm heals. He chose to use alternative clothing rather than use an alternative technique to button the buttons or to use a button aid or other adaptive device to help with the task. Jon also said that he was going to switch to boxer shorts because briefs are too difficult for him to manage with one hand. If the therapist did not address toileting, Jon may not have developed compensatory strategies for this activity. Grace preferred not to change the type of clothing she likes to wear. Instead of wearing sweat pants with an elastic waist, she learned to use a button aid and zipper pull to fasten her pants after toileting. Activities are rarely addressed individually. By addressing toileting, both clients (and both occupational therapists) addressed dressing as well.

Where to Start

In many instances, it makes the most sense to start intervention by addressing the body structure and body function. By improving the status of the structure, performance of ADL is improved. If this is the case, it is important for the therapist to discuss the relation of the body structure to the performance of ADL. Clients may then be better able to articulate the relationship and may be able to perform ADL that are not addressed during treatment. This generalization of learning helps the client to become even more able to participate in activities.

Choosing the approach to treatment is a decision that therapists can make, depending on the client, the limitation, the environment, and all the other factors influencing participation. With ADL, the intervention is usually based in some combination of improving function and compensating for disability that cannot be changed. The compensation usually comes in two forms: changing the strategy used to complete the activity or adding adaptive equipment or technology. In Figure 15.3, notice that the client is using a universal cuff to hold the toothbrush. Because of paralysis following a spinal cord injury, he is unable to hold his toothbrush in the usual

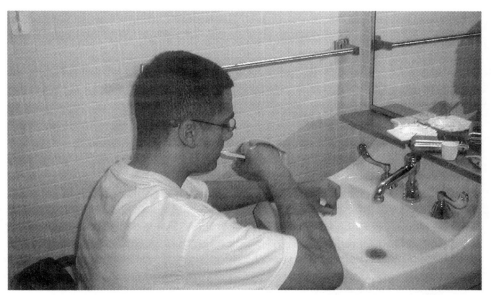

Figure 15.3. Brushing teeth while seated in a wheelchair. Notice the universal cuff on the young man's hand into which the toothbrush is placed. Additionally, lever faucets make it easier to set water force and temperature.

way. He also is unable to use an alternate technique to hold the toothbrush securely. Instead, the client uses adaptive equipment to compensate for the paralysis.

Use the Information Gained During the Evaluation

Body structure information tells the occupational therapy practitioner about diagnosis. The anatomical structure, including the presence and extent of impairment, sets the stage for occupational therapy intervention. It is easy to see that a person with missing body parts may have difficulty performing ADL or will perform ADL using an alternative technique. The same goes for impairment of any body structure. During the evaluation, the extent of the impairment is identified, and the expected recovery is determined. Goals are set according to the expected recovery and the expected ability of the person to compensate for any residual impairment.

Related to body structures are body functions, how is the person able to function within the confines of the extent of impairment in any of the body structures? Occupational therapy practitioners focus their treatment at this level. Practitioners use purposeful activities to heal body structures and improve body functions.

Case Scenario, Part 10: Grace's Intervention

Because Grace had a hemorrhagic stroke during surgery, there is no way to know how much of the blood will be reabsorbed or how much residual damage there will be. The expected recovery of the neurologic system is not known. Brain function may come back as the blood is reabsorbed and the swelling resolves. Associated areas of the brain may take over for the damaged areas. The therapist may have difficulty knowing how much recovery will occur in Grace's flaccid right arm and in her cognitive functioning. Grace's overall treatment is designed to allow medical recovery of body structures to occur. Occupational therapy intervention will include purposeful activities to attempt to improve Grace's ability to use her right arm. She will learn alternative techniques, such as using her left arm to put her right arm in a position to act as a stabilizer when, for example, stabilizing her toothbrush while applying toothpaste with her left hand.

Case Scenario, Part 10: Jon's Intervention

Jon has a mostly temporary disability. In all likelihood, the bones will heal. He should recover fully, although a chance exists that he will have limited mobility in his forearm, affecting his ability to supinate and pronate. Jon also is at risk for developing infection at the wound sites.

Both Grace and Jon will use alternative techniques to complete their ADL. Part of the intervention for both clients may include training in upper-extremity self-range of motion exercises. To have the potential for the highest level of independence, both Jon and Grace need to maintain the structural integrity of their arms in order to allow them to use their arms as fully as possible when they are able.

As stated earlier, the evaluation also provides information about the contextual factors affecting a client's participation in ADL. How so? Think about how the physical environment could influence participation. The person pictured in Figure 15.4 has been paralyzed for many years and has always dressed himself independently. Recently, however, he started using an alternating pressure mattress to decrease the pressure over his bony prominences following flap surgery for a Stage III pressure ulcer. The softness and dynamic qualities of the alternating pressure mattress made it nearly impossible for him to position himself and to move to dress. The solution was to fully inflate the mattress and to stop the alternating airflow while he dresses his lower extremities and performs transfers. The motor for the alternating pressure mattress is next to him on his bed, and he can manage the switch independently.

As depicted in Figure 15.5, a young man uses an alternative technique to hold a pen. He weaves the pen in between his fingers and uses tenodesis to hold the pen tightly. This technique allows him to write with enough force to see the ink. He prefers this method to using an adaptive device because he can use any pen or pencil available and does not have to remember to carry another piece of equipment with him.

Case Scenario, Part 11: Grace Summary

Grace is now on a rehabilitation unit in an acute care hospital and is likely to stay for about 3 weeks before she goes home. This environment is not similar to her home, as Grace lives in a small apartment.

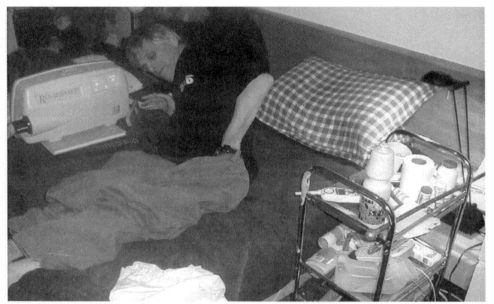

Figure 15.4. Dressing on an alternating pressure air mattress.

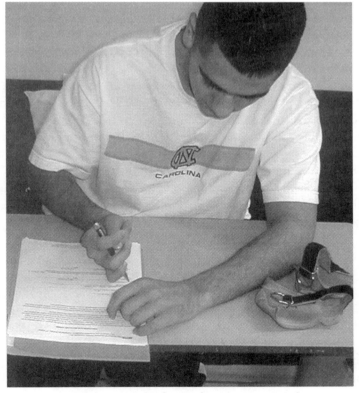

Figure 15.5. Pen is woven between the fingers for stronger control.

Case Scenario, Part 11: Jon Summary

Jon is treated in an outpatient occupational therapy setting. This environment is not similar to his home either, as Jon lives in a large home.

How will you develop your interventions to be meaningful for Grace and Jon? How can you simulate their home environments in an inpatient or outpatient clinic? Therapists process these concepts in order to develop interventions that are going to be the most useful. There are many other factors to think about. Age and gender influence the types of activities the practitioner brings into treatment. They also may influence the client's priorities. Even though Grace is a female adult and Jon is a male adolescent, both have stated that hair care is high on their lists of priorities.

Other personal factors also will influence the focus of treatment and the purposeful activities used during treatment. It would be important, for example, to know that a client is a vegetarian so that cooking activities would include ingredients that the client will eat. It is just as important to know whether there are dietary restrictions related to religion or, for that matter, because of personal taste and preferences. Tying personal factors to body functions and structures, a practitioner can see that a client wears dentures or is dysphagic and would prefer soft food that is easy to manage.

Group vs. Individual Treatment

Many facilities encourage group treatment. ADL can be addressed very effectively in groups. A common example is the existence of self-feeding groups in many facilities. A group of clients with dysphagia may eat together, with a speech–language pathologist, occupational therapy practitioner, or nursing assistant available for cuing and assistance. Routine participation in a grooming group may be effective in helping a client with mental illness resume these activities. This routine group daily life activity uses Slagle's concept of rebuilding routines and allows each participant to develop and refine interpersonal communication skills and appropriate social behaviors. Whether working on interpersonal interactions and relationships, domestic life, mobility, or communication, a cooking activity can be developed to allow each member to work on his or her individual goals.

Summary

Good ADL intervention "gets the most bang for the buck." The occupational therapy practitioner can treat many body structures and body functions by focusing on the activities of daily life. Identify the factors that influence the person's ability to participate in ADL. Make the most of the factors that facilitate participation, and figure out ways to lessen the impact of those that are barriers. The end result should be the highest level of independence, or the highest degree of participation in the ADL, that you address. ■

References

American Occupational Therapy Association. (1994). Uniform terminology for occupational therapy—Third edition. *American Journal of Occupational Therapy, 48,* 1047–1059.

Arnadottir, G. (1990). *The brain and behavior: Assessing cortical dysfunction through tasks of daily living.* St. Louis, MO: Mosby.

Heinemann, N. E., Allen, C. K., & Yerxa, E. J. (1989). The Routine Task Inventory: A tool for describing the functional behavior of the cognitively disabled. *OT Practice, 1*(1), 67–74.

Jette, A. M., Davis, A. R. Cleary, P. D., Calkins, D. R., Ruberstein, L. V., Fink, A., et al. (1986). The Functional Status Questionnaire: Reliability and validity when used in primary care. *Journal of General Internal Medicine, 1,* 143–149.

Klein, R. M., & Bell, B. (1979). *The Klein–Bell ADL Scale manual.* Seattle, WA: Educational Resources, University of Washington.

Kohlman-Thompson, L. (1992). *Kohlman Evaluation of Living Skills (KELS)* (3rd ed.). Rockville, MD: American Occupational Therapy Association.

Leonardelli, C. (1988). *Milwaukee Evaluation of Daily Living Skills (MEDLS).* Thorofare, NJ: Slack.

Rogers, J. C., & Holm, M. B. (1994). *Performance Assessment of Self-Care Skills–Revised (PASS)* (Version 3.1). Unpublished functional performance test, University of Pittsburgh, Pennsylvania.

Smith, R. (1990). *Occupational Therapy Functional Compilation Tool (OT FACT): Administration and tutorial manual.* Rockville, MD: American Occupational Therapy Association.

Williams, J. H., Drinka, T. J. K., Greenberg, J. R., Farrel-Holtan, J., Euhardy, R., & Schram, M. (1991). Development and testing of the Assessment of Living Skills and Resources (ALSAR) in elderly community-dwelling veterans. *Gerontologist, 31,* 84–91.

World Health Organization. (2001). *ICF: International classification of functioning, disability and health, short version.* Geneva, Switzerland: Author.

16

Range of Human Activity:
Care of Others

Dalia Sachs, PhD, OT
Deborah R. Labovitz, PhD, OTR/L, FAOTA

Caring is a basic relationship between people and is the activity that structures most of the primary and ongoing forms of connection between human beings. Caregiving directed to appropriate receivers of care is one of the important activities responsible for the survival of human beings and society. Without being cared for, humans cannot survive during many critical periods of their lives, such as infancy and childhood, times of temporary or permanent illness or disability, and extended old age. Without caring and being cared for, people cannot have a fully meaningful day-to-day existence throughout their lives. Caring for the self and caring for others are, therefore, essential activities of human existence and as such can be considered part of the primordial structure of human life. These dual forms of caring, self-care, and caregiving to others are expressed in a variety of ways and function at the physical, cognitive, interpersonal, psychological, emotional, and moral and spiritual levels.

Caregiving has not always been so clearly recognized as one of the activities that is immensely significant to our own lives and to the lives of so many of our clients. But recently, with a focus on client- and family-centered care and occupational performance models, occupational therapy practitioners have focused on caregiving as part of the profession's domain of concern. We acknowledge that caregiving is an occupational role that not only involves care given to the client by professionals but also includes the clients themselves, the clients' family members, and their formal and informal caregivers (Clark, Corcoran, & Gitlin, 1995; Gitlin, Corcoran, & Leinmiller-Eckhardt, 1995).

What Is Caregiving?

The main human populations that require care are children, older adults, and people who are limited in their daily activities by acute or chronic physical, psychosocial, and cognitive conditions. Caregiving, however, is not limited to those who need long-term assistance in their daily activities. Caregiving also is appropriate for family members, other loved ones, and friends who have temporary needs for some kind of care. Think of the times when friends turned to you during difficult periods and asked you to help them do their shopping, clean their house, listen to and advise them, or care in some way for them. How did you feel when you did it? Was it a challenging, difficult, or satisfying activity, or was it some or all of these? Think of yourself when you had the flu and your mother or friend or partner prepared hot soup to comfort you. How did you feel when it happened?

Caregiving and care receiving are the two parts of caring. Both caregiving and care receiving are important for the survival of the person in need and it also can be satisfying to both the person receiving care and the caregiver. But it is important to recognize the complexity of both roles and to understand some confusion about the concept that forms their basis (i.e., caring). The word *caring* has been used to describe many things and to stand for some often seemingly contradictory concepts. For example, caring for a child or a family member is supposedly a very valuable activity, and those who do so are considered loving and responsible; yet, in most companies, staying home from work to care for a sick child or to take an elderly parent to a physician appointment is not generally accepted as a legitimate excuse to receive pay for the day as a "sick" day.

Similarly, although we recognize that they are vital to the survival of their clients and the rest of the client's family members, home health aides who care for people who are very ill often are not paid for by insurance companies or by governmental medical assistance programs. Despite the fact that the work can be unpleasant, constantly demanding, physically taxing, and emotionally stressful, such jobs are considered menial labor, are available to people with no specific training for the work, and offer minimum wages. Therefore, caring connotes on the one hand a meritorious attitude and virtue, and on the other hand, it denotes activities that sometimes seem to earn little appreciation in society, that are associated with much burden, and that may even be penalized.

Another common example of these contradictions can be found in descriptions of motherhood. Mothering is a role associated with caring. It must be done correctly, with enthusiasm and love. Mothering is not only the most fundamental of caring relations but also the prototype of professional caring (Sachs, 1988). Yet at the same time, caregiving related to mothering often is trivialized, considered less important than other careers available to women, and described as a burden and hardship (Fisher & Tronto, 1990). In addition, like much of the work that takes place within the home, caregiving, done within and for the family, is usually unpaid labor and done without formal education or training. Similarly, the skills and knowledge required for formal, informal, and professional caregiving in the workplace, regarded possibly as an extension of women's activities at home with their families, are not always appreciated on a societal level, and the pay is generally low for those who do such work.

Nevertheless, the satisfaction related to caregiving often is immeasurable and priceless to those who engage in it. We recognize caring as a relationship and an occupation that may consume a large part of our clients' time and as a role that constitutes an important part of their self-images while providing meaning for their lives. An occupation this complex and long lasting has definite value to the people who do it. We also believe that for many women as well as for some men, the decision in general to join a health care profession, and specifically to become an occupational therapy practitioner, is related to a strong caring commitment and a sense of satisfaction derived from caregiving. A study of female occupational therapists found that self-perception as caregivers affected these women's professional choice and that their perception of caring shaped their role definition as therapists (Sachs, 1988; Sachs & Labovitz, 1994).

We care for larger groups in our communities as well when we volunteer to cook for the local Meals on Wheels program, help out at a shelter for people who are homeless, or volunteer to help in a town cleanup. As a community, we provide education for our children, programs for people with special needs, homeless shelters, transportation systems for people with disabilities, and day centers for elderly people. Thus, the concept of care and caring is interwoven with and forms the basis for our attitude of responsibility and concern for other people, nonhuman living things, social issues, and environmental concerns.

——— ▦ ———

Exercise 16.1—Personal Care

Think about and list the occasions during the past month when you gave and received care. What caring responsibilities do you have that are probably shared by many of your classmates? What unique caring responsibilities do you have? How do these activities relate to your daily occupations? Are your caring responsibilities related to your decision to become an occupational therapy practitioner? In what ways do they enhance your occupational therapy education, such as by providing you with case examples or by creating empathy? In what ways do they interfere with your occupational therapy education, such as by being very time consuming or by creating role conflict (e.g., having to choose between performing your child care responsibilities and studying for an exam)?

———————

Definitions of Caregiving

Caring is a special relationship that encompasses a sense of attachment and commitment to others' well-being. Caring, or as Graham (1983) named it, "the labour of love," can be defined as that range of human experiences that have to do with feeling concern for and taking care of the well-being of others. Caring is the commitment that the lives of those receiving care be made meaningful. Caregiving includes

■ Physical activities such as feeding, washing, cleaning, dressing, shopping, and transporting

- Cognitive activities such as solving problems of finances, logistics, scheduling of services, and organization of the overall care plan

- Psychological activities such as understanding, protecting, comforting, and reassuring

- Emotional activities such as forming bonds with and worrying about the welfare of those who receive care

- Interpersonal activities such as helping care receivers and their families to cope with their new or progressively worsening circumstances while maintaining their roles, relationships, and activities

- Moral and spiritual activities such as ensuring that the recipients of care get the sensitive and compassionate care they need based on the entire situation while not exploiting the resources and capabilities of the caregiver.

Some of the physical activity required in caregiving can be taxing and burdensome. Conversely, some emotional and cognitive activities of caregiving do not require physical activity or exertion. Examples are when we sit and listen to people and hold their hands, talk to them on the telephone, give them advice to help them organize their lives, or make telephone calls to arrange services for them. Yet these nonphysical activities can be very burdensome to caregivers if they are perceived as excessive demands, if they occur at a time of unusual and competing stress for the caregivers, or if they are being demanded by those with whom the caregivers do not feel positively emotionally connected. Therefore, it is not always clear cut or easy to determine when and under what circumstances caregiving is joyously given and when it is a burden. Sometimes both feelings can be present sequentially in the same caregiving relationship, and sometimes ambivalent and contradictory feelings can be present simultaneously.

Case Scenario

There are times when caring for a loved one with a chronic condition that becomes progressively more debilitating can start out as a labor of love and necessity. But over months or even years, providing care can become an overwhelming burden that taxes the physical and emotional strength of even the most loving family member. Although the positive feelings of love and respect for the care receiver may not change, as time goes on the physical and psychological burden may increase beyond the endurance of the caregiver. In such situations, the occupational therapy practitioner or other medical professional may recognize that the well spouse or the adult son or daughter caregiver's physical or psychological health has deteriorated to the point that he or she or the entire family is in "dire straits." Such professional awareness can lead to support for seeking alternative care arrangements, such as nursing homes or other long-term-care facilities (Cohen, 1996).

Caregiving can embody the various components of caring in many different ways. We can give the care without the feelings associated with or seemingly required in the special caring relationship. For example, we can be skillful caregivers to our clients even if we do not always feel the positive caring quality in our relationships with all of them (Grott, 1998). At the same time, we can love our grandparents very positively and strongly and feel intensely committed to their well-being, yet because of our lack of skills and knowledge, geographic distance, or someone else (e.g., our parents, siblings, a professional caregiver) who has the primary daily caregiving responsibility, we can participate very little in the actual instrumental activities required in daily caregiving. We can talk with our grandparents, be sensitive to their needs, feel responsible for them, and include them in family life, thus participating on the emotional or interpersonal level of caregiving. Although in caregiving in the personal sphere, more emphasis is placed on feelings and relationships, and in caregiving in the public sphere, more emphasis is placed on skills and instrumental knowledge, the ultimate quality of caregiving relies very much on the balance among all components of caring (Sachs, 1988). Often, caregiving is a paid job that provides employment to many people, usually women with little training.

Literature in other professions such as nursing often strongly emphasizes the physical requirements of caregiving to children, older adults, and people with disabilities, thus stressing the burden associated with these activities. Although it is true that many of the activities that we associate with caregiving demand the use of motor skills such as lifting, cleaning, feeding, carrying, and transporting, caregiving as a total activity encompasses all of the components discussed in the previous paragraphs and those to follow. Therefore, as occupational therapy practitioners, it is important that we consider all of these aspects when analyzing caregiving activities and using them therapeutically.

Caregiving also requires an ongoing cognitive process of thinking and problem solving. In real-life situations, faced with the challenging needs of others, caregivers must be involved in planning and problem solving while providing care. It is sometimes difficult to find ways of giving care that will both satisfy the caregivers' needs for effective action to resolve a situation or achieve a goal and, at the same time, fulfill the needs of the person being cared for (Hasselkus, 1998). Thus, caregivers are involved in using task modification strategies to deal with caregiving requirements and, most of all, to ensure their own safety and well-being (Corcoran & Gitlin, 2001).

Caregiving is involved with interpersonal relationships. Therefore, it requires a special sensitivity and attentiveness to the needs of the person receiving care. The caregiving dyad can be intimate and, hence, may require emotional and physical closeness. In certain caregiving situations, you may be devoted to fostering the growth and development of the person receiving care, and thus, you may experience the other person "both as part of you and as apart from you" (Moroney et al., 1998, p. 8). On the interpersonal level, caregiving is not only a skill but also an art. The art consists of developing a mutual interpersonal relationship with someone who needs our care and of being sensitive to the verbal and nonverbal cues with which they communicate their emotional and physical needs.

A dimension of caregiving that is frequently neglected is its being a work of emotions (McRae, 1998). Often in personal caregiving, but many times in professional caregiving, we become emotionally attached to the person receiving care and are thus more able to engage positively in the caregiving situation. It can be even more stressful in complex situations and when success is hard to define, such as in the case of giving care to people who are dying (Hasselkus, 1993). The continuing responsibility to care for a child with disabilities or a young adult whose illness or disabilities are chronic and have no end in sight may cause a much higher level of stress precisely because there is no way to predict how long the caregiving situation will last (Cohen, 1996).

There are times when the client, the caregiver, the family, or the practitioner develop negative feelings about one another. Negative feelings can arise when clients project their anger and disappointment about having a disability or about not succeeding in achieving successes in the treatment process onto the caregiver or onto the occupational therapy practitioner. Conversely, the caregiver or practitioner can begin to dislike an uncooperative, unsuccessful, or unappreciative client such that the caregiving or therapeutic relationship is difficult to maintain (Abbot, 1990).

Exercise 16.2—Caregiver Situation

Imagine that you are the caregiver in the following situation. You are an adult caring for your dying father with whom you have a warm and loving relationship. He lives by himself in his own apartment a short distance from your home and has only a few months left to live because he is in an advanced stage of cancer. Describe how the various levels of caregiving defined previously relate to your activities and responses as a caregiver. What would you do, and how might you feel?

Caregivers and Care Receivers

Most human beings spend parts of their lifetimes performing the normal kinds of caring activities that make life possible. Informally, parents care for children, children care for siblings and pets, people care for family and friends, and adult sons and daughters care for elderly parents. Formally, paid professional caregivers care for those in need of such attention. The population of people receiving care varies widely. In general, children, people of all ages with disabilities, and elderly people are the broadly identified target groups. Elderly people with Alzheimer's disease are a large group needing both informal and formal caregivers. A working-age adult population needing care is persons with HIV/AIDS. In many instances foster parents care for infants and children born with HIV/AIDS, and friends and acquaintances of both genders care for adults.

The caregiving responsibilities that take up the most time are activities of daily living (e.g., feeding, dressing, housework, meals, laundry, groceries, emotional support), guardianship, legal responsibilities, financial management, health care tasks

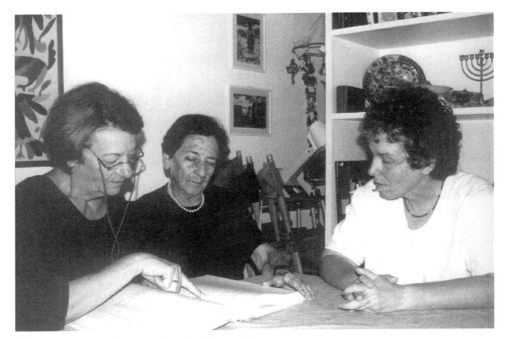

Figure 16.1. Daughters caring for their mother.

(e.g., bandaging, giving medication), and transportation. Generally, women provide the majority of the care at home and in the paid market. Gender is strongly related to caregiving; caregiving is associated with women's occupations. Historically and still to a very large extent today in most Western societies, responsibility for caring is assigned to and assumed by women. Much of the caregiving occurs in the home as unpaid work performed by wives, mothers, daughters, daughters-in-law, grandmothers, and granddaughters. Paid caring occurs in the workplace, done mainly by female nurses, nurses' aides, teachers, teachers' aides, day care workers, social workers, and various health professionals, including occupational therapy practitioners. Much of this paid caring activity is considered the natural work of women, requiring little or no formal training or skill. Many believe women enjoy helping others because they enjoy the role of helper (Fisher & Tronto, 1990).

Case Scenario

One unique group of caregivers is grandmothers, who assume primary caring responsibility for very young children as more younger women with children enter the workforce. A large number of African American grandmothers have taken responsibilities for their grandchildren, seeking to ensure family stability and well-being (Brown, 1999). More than 4 million American children live with grandparents, mainly grandmothers, and many do so under stressful circumstances ("Event Aids Grandparents," 1999).

Culture and social organization affect the expectations, form, and performance of caregiving activities. For example, it is deeply imbedded in the culture of African Americans that care will be given by and to family members and care, in turn, will be received at the hands of family or extended family when the caregiver's turn comes (Wilson et al., 1995). Other cultures around the world have developed varying methods of providing care to those in need; some support the view that caregiving is a family's responsibility only. The absence of formal caregiving mechanisms in such societies may result from that orientation. Other countries pride themselves on their elaborately designed social services that function as a "safety net" to take care of categories of their population who cannot make it on their own in the economic or social system. In westernized or industrialized countries, people living in cities, in poverty, or far away from their families tend to follow this pattern to a greater or lesser degree, depending on their blend of cultural and religious traditions that influence their attitudes about helping others (Kohn & Wilson, 1995).

In American society, children are cared for informally by parents and other family caregivers. A parallel formal child care network of paid caregivers has expanded in response to the increase in two-wage-earner families and to welfare reforms that stress reducing the welfare rolls by mandatory employment. Formal child care for infants, toddlers, and preschool children is provided by paid babysitters and family day care providers in private homes. Day care centers for infants and toddlers, private preschools and nursery schools, and government programs that employ day care staff also exist.

Occupational therapy practitioners can be employed as consultants for day care workers, preschool aides and teachers, and paid family day care providers who may need advice about developmentally appropriate play and toys, the use of creative activities, the reduction of behavior problems, and the identification of children at risk for physical, emotional, or social problems. Practitioners also can provide therapeutic interventions in such settings for children already identified as needing these professional services.

Adults and elderly people needing care are served by a plethora of paid and professional caregivers and care agencies. Paid companions provide one-on-one attendant care in homes and hospitals. Senior centers and other such facilities run day programs with activities and meals for those who are mobile enough to attend. Home health aides and volunteers visit people who are homebound to provide medical treatments, assist with self-care activities, and help with cleaning and household tasks. Agencies who supply such home caregivers are part of a growing care industry.

Occupational therapy practitioners may be called on to instruct such formal caregivers and paid staff in performing the instrumental tasks of daily living in ergonomically sound ways. They also help caregivers to understand the importance of meaningful activities in their clients' lives and assist them in helping clients to use activities more successfully (Hasselkus, 1998). Moreover, they assist caregivers in improving caregiving strategies and in balancing caregivers' and the recipients' well-being (Corcoran & Gitlin, 2001; McGrath, Mueller, Brown, Teitelman, & Watts, 2000). Occupational therapy practitioners also can help clients and families to make transitions to a caregiver role and, when necessary, from one level of care to another.

Caregiving and Human Occupation

When we come to look at how caregiving is related to human occupation, we must show how different people in various caregiving roles attribute meanings to caregiving and how the diverse context in which the occupation is taking place affects its performance and how gender, age, physical and mental disability, class, sexual orientation, culture and social organization affect the form, process, and meanings of caregiving. To understand caregiving as a significant occupation that involves purposeful activities used in the occupational therapy intervention process, we must demonstrate how the interaction between the caregiver and the recipient of care, the caregiving task, and the environmental context influence caregiving's meanings, form, and performance for the individual client.

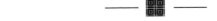

Exercise 16.3—Feelings Toward Caregiving Tasks

Look at the possible meanings of caregiving in the following situations:

- A single mother of three children who is working outside her home and is taking care of her elderly parents

- A paid aide who is taking care of a lonely and frustrated elderly man

- An adult son helping his elderly mother, who needs assistance in everyday life activities

- A paid day care worker or babysitter caring for a young child during the day

- A 37-year-old woman who has had total responsibility for the past 5 years for her 40-year-old husband of 15 years who has progressively more extensive permanent disabilities caused by multiple sclerosis

- An elderly man taking care of his dependent wife after 45 years of marriage

- A 60-year-old daughter caring for her 90-year-old mother, who is in a hospice facility dying of cancer

- A religious leader who is taking care of his or her community.

We can assume that, because of the different personal, occupational, and environmental circumstances, the meanings and forms of caregiving to each of these people will be very different. Identify possible feelings for each scenario and the caregiving tasks required.

———————————

Thus, caregiving can be a stressful human occupation for both informal and formal caregivers, including occupational therapy practitioners. A certain amount of stress is inherent in the caregiving situation and is to be expected. But prolonged or inordinately high levels of stress can lead to burnout, a condition in which the caregiver is completely overwhelmed by the negative aspects of the situation to the point of being unable to continue without incurring serious physical or psychological damage. Giving care to a family member is associated mainly with an increase in depressive symptoms and a feeling of isolation (Marks, Lambert, & Choi, 2002). Therefore, support groups for caregivers, clients and families, and professionals are generally an important protective action that occupational therapists can develop (Cohen, 1996). At the same time, caregiving is associated with positive effects, such as finding purpose in life and strengthening the relationships among family members.

The Development of Caregiving Skills

As human beings, first we receive caring, then we learn how to care for ourselves, and last we discover how to care for others. How do we discover it? Is it part of our nature? Is it a personal tendency? Does it come with our gender, or do we learn it through training and modeling? As it is with most other human occupations, caring must be a combination of all of these. The important questions are, How can we foster the acquisition of a caring attitude? and How can we facilitate the learning of the skills and the knowledge required for caregiving activities for both girls and boys as they are growing up?

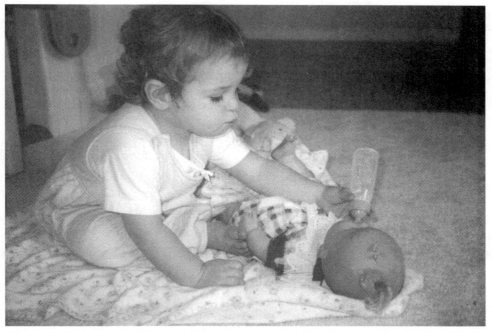

Figure 16.2. For nearly 200 years, little girls have learned to take care of their baby dolls by imitating their mothers.

Parents' caregiving behaviors foster the development of children as occupational beings (Humphry, 2002). Young children, mainly girls, imitate their parents' caregiving behavior by playing with dolls or with younger siblings or friends. They feed and clean their dolls, play house, and role-play parenting with other children. In many cultures and in large families, children may be required to take some caregiving responsibilities while still quite young. In Western cultures, children generally are first encouraged to take care of pets and plants. As school-age children or as adolescents, they may then be expected to share caregiving responsibilities for their younger siblings, such as feeding them; helping them with homework; playing with or otherwise occupying them; seeing that they get home from school safely; babysitting for them in the afternoon while the parents are at work or in the evening while the parents are out; or, when they are old enough, driving them or accompanying them on public transportation to after-school activities.

Children and adolescents have to be taught, encouraged, and given the opportunities to develop their caregiving roles. Sometimes, it is sheer necessity that draws adolescents into being involved in caregiving because they have a grandparent in their home; a sibling with a disability; a parent with problems, such as alcoholism, drug abuse, mental illness, or domestic abuse; or traumatic experiences, including stress, unemployment, or poverty. In extreme cases, some children may have to assume parental caregiving responsibilities at an even earlier age. In such situations, training for the teenagers and other family members and support to prevent the stress levels from becoming so high that burnout occurs are critical areas that occupational therapy practitioners can address.

Adolescents' involvement in caregiving encompasses the gamut of life experiences that includes burden, stress, sensitivity to others, responsibility, wage-earning opportunities, change of attitudes, sharing, and developing intimate relationships. On one hand, caring for parents and assuming many parental responsibilities can be a burden; on the other hand, sharing caregiving responsibilities for grandparents results in many cases not only in the development of greater empathy on the part of the teenagers for older adults but also in improving relationships and strengthening the adolescents' degree of bonding with family (Beach, 1997). Apparently, when the burden and stress of caregiving are not too overwhelming, such as with grandparents and community projects, caregiving can be an enriching role that contributes to adolescent growth and development. Caregiving also prepares the adolescent to enter adulthood as a person with enhanced responsiveness to the needs of others.

Similarly, the development of social caring and community responsibility is related to early experiences with caring and with positive role models of caregiving. People who respond to community needs by becoming adolescent or adult volunteers on projects to help others who are less fortunate in their communities or in religious and charitable organizations tend to have learned these values earlier in their lives. Performance of good deeds and acts of kindness and charity has been linked to a strong sense of empathy for others, which is a basic foundation of the caring relationship. Even the ability to act morally when faced with difficult decisions in exten-

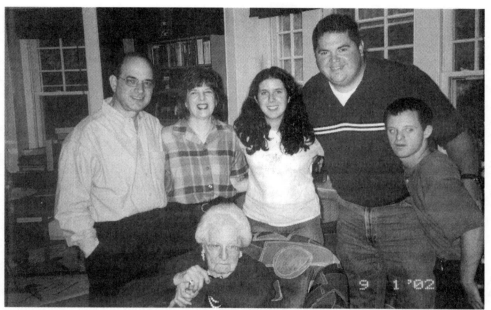

Figure 16.3. Extended families take care of one another, particularly if they include a member with special needs and a 95-year-old grandmother.

uating circumstances, such as wartime, has its roots in a well-developed commitment to caring.

Caregiving: A Human Occupation

Caregiving is a critical occupation, and the caregiver role is one that is significant and necessary in the lives of many of our clients and their families. In addition, the valuing of and active engagement in caregiving are essential to the development of an emotional and moral commitment to the well-being of others and to enhancing one's ability to acquire the skills necessary to perform the tasks involved. At the same time, and sometimes for the very same people, caregiving can be very hard and stressful labor, especially for those responsible for the daily functioning of children, elderly people, or people with severe disabilities. Occupational therapy practitioners can help clients to engage in caregiving as an occupation. Occupational therapy can help family and paid caregivers to be efficient and effective in their tasks and reduce the physical and emotional burden associated with the role.

Interventions with informal and formal caregivers involve helping them to develop successful and satisfying ways of giving care and helping them to prevent or deal with stress. Another group of clients are potential caregivers who can be helped to develop caring attitudes or can be taught caregiving skills. These clients include children, people with developmental disabilities, people with mental illness, or new teenage mothers. Another set of clients are people who are caregivers or who have been caregivers but whose caregiving role has been lost. For elderly people; those with newly acquired, chronic, or progressively worsening disabilities; or anyone whose opportunities for caregiving have been reduced or eliminated, occupational therapy practitioners can offer guidance in relearning lost caregiving skills or in finding alternative ways to fulfill caregiving needs.

Occupational Therapy for Family and Other Informal Caregivers

Occupational therapy can be very valuable for family members, friends, or paid helpers who give care to people who cannot live independently because of cognitive, developmental, or physical disabilities. Because most caregiving for the frail population is done in the home, informal caregivers have become a major group of clients needing and receiving professional services. These caregivers may include spouses, parents, children, neighbors, and friends who share only a few caregiving responsibilities, or paid caregivers in the home or in day care facilities and nursing homes. The skills and hard labor needed to give ongoing quality care daily have transformed these caregivers into a significant group needing occupational therapy services. Understanding the multiple meanings of caregiving to these caregivers and analyzing the way they provide care can help us to design appropriate occupational therapy intervention strategies that will enhance caregivers' performance and reduce their stress (Corcoran & Gitlin, 2001; McGrath et al., 2000; Perkinson & LaVesser, 2000).

Research on the interaction between families and occupational therapy practitioners has revealed that one of the first difficulties that practitioners encounter in working with family caregivers is accepting them as the ones responsible for the well-being of the care receivers and respecting their knowledge (Gitlin et al., 1995; Perkinson & LaVesser, 2000). Hasselkus (1988) found that occupational therapy practitioners differ from family caregivers in their values, beliefs, and ethics. For example, occupational therapy goals were not always compatible with family caregiver priorities. Whereas practitioners focused on enhancing independence of those receiving care in activities of daily living, family members were more concerned with safety and sense of identity and with maintaining daily routine (Gitlin et al., 1995). As a result, family caregivers did not always cooperate fully with occupational therapy intervention programs. At the same time, occupational therapy practitioners perceived family caregivers as obstacles to their own intervention (Gitlin & Corcoran, 1993). This research demonstrates the importance of understanding the meanings of caregiving to individual caregivers and those receiving care, considering their knowledge and skills, and respecting their personal and cultural values when designing caregiver interventions.

Family members or other informal caregivers may vary. Because all caregivers are different and all those receiving care are different, caregiving situations vary immensely. In designing an intervention plan with caregivers, occupational therapy practitioners first and foremost must take into consideration the characteristics of those giving and receiving care; the social and physical environment in which the caregiving task is taking place; and the caregivers' preferences, values, and experience.

Client-Centered Approach in Caregiving

Partnership in designing the intervention plan with caregivers, based on the client-centered approach, can help in adapting the plan to the individual caregiver's needs and values (Corcoran & Gitlin, 2001; McGrath et al., 2000; Perkinson & LaVesser, 2000). A number of tools to plan intervention with caregivers, based on a client-centered approach and aimed at identifying caregiver needs and priorities, are suggested in the occupational therapy literature as follows:

■ Use of the Canadian Occupational Performance Measure (Law et al., 1994) to enable caregivers to identify and define their own needs and priorities (Corcoran & Gitlin, 2001; Perkinson & LaVesser, 2000).

■ Use of ethnographic interviewing methods to get an understanding of the caregiver's point of view (Perkinson & LaVesser, 2000). Hasselkus (1992) described the process of ethnographic interviewing to ascertain exactly what the caregiving experience means to each person in the situation.

■ Use of interviews such as Weinstein's (1997) semistructured interview designed to discover the level of caregivers' knowledge and comfort with their role.

All these tools can help therapists to design interventions with caregivers that are unique to every caregiving situation and to each caregiver and promote partnership and collaboration between practitioners and clients.

Plan for Intervention

Based on the understanding of the uniqueness of every caregiving situation, the importance of understanding caregivers' perspectives, and the client-centered approach, Gitlin et al. (1995) provided an approach for occupational therapists to use in order to develop a plan for intervention. Although the specific example that follows is about caregiving for elderly people, the principles are adaptable to all caregiving situations. Four principles represent four stages of intervention. We briefly present the principles with case examples in order to demonstrate how the understanding of caregiving as a human occupation can be translated into an effective intervention program in occupational therapy.

STAGE 1

The first stage involves identifying the main person responsible for providing the care. When we come to a home visit, we must recognize that an organization of caregiving already exists. Out of necessity, the family members have probably already developed their own strategies, practices, and skills of caregiving. For example, an elderly wife may be the primary caregiver for her husband with dementia, being responsible for managing the care and providing most of it by herself.

STAGE 2

The second stage involves making an attempt to understand the caregivers' unique perspective that shapes the caregiving practice. We observe the caregiving situation and pay attention to how caregivers organize the environment; we listen to caregivers' stories of their daily routines and their past experiences; and we ask them questions that will help us to understand their attitudes, beliefs, concerns, and priorities. During the following visits we can observe the woman helping her husband getting dressed, walking to the dining room, eating, and sitting to watch television. We can listen to her describing what she is doing on a typical day and her concerns regarding her caregiving activities. We can ask her how she perceives her husband's situation, what his main difficulties are, how he was in the past, how she would like to plan their future, and in what areas she would like us to help her.

STAGE 3

The third stage involves self-questioning and evaluation of how much good insight we, the occupational therapy practitioners, obtained about the caregiver's perspectives and the caregiving situation and to what extent our professional and personal goals, beliefs, and values are congruent with those of the caregiver. We can ask some of the following questions: Do we know what the wife's main physical and psychological difficulties are in providing the care? Whom does she trust and consult when she encounters difficulties? How much are the grown children accessible, and in what ways do they participate in providing care to their father (and mother)? How would she like to see her daily activities organized? How does she perceive her husband's situation, and what does dementia mean to her? Furthermore, we should then examine ourselves and ask whether we could accept the wife's priority to dress her husband so that he appears well groomed rather than take the time to let him get dressed independently and refrain from helping, if independent dressing is time consuming and tiring for both of them and ultimately produces fewer successful results.

STAGE 4

The occupational therapist in the fourth stage analyzes and interprets the caregiver's point of view in order to design an intervention that will best suit the unique caregiving situation. Therapists can plan to teach the wife grooming techniques that will facilitate the physical efforts required for the task, to teach her how to engage her husband in an activity that she perceives as respectful to his image and that is manageable and meaningful to him, and to help her plan a weekly schedule and include in it times in which a paid helper or her children will take over the caregiving responsibility to give her some relief and to enable her to engage in activities that are necessary to run her household and other activities that are important to her.

Intervention Strategies to Enhance Caregivers' Performance

Corcoran and Gitlin (2001) identified hundreds of strategies that caregivers used to deal with caregiving requirements. The large number of strategies resulted from the uniqueness of every caregiving situation. They categorized all the strategies into three groups: object modification, task modification, and social groups. In the first group, objects were modified to ensure the care receivers' safety, to enhance their activities of daily living, to facilitate handling techniques, and to enable communication with assistive technology devices. Task modification included task breakdown and grading of activities to simplify self-care. Modifications also included guidance in providing clear and brief instructions to those receiving care. Social groups were used mainly to support caregivers and to address special and catastrophic reactions.

Intervention Strategies to Support Caregivers and Reduce Their Stress

Individual support and support groups for caregivers, clients and families, and professionals are generally an important protective action that occupational therapy practitioners can develop (Cohen, 1996).

Social groups can be designed, or preexisting groups can be identified, to support caregivers. These groups can help caregivers to expand and coordinate a network of helpers, have some rest and time to enjoy, and identify and meet caregivers' own needs (Corcoran & Gitlin, 2001). Occupational therapy practitioners can organize and run such support groups and inform families about groups run by local hospitals, agencies, or volunteer organizations devoted to various illnesses. Recognition of the limits of family caregiving, provision of professional advice about alternatives, and support for the difficult decisions that families face surrounding the need to institutionalize their loved ones also can be part of the practitioner's treatment responsibility because he or she can offer valuable insight to the families about evaluating nursing homes and other long-term-care facilities.

Occupational therapy practitioners can help with situations that present particularly stressful conditions for families and individual caregivers. For example, the birth of a child with disabilities can be a trauma for the entire family. Bringing home a high-risk infant and adapting the family to accommodate the needs of the baby can try the patience and challenge the emotional resilience of even the strongest and most stable families. Major stress may result from fear of the frail physical condition of the infant, uncertainty about how to perform medical or other procedures needed by the infant, and realization of the amount of time needed for and the inconvenience of repeating such daily routine tasks as feeding, changing, dressing, and transporting the baby. Moreover, the inability to pay attention simultaneously to other children or to

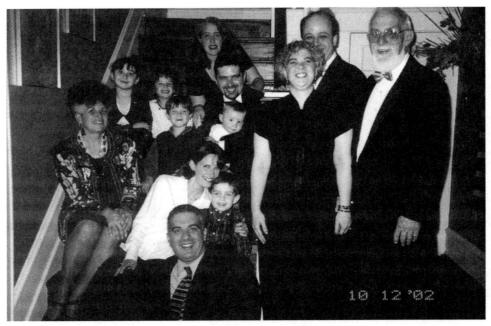

Figure 16.4. Families take care of their children, and grandparents take care of their grown children and spouses and grandchildren.

respond to their and other family members' needs can cause major distress to the entire family. Realization that this problem might be a lifelong one that will require major reorientation of the family's patterns of functioning can be a shock. Furthermore, the financial burden of special equipment, repeated medical consultations or procedures, and specialized sitters or paid caregivers, coupled with the possible loss of income if one of the parents must leave paid employment in order to assume caregiving tasks, may prove impossible for the family to sustain (Vergara & Angley, 1990).

Case Scenario

Families with a child with a disability must work out their own accommodations to meet their unique needs. They may need help with the psychological tasks of acceptance of the disappointment and anger about having the disability, adjustment to their altered roles and perceptions of themselves as parents and family members, and recognition of their uncertainties about the future expectations for their child with disabilities. They must also deal with the disappointments of other extended family members and the reaction of friends, neighbors, and colleagues who may or may not be helpful in their responses to the situation. Families may need guidance and reassurance about the physical procedures and adaptations that they must learn to participate in the various treatments that their child will need. They must learn to cope with the parade of therapists and medical personnel who will become a part of their households either daily or periodically. Moreover, they may require help finding the resources to deal with the financial burdens that dealing with the child with disabilities will impose (Humphry & Case-Smith, 1996).

— ▦ —

Exercise 16.5—Interdisciplinary Care

Imagine that you are an occupational therapy practitioner working as part of an interdisciplinary health team with a family who has a child for whom it is difficult to provide care. You are supposed to be providing the therapeutic handling that is the focus of the occupational therapy intervention, but you realize that the family is not cooperating with the child's treatment program. What are the contextual and psychosocial aspects of the caregiving situation that you would analyze in order to understand the family's attitude? What are your responsibilities to the family members? How would you try to enlist the family's cooperation?

In this situation, the practitioner must be sensitive to the family's priorities and the other children's needs and be sure to include both parents in the discussions. Parents should be kept informed and the treatment priorities jointly negotiated and agreed on. Goals and activities should be developed cooperatively so that the therapy fits the family's needs, goals, and schedules. The practitioner ascertains with the parents how much time, energy, and funds the parents plan to invest in this child and takes the family members seriously as the ones who know the child best. The practitioner may coordinate services with all the other team members and be aware of everything they are doing and what their goals are. The treatments should be scheduled so as to be sensitive to the family's time constraints. Practitioners should not make the parents take time from work to meet with them; take up room in the family's house; or come at mealtimes, which can disrupt the family's routine. There should be suggestions of ways to make the daily chores easier, if possible. The practitioner teaches the family members the treatment techniques, listens to their feedback, and acts on it.

Engaging Clients in Caregiving

Many people who have chronic physical, mental, cognitive, or developmental disabilities are not given the opportunity to be engaged in caregiving. Similarly, young people with physical and developmental disabilities are many times denied initial access to any caregiving responsibility. In addition, people who are injured may suddenly lose their caregiving abilities and unexpectedly lose their customary caregiving roles. Finally, older people often renounce their role as caregivers, even though it is a role that may have been central to their lives. Moreover, if their health deteriorates as a result of illness, stroke, a mental condition, or cognitive deterioration, the remaining activities and responsibilities of caregiving are generally taken away from them.

In this way, caregiving seems to be considered incompatible with receiving care, as quite frequently people with disabilities are denied the right to give care to others. For some of these individuals, especially women, taking care of the welfare of their family and neighbors had been a central part of their existence. With others, especially the younger people with developmental, cognitive, or physical disabilities, we recognize the significance of helping them move from receiving care to caring for themselves, but we often fail to consider the advantages and consequences of moving them further along to giving care to others. Therefore, it is significant to be aware of the importance of caregiving as a developmental and empowering experience to many people and to give them opportunities to engage in the tasks involved in caregiving.

Yet another potential benefit to clients engaging in caregiving exists. Because caregiving is such a complex activity that requires multilevel skills, through involvement in the required tasks, clients possibly can improve their level of functioning in other areas. Moreover, involvement in caregiving activities usually has enhanced meaning because in the past, caregiving has been significant in most peoples' lives. Therefore, although it is important to make caregiving available to clients, practitioners must always give them the choice of whether and how to get involved in it.

Occupational Therapy Interventions to Engage Clients in Caregiving

The following examples illustrate how caregiving can be used in the treatment of different groups of clients. Much of the emphasis in this chapter thus far has been on the caregiver, both informal (family) and formal (paid nonprofessional or professional); the caregivers' needs for skills specifically used in the caregiving process; and the strategies to deal with stress and to prevent possible burnout. Occupational therapy practitioners provide information and activities as interventions for both of these groups of caregivers as clients.

This section deals with perhaps the more obvious, but often unserved, population of clients who because of age, impairment, or lack of opportunity have reduced or eliminated the element of caregiving in their own lives or have been forced by others to relinquish it. Whether the occupation of caregiving to others was an important part of their previous life roles, or in situations in which this occupation was never fully developed, having the opportunity to give care to others is a fundamental and important part of being human and living a meaningful life. Therefore, it is critical that we as occupational therapy practitioners provide such opportunities for caregiving to our clients. We can also provide education or reeducation in caring as an occupation when needed, and the supportive environment for this caregiving to occur, by structuring appropriate activities in which our clients can participate. Accordingly, following are some examples of the kinds of activities that will accomplish this objective.

Case Scenario

There are many ways in which even young children can become involved in being sensitive to and providing care for the needs of others. When children see their teachers or therapists being sensitive to the feelings of others and doing small caring actions, such as making sure that they are comfortable in their wheelchairs, that they can reach all of the supplies they need while doing a project, or that none are left out of the conversation in a social situation, the children learn appropriate attitudes and behaviors. Children can participate in a toy or book drive by selecting one of their own toys or books or holiday gifts to give away, or they can make gifts during the holidays to donate to less-fortunate children. They can "adopt" an elderly nursing home resident and send drawings, photographs, or small gifts to their adopted grandparent; they can then be encouraged to visit the nursing home in a group to sing songs or to bring their pets or a favorite object to talk about with the senior.

Case Scenario

We can work with adolescents with cognitive, physical, or mental disabilities toward getting involved in taking care of others. Frequently, no one in the family will consider involving these adolescents in the family caregiving tasks, denying them the opportunity of developing a caring attitude, acquiring the skills that are within their capability, and experiencing the satisfaction and social recognition connected to the role. Altering the social and physical environment and creating opportunities for these young people to practice some caregiving tasks, such as feeding or cleaning their pet and taking the responsibility for its well-being, might change their self-perception and their parents' perception from being only care receivers to being caregivers.

Case Scenario

People who lose their caregiving ability because of injuries or illnesses feel a double loss when they realize the hardship or difficulties of those who relied on their care. This situation could arise when a parent with young children is injured or when the caregiving spouse of an elderly person suddenly has a stroke. In such situations, the occupational therapy practitioner can help the person to evaluate the extent of the injury and the likelihood of his or her being able to resume caregiving responsibilities with appropriate training, assistance, or assistive devices. If the person is not going to be able to resume these activities, helping to make appropriate alternative caregiving arrangements would solve the immediate situation and would alleviate worry and guilt. Finally, clients should be helped to find alternative ways of expressing caregiving, if necessary. For example, the injured parent can talk and read to his or her children when performing physical caregiving activities is no longer possible.

Case Scenario

The occupational therapy practitioner's caregiving role during the dying process has been described by Hasselkus (1993) in her moving description of her own personal experience with caring for her dying mother. Her situation involved a very old person who was physically frail but cognitively alert and staying in a hospital where her physical care was being done by others on the hospital staff. Not all deaths take place in this manner, of course. In this situation, Hasselkus described the stages of care that she went through, suggesting that whatever the actual time sequence, caregiving for people who are dying may start out as what she terms "caregiver from a distance" (p. 717), which involves watching, monitoring, and offering suggestions. She then progressed to more frequent caregiving in which she began taking responsibility for household matters. Then during the dying phase, her caregiving tasks changed to listening, talking, helping her mother conduct life reviews, funeral planning, and helping her mother face dying and the death process.

Summary

This chapter explores the meaning of caring, caregiving, and care receiving as human occupations. It discusses the importance of maintaining our opportunities to be caregivers throughout our lifetimes and gives examples of the ways in which people can care. Finally, the chapter presents some ways in which occupational therapy practitioners can encourage caregiving for people of all ages with all kinds of disabilities through the use of purposeful activities to help them to participate in such a meaningful occupation. ■

References

Abbot, N. (1990). The caregiving alliance. *OT Practice, 2*, 60–65.

Beach, D. L. (1997). Family caregiving: The positive impact on adolescent relationships. *Gerontologist, 37*, 233–238.

Brown, A. C. (1999). Grandmothers raising grandchildren in African-American families: Predictors of coping strategies. *Dissertation Abstracts International, 59(9-B)*, 5163. (UMI No. AAT 9907431)

Clark, C. A., Corcoran, M., & Gitlin, L. N. (1995). An exploratory study of how occupational therapists develop therapeutic relationships with family caregivers. *American Journal of Occupational Therapy, 49*, 587–594.

Cohen, M. D. (1996). *Dirty details: The days and nights of a well spouse.* Philadelphia: Temple University Press.

Corcoran, M., & Gitlin, L. M. (2001). Family caregiver acceptance and use of environmental strategies provided in an occupational therapy intervention. *Physical and Occupational Therapy in Geriatrics, 19(1)*, 1–20.

Event aids grandparents who raise young children. (1999, January). *NRTA Bulletin, 40*(1), 20.

Fisher, B., & Tronto, J. (1990). Toward a feminist theory of caring. In E. K. Abel & M. K. Nelson (Eds.), *Circles of care: Work and identity in women's life* (pp. 35–62). Albany: State University of New York.

Gitlin, L. N., & Corcoran, M. (1993). Expanding caregiver ability to use environmental solutions for problems of bathing and incontinence in the elderly with dementia. *Technology and Disability, 2*(1), 12–21.

Gitlin, L. N., Corcoran, M., & Leinmiller-Eckhardt, S. (1995). Understanding the family perspective: An ethnographic framework for providing occupational therapy in the home. *American Journal of Occupational Therapy, 49,* 802–809.

Graham, H. (1983). Caring: A labour of love. In J. Finch & D. Groves (Eds.), *A labour of love: Women, work and caring* (pp. 13–30). Boston: Routledge & Kegan Paul.

Grott, G. (1998, March 16). The caregiving therapist. *Advance for Occupational Therapists*, p. 19.

Hasselkus, B. R. (1988). Meaning in family caregiving: Perspectives on caregivers' professional relationships. *Gerontologist, 28,* 686–691.

Hasselkus, B. R. (1992). The meaning of activity: Day care for persons with Alzheimer disease. *American Journal of Occupational Therapy, 46,* 199–206.

Hasselkus, B. R. (1993). Death in very old age: A personal journey of caregiving. *American Journal of Occupational Therapy, 47,* 717–723.

Hasselkus, B. R. (1998). Occupation and well-being in dementia: The experience of day-care staff. *American Journal of Occupational Therapy, 52,* 423–434.

Humphry, R. (2002). Young children's occupations: Explicating the dynamics of developmental processes. *American Journal of Occupational Therapy, 2,* 171–179.

Humphry, R., & Case-Smith, J. (1996). The development process: Prenatal to adolescence. In J. Case-Smith, A. Allen, & P. Pratt (Eds.), *Occupational therapy for children* (3rd ed., pp. 46–66). St. Louis, MO: Mosby.

Kohn, L. P., & Wilson, M. N. (1995). Social support networks in the African American family: Unility for culturally compatible intervention. In M. N. Wilson (Ed.), *African American family life: Its structural and ecological aspects* (pp. 35–58). San Francisco: Jossey-Bass.

Law, M., Baptiste, S., Carswell, A., McColl, M. A., Polatajko, H., & Pollock, N. (1994). *Canadian Occupational Performance Measure* (2nd ed.). Toronto, Ontario: Canadian Association of Occupational Therapists.

Marks, N. F., Lambert, J. D., & Choi, H. (2002). Transitions to caregiving, gender, and psychological well-being: A prospective U.S. national study. *Journal of Marriage and Family, 64,* 657–667.

McGrath, W. L., Mueller, M. M., Brown, C., Teitelman, J., & Watts, J. (2000). Caregivers of persons with Alzheimer's disease: An exploratory study of occupational performance and respite. *Physical and Occupational Therapy in Geriatrics, 18*(2), 51–69.

McRae, H. (1998). Managing feelings: Caregiving as emotion work. *Research on Aging, 20,* 137–160.

Moroney, R. M., Dokecki, P. R., Gated, J. J., Haynes, K. N., Newbrough, J. R., & Nottingham, J. A. (1998). *Caring and competent caregivers.* Athens: University of Georgia.

Perkinson, M. A., & LaVesser, P. (2000). Therapeutic partnerships: Caregiving in the home setting. In C. Christiansen (Ed.), *Ways of living: Self-care strategies for special needs* (2nd ed., pp. 383–397). Bethesda, MD: American Occupational Therapy Association.

Sachs, D. (1988). *The perception of caring held by female occupational therapists: Implications for professional role and identity.* Unpublished doctoral dissertation, New York University.

Sachs, D., & Labovitz, D. R. (1994). The caring occupational therapist: Scope of professional roles and boundaries. *American Journal of Occupational Therapy, 48,* 997–1005.

Vergara, E. R., & Angley, J. C. (1990). Preparing families to take home a high-risk infant. *Occupational Therapy Practice, 2,* 66–83.

Wilson, M. N., Greene-Bates, C., McKim, L., Simmons, F., Askew, T., Curry-El, J., et al. (1995). African American family life: The dynamics of interactions, relationships, and roles. In M. N. Wilson (Ed.), *African American family life: Its structural and ecological aspects* (pp. 5–21). San Francisco: Jossey-Bass.

Weinstein, M. (1997). Bringing family-centered practices into home health. *OT Practice, 2*(7), 35–38.

17

Occupation, Purposeful Activities, Activities, the Empowerment Process, and Client-Motivated Change

Paula McCreedy, MEd, OTR
Prudence Heisler, MA, OTR

S ince the profession's inception in the early 1900s, occupational therapy practitioners have observed that engagement in occupations and purposeful activity facilitates a sense of competence or empowerment (Clark et al., 1991; Dunton, 1919; Kielhofner, 1995; Meyer, 1922; Mosey, 1986; Reilly, 1974). The process by which occupation is able to facilitate empowerment, however, has not been as thoroughly articulated. This chapter explores the use of occupation and purposeful activity to empower people with disabilities, delineates the principal elements involved in the empowerment process, and uses case examples to illustrate the role of client-motivated change.

The Empowerment Process

Empowerment is the process through which people obtain the competence necessary to exert positive influence over the social systems, groups, people, and personal behaviors that affect their quality of life (Wilson, 1996). *Quality of life* is the extent to which people believe that life is meaningful, manageable, and comprehensible and holds opportunities for personal growth and goal attainment (Hood, Beaudet, & Catlin, 1996). Quality of life often is measured by the degree to which people have been able to establish (a) satisfying interpersonal relationships (and the internalization of acceptance by a family member or friend), (b) the presence of a supportive social network for needed resources and guidance, and (c) the participation in activities and occupations that provide a sense of meaning and personal gratification (Antonovsky, 1992). *Activity* is defined as the execution of a task or action by a person (World Health Organization [WHO], 2001), and *participation* is involvement in a life situation (WHO, 2001). According to the WHO's (2001) *International Classification of Functioning, Disability, and Health* (ICF), a person's behaviors in activities and participation must be understood in terms of performance and capacity qualifiers. These qualifiers can limit, restrict, or enhance activity and participation. *Contextual factors* represent the person's complete background and can create barriers or provide facilitators that will influence the person's performance in life situations. This context includes society, which also can create barriers or provide facilitators (WHO, 2001). In the case examples cited in this chapter, both environmental and personal contextual factors are illustrated.

Empowerment often is measured by the presence of five fundamental elements (Gutierrez, 1995):

1. *A repertoire of skills:* People need to establish a repertoire of skills that will help them to meet environmental challenges and demands.

2. *A sense of competence:* A sense of competence is the belief that one's skills are sufficient to achieve desired goals.

3. *Feelings of self-determination:* Self-determination is the belief that one can exert volitional control, or personal will, over life circumstances to enhance his or her quality of life.

4. *A sense of belonging:* A sense of belonging involves the recognition that one deserves to be accepted as a member of the community (or larger society) rather than ostracized because of disability. Recognizing that one deserves to be accepted as a member of the community involves the corollary beliefs that one is entitled to participate in and contribute to the community—as would any other group member—and that one's contributions are valuable to the society.

5. *A sense of equality:* A sense of equality is the belief that one has the same rights as all others to strive for and achieve a personally satisfying quality of life.

These elements underlie the empowerment process and are present when people believe that they can exert positive influence over their life circumstances in order to enhance their quality of life.

The empowerment process also requires the person to make four attitudinal and behavioral changes (Wilson, 1996):

1. *The belief in personal change:* The first change necessitates that people accept the belief that they have choices and can act on them. Recognizing that one has choices is the first step in the empowerment process and is necessary for people to replace stagnation with action.

2. *Internal motivation:* A second change requires that people mobilize their internal resources to take action. To mobilize one's internal resources, one must become internally motivated to engage in the change process. Such internal motivation depends on the belief in both personal choice and in one's competence to implement desired change.

3. *The belief in self-efficacy:* A third change mandates that people obtain a repertoire of skills needed to meet environmental challenges and demands. Self-effi-

cacy requires the initial belief that one can learn and master the skills needed to implement desired change.

4. *The establishment of external support:* The fourth change requires people to develop a supportive social network (consisting of family members, peers, and health care providers) to rely on during the natural setbacks and gains that occur in every change process. People must internalize such external support in order to use effectively the material and emotional resources offered by the support system when members of the support network are not present.

Disempowerment as a Result of Disability

To understand fully the components of the empowerment process, an exploration of the factors that precipitate disempowerment also must be made. Disability often is disempowering because it limits a person's capacity to perform the skills needed to function competently in family systems, school and work sites, and communities. Disability disrupts long-established roles and relationships among people and their family members, friends, and coworkers, causing role strain and role loss (Goffman, 1963; Mosey, 1986; Pearlin & Schooler, 1978). As a result of such role strain, these individuals often lose their predisability identity and are forced to re-create and renegotiate roles and relationships that once were familiar and stable.

For example, a change in one family member's roles, abilities, and identity affects and alters the family system as a whole. Other family members may be required to adopt new roles to maintain the family system's functioning. Practitioners must understand the effects of change on all family roles and relationships in order to help the family system adapt to and survive the disruptions brought on by a loved one's disability. Family members should be encouraged to collaborate with and participate in their loved one's treatment planning and therapy.

It is important for practitioners to recognize that such change processes are forced on people and their family members by an unwanted disability. All change processes are difficult and frequently require protracted periods of time. Change processes that are thrust on the person by disability are disempowering particularly because one's sense of control and volition have been disrupted or lost.

Practitioners also must recognize that the traditional medical model in which the client is asked to assume a passive sick role while the medical authority assumes a position of dominance and control often disempowers people with disabilities. People who become clients in a traditional medical model often are enjoined to believe in their inefficacy and powerlessness. This in turn produces feelings of alienation, loss of self-esteem, and loss of dignity (Mattingly & Fleming, 1994).

Disempowerment can be measured by the presence of six elements:

1. *Loss of self-determination:* Loss of self-determination occurs when the person believes that volitional control and personal choice have been stripped away by disability.

2.   *Loss of competence:* Feelings of lost competence—and the concomitant feeling of inadequacy—occur when the person loses the skills needed to meet the demands of the environment and, consequently, feels a lack of proficiency regarding previously mastered daily life activities.

3.   *The experience of stigmatization:* Stigmatization occurs when the person feels ostracized, or set apart from the larger community, because of disability, appearance, or a difference in functional abilities.

4.   *Feelings of devaluation:* Feeling devalued occurs when the person perceives that his or her contributions are neither accepted nor respected by the community, work site, or family system.

5.   *Feelings of inequality:* Feeling unequal with other community members occurs when the person believes that, as a result of disability, the community, work site, or family system no longer considers him or her entitled to the same rights as all others to strive for and achieve a personally satisfying quality of life.

6.   *Loss of self-identity:* A loss of self-identity occurs when the person no longer understands him- or herself in relation to familiar people and objects in the environment. Loss of self-identity occurs as a result of the disruption in predisability occupations, activities, roles, and relationships. Health care practitioners must understand and acknowledge that people often experience even the loss of dysfunctional occupations, activities, roles, and relationships as a disempowering loss of identity. Nonidentity anxiety is a powerful barrier to the change process.

The Therapeutic Facilitation of Client-Motivated Change

Understanding how to address therapeutically the components of disempowerment is a critical skill that often differentiates the experienced practitioner from the novice (Benner, 1984; Benner & Tanner, 1987; Mattingly & Fleming, 1994). The ability to assist people who feel disempowered to mobilize their internal resources requires the practitioner to both instill hope and confront the defense mechanisms that enable the person to remain in a disempowered state. Denial; rationalization; and attachment to dysfunctional occupations, activities, roles, and relationships are defense mechanisms that may hinder a person from mobilizing the internal resources necessary to positively alter the quality of life (Horney, 1950). Therapists must be aware of a client's use of defense mechanisms and understand how to confront their operation therapeutically in a client's life.

The concept of ambivalence also is critical for practitioners to understand when helping clients through a change process brought on by a disability. Ambivalence occurs when people hold opposing or contradictory affective orientations toward a specific person, object, or event (Smelser, 1998). Clients commonly experience ambivalent emotions toward their disability, their therapists, and their treatment process. It is important for practitioners to understand that, although ambivalence hinders motivation, it is a normal experience in the range of human responses to disability. Practitioners must learn to tolerate a client's ambivalence in order to help the client to use his or her ambivalent feelings to effect positive change. Helping a client to consciously recognize and accept ambivalence is a critical step in the facilitation of motivation.

The instillation of hope—or the ability to persuade people to believe that they either possess or can develop the skills necessary to enhance their life satisfaction—often can be more difficult than confronting defense mechanisms and ambivalence and is significantly influenced by the degree of resilience, tenacity, and perseverance possessed. Why some clients experience successful rehabilitation courses whereas others lose motivation depends on both genetic traits and life experiences, among other factors. Regardless of whether a person possesses high or low levels of resilience and perseverance, practitioners can use specific techniques to facilitate motivation when clients feel disempowered. Bandura (1977) described motivation as derived from four principal sources: (a) performance accomplishments, (b) vicarious experience, (c) verbal persuasion, and (d) optimal emotional states.

Performance accomplishments are the success experiences that clients need to encounter in order to develop the motivation to change. When clients who participate in new occupations and activities experience a series of successes, they are more likely to develop the confidence and skills necessary to eventually accomplish feared but desired life goals (Bandura, 1977). Occupational therapy practitioners grade purposeful activities in accordance with a client's skill level to facilitate successful experiences. They choose purposeful activities that allow the client to practice needed skills in a safe, nonthreatening environment. The participation in purposeful activities may begin in simulated settings (e.g., the occupational therapy clinic) and move to the natural environment (e.g., a community shopping center, the work site) as the client gains competence. Expectations and purposeful activities are continually made more demanding or complex, graded until the client is practicing the actual set of skills required to enhance his or her quality of life and enable participation in occupations.

For example, a client may need to obtain the skills necessary for a job interview. The practitioner and client may role-play the job interview scenario, first in the safety of the occupational therapy clinic and then in applying for a role in a sheltered job program. The client initially may be asked to practice one skill, such as maintaining eye contact while answering interview questions. When this skill is mastered, the purposeful activity is expanded so that the client then may be required to maintain eye contact while answering questions, dress appropriately for an employment interview, and shake hands with the employer both before and after the interview. Later in the therapy sequence, the client may practice interviewing skills in a series of real-life employment interviews for jobs that represent reduced stress because they are mere stepping stones to a highly desired job. The therapist continually provides feedback so that the client can incrementally make improvements in skill level and adapt to change. In this way, the therapist sets up the optimal conditions through which a client can gradually experience successes. The need for feedback from the therapist is replaced by the client's integration of new identities until the highest level of desired skill is mastered, and participation in occupations is self-motivated.

Vicarious experience involves learning from observing others or modeling (Bandura, 1977). Providing opportunities for clients to observe others who have similarly struggled to successfully gain the skills the client desires can enhance motivation. Opportunities for clients to observe how others, with whom the client identifies, engage in specific skill behaviors often is enacted in both virtual (e.g., television, film) and natural environments (e.g., the community shopping center) to provide optimal learning experiences in more challenging settings.

Vicarious experience also can be gained by providing the opportunity for clients to receive mentorship from a peer who has experienced a successful rehabilitation course. Alcoholics Anonymous and many consumer service organizations have used the peer mentorship or buddy system effectively to provide clients with one other person who, through vicarious experience, can model appropriate behaviors that the client needs to adopt in order to enhance his or her quality of life (Caron & Bergeron, 1995; Hutchison, Osborne-Way, & Lord, 1986). For example, Gutman and Swarbrick (1998) described a woman, Eli, who sustained a head injury as a result of abuse perpetrated by a male partner. As part of her participation in an occupational therapy group, Eli was paired with a woman who had successfully extricated herself from prior abusive relationships and had learned the skills necessary to lead a more healthful lifestyle characterized by positive self-regard. Through peer mentorship, this woman was able to both challenge Eli's risk-taking behaviors and model the positive skills Eli needed to acquire to end her pattern of participation in abusive relationships.

Vicarious experience often is a powerful method of learning. It offers a safe emotional distance from the arousal of doing, and it offers the client an opportunity to observe that others sharing similar life circumstances are able to make the positive life changes that the client presently desires. Such an observation can be highly motivating because people often find greater credibility in peer mentors having lived similar experiences than in practitioners who may not share the same gender, race, socioeconomic status, or cultural belief systems as those of the client (Krefting, 1991; Mattingly & Fleming, 1994).

An effective motivator, vicarious experience allows clients to observe the accomplishments of those with whom the client identifies, providing hope and inspiring belief that the desired positive outcomes can be achieved. Vicarious experience becomes most effective when the client is able to internalize the modeled behaviors and, through purposeful activity, use the stored images as a resource to guide participation in activity when the peer mentor is not present.

Verbal persuasion is a form of motivation in which people are persuaded to believe that they possess the abilities to master difficult skills (Bandura, 1977). In the initial uses of verbal persuasion, the practitioner (or peer mentor) seeks to encourage confidence in the client by verbally coaxing the client and providing support and organization while the client attempts to perform new and often-feared activities. As the client begins to practice desired skills consistently, verbal persuasion can be less direct in the form of a set of instructions regarding the expectation and sequence of performance of specific behaviors. Such instructions act as a reference for the client to follow independently when the practitioner is not present. When the client has internalized the verbal coaching and instructions, he or she can use self-talk to guide him- or herself through a particular activity, gaining a newly learned skill linked to the positive affect required for participation in occupation.

For example, a client who chooses to learn assertiveness skills to cope more effectively with demanding employers and coworkers may initially need the verbal coaxing of a practitioner or peer mentor to believe that he or she can indeed learn and use desired assertive behaviors. The practitioner and client may role-play the use of assertiveness techniques within specific scenarios that the client is likely to encounter, whereas co-group members may verbally encourage the client as he or she practices the use of new assertive behaviors. The practitioner may coach the client through a specific scenario requiring assertive behaviors as the client engages in role-playing activities with another client. A goal of therapy is that verbal persuasion would become incorporated into a skill repertoire that the client calls on in occupations when the practitioner and co-group members are not present. For such participation in activities to occur, the opportunity for a sufficient amount of role-playing balanced with real-life practice must be provided until the client demonstrates comfort with and competence in using desired occupational skills in the context of the original conflict.

Because high degrees of arousal often reduce one's performance level, it is critical that practitioners help clients to achieve optimal emotional states (Bandura, 1977) through reparative experiences using stress reduction techniques. People partly rely on motivating anxiety level and physiological arousal when assessing and initiating their ability to perform feared or novel activities. When clients experience excessively high degrees of anxiety in response to specific feared or novel activities, they are likely to believe that they are unable to learn the skills necessary to perform those activities effectively or to participate in the desired occupations. Shutdown or withdrawal can result from the sustained experience of excessive anxiety. Until a client achieves a manageable physiological state and an optimal comfort level, that is, a level in which the client can engage in the practice of feared activities or desired occupations, new learning is unlikely to occur. The experienced practitioner will help the client to acknowledge the effects of anxiety and take responsibility for using means to manage and reduce anxiety before participating in desired therapeutic and purposeful activities. Stress reduction techniques may take the form of breathing exercises, meditation, guided imagery, and biofeedback. With children, stress reduction techniques may take the form of play in activities with high degrees of calming tactile or proprioceptive input. If such therapeutic techniques are not effective, the client may need a referral for pharmacological intervention to reduce anxiety (American Psychiatric Association, 1994). The therapist must be able to assess when pharmacological intervention may be necessary and make a timely and appropriate referral.

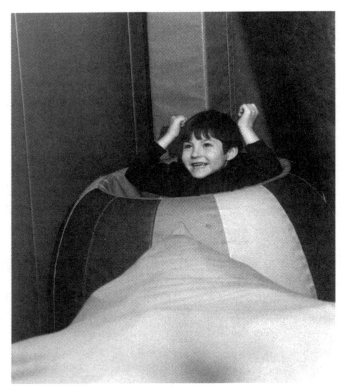

Figure 17.1. A tiny space provides comfort and security for a young boy.

One of the most effective forms of stress reduction is desensitization therapy (Wolpe, 1958, 1981). Before actually practicing the skills needed for a specific feared or novel activity, the client engages in a series of visualization techniques in which he or she imagines participating in the feared activity within the safety of the therapy setting. With children, the practitioner may become a partner in a playful game of "dragon slayer" to help the child visualize the particular "demon." Support in defeating the "fear" may take the practitioner's play-acting the assertive role for the child while encouraging the child to join in as a trusted "assistant dragon slayer." Desensitization therapy is practiced until the client is able to visually imagine him- or herself participating in the feared activity without concomitant feelings of anxiety. At this time, therapeutic activities can be directed toward role-playing and, later, real-life practice. For example, John, a young adult client with a history of depression, panic disorder, and substance abuse, reported that he experienced anxiety in response to a constellation of job stressors, including the need to make presentations for his job. John's attempt to alleviate his performance anxiety through alcohol intake caused him to be temporarily suspended from his employment and required to participate in a compulsory drug and alcohol abuse program before returning to work. As part of his rehabilitation, John participated in an occupational therapy group in which he was taught stress reduction techniques using meditation and biofeedback. John also received one-on-one desensitization therapy with an occupational therapist that enabled him to practice public speaking both in rehearsal and in actual circumstances within the safety of the therapeutic setting. When John reported that he could imagine himself engaged in the activity of public speaking outside the therapy setting without experiencing debilitating levels of anxiety, he began to practice making short presentations aloud in front of the occupational therapist. Shortly thereafter, John attempted to present in front of his five-member occupational therapy group. At this time, John reexperienced high degrees of anxiety that rendered his presentation skills nonfunctional, so the facility's psychiatrist prescribed an antianxiety medication. This medication helped John to continue his practice of public speaking in front of the occupational therapy group without feelings of extreme apprehension. As a result of continued practice with reduced, but motivating anxiety, John was able to learn the skills of public speaking needed to succeed in meeting the activity demands of his employment.

Knowing when to use performance accomplishments, vicarious experience, verbal persuasion, and stress reduction techniques to motivate clients is a skill that develops with clinical experience. A practitioner who pushes the use of such techniques too quickly in the intervention process without respecting the client's need to grieve over losses may unwittingly dissolve a client's trust and further inhibit motivation. Before initiating motivation techniques, practitioners must understand that a period of grieving about lost roles and relationships (even dysfunctional ones) must occur before clients can mobilize their internal resources to re-create meaningful lives.

Practitioners also must recognize that change processes are difficult and that each client will require varying lengths of time to grow more comfortable with changes forced by disability or illness. It is important too that practitioners help their clients to understand that rehabilitation often is characterized by a series of gains and setbacks. Setbacks that occur in a rehabilitation course are not indications of failure but, rather, are a natural occurrence of all change processes. Some setbacks in performance are the direct result of barriers in the client's social and environmental factors and do not result from a client's disability. Lack of products or technology, attitudinal factors or services, and system and policy problems are qualifiers that must be evaluated for their impact on or restriction of participation in activities (WHO, 2001). Practitioners who are able to convey an understanding of these ideas to their clients have made significant strides in the initial stages of the motivation process.

Use of Occupation and Purposeful Activities in the Empowerment Process

One of the principal philosophical assumptions of occupational therapy is that participating in meaningful occupation is necessary for people to gain a sense of mastery over their environment and life circumstances (Mosey, 1986; Reilly, 1974). Occupational therapy practitioners assist people with disabilities to perform desired occupations that are necessary for them to function as members of a community and family system. Participation in occupations is empowering because it provides the opportunity for humans to interact meaningfully with the objects and people in their surroundings. Occupation is the primary medium through which people seek a human experience; that is, it is the medium through which people experience themselves in relation to the human and nonhuman environment. People know themselves through their engagement in activities that support their roles and relationships. Occupation is innately empowering because it almost always is the medium around which humans communicate and socialize with one another. Thus, because humans are interdependent beings who know themselves through their interactions with the people and objects in their environment, engagement in occupation is necessary to form a human identity.

The formation of human identity can be delineated as a tiered process involving three steps (see Figure 17.2):

1. In the first stage of identity formation, people participate in specific chosen occupations that can support the assumption of desired social roles.

2. The assumption of specific social roles provides the opportunity for people to engage in relationships with others.

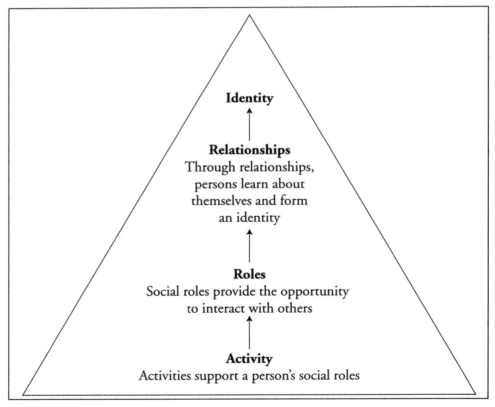

Figure 17.2. Activities support the roles and relationships that form a human identity.

3.   Through engagement in relationships and the occupations and roles that support those relationships, humans come to know themselves as people who are part of larger communities.

When disability causes the loss of meaningful occupations, activities, roles, and relationships, people lose an understanding of who they are in relation to others in their environment. Consequently, one's sense of self, or identity, often becomes displaced as the person struggles to maintain familiar activities and roles that have become jeopardized by the onset of disability. For example, a 40-year-old woman with multiple sclerosis found that she could no longer participate in many of the caregiving occupations and activities required by her 4-year-old child. As a result of the lost ability to participate in parenting occupations, the client believed that she was losing her role as a mother and that her relationship with her husband had become strained and uncomfortable. Because multiple sclerosis had disrupted the occupations that supported her roles and relationships as a wife and mother, the client experienced a loss of the predisability identity she had established before her medical condition was diagnosed. Disability strips persons of familiar occupations, roles, and relationships and forces them to surrender long-established and often comfortable identities.

Use of Activity to Empower People With Disabilities

By assisting persons with disabilities to engage in the daily life activities that support their occupations and roles within communities, family systems, and work and school settings, occupational therapy practitioners provide one of the first opportunities for these persons to feel empowered after the onset of disability. Practitioners address two primary categories of activity: (a) activities of daily living (ADL), or basic self-care tasks, and (b) instrumental activities of daily living (IADL), or complex multistep activities requiring the integration of higher level cognitive skills (e.g., meal preparation, money management, community travel). In a broader sense, ADL and IADL can be compared with Maslow's (1968) categorization of basic needs (or deficiency needs) and "meta-needs" (or growth needs) (see Table 17.1). Basic needs include both physiological needs and safety needs and are akin to the basic self-care ADL that occupational therapy practitioners address (e.g., eating, bathing, dressing, home safety). Meta-needs consist of the human need to experience (a) a sense of belonging; (b) self-esteem, or personal competence; and (c) self-actualization, or feeling empowered in one's ability to accomplish life goals. The occupations that support meta-needs are most related to the IADL that people must acquire to participate in complex social relationships and societal organizations. For example, the need to feel a sense of belonging requires a person to obtain the skills necessary to reintegrate into the community and to develop a supportive social network that provides needed resources and guidance. Self-esteem and competency needs require the person to develop a set of skills sufficient to meet specific environmental challenges and demands, for example, being able to adhere to a monthly budget to maintain independent apartment living. Self-actualization needs require a person to develop the skills necessary to rebuild a personally satisfying quality of life in which desired life goals can be accomplished despite the presence of disability. For example, a person with quadriplegia may desire to develop the skills necessary to return to school to embark on a more satisfying postinjury career.

Occupational therapy practitioners help clients fulfill both basic and meta-needs through participation in purposeful activities that can support the roles and relationships disrupted by disability. The process through which practitioners use purposeful activity to help clients rebuild desired roles and relationships can be delineated as a sequence of five steps:

1. The therapist and client identify the specific roles and relationships that the client has lost as a result of disability or never gained as a result of developmental delay.

Table 17.1
A Comparison of Activities of Daily Living and Maslow's (1968) Needs Hierarchy

ADL	Basic needs	Physiological needs	• The person can transfer from a bed to a commode. • The person can prepare a cold meal.
		Safety needs	• The person is safe and can live independently in his or her environment.
IADL	Meta-needs	Belongingness	• The person has reintegrated into the community and become a participating group member whose contributions are valued. • The person has developed a supportive network that provides resources and guidance.
		Self-esteem	• The person feels competent that his or her skills are sufficient to meet environmental challenges and demands.
		Self-actualization and empowerment	• The person possesses the skills necessary to exert positive change to create a meaningful quality of life.

Note. ADL = activities of daily living; IADL = instrumental activities of daily living.

2. The client and therapist indicate the specific activities that the client used to support lost roles and relationships. For people who never obtained desired roles and relationships as a result of developmental delay, it is important for the therapist to help these clients to identify activities that could support desired, but never obtained, occupations, roles, and relationships.

3. The therapist then encourages the client to determine which roles and relationships he or she wishes to rebuild, or build anew, after the onset of disability or delay.

4. The therapist and client choose occupations and purposeful activities that will support the rebuilding of desired roles and relationships: The therapist should (a) assist the client in the adaptation of predisability activities in accordance with sequelae secondary to the client's disability and (b) help the client to explore occupations and novel activities that also could support the client's desired participation in activities impaired because of the onset of disability or delay. In this way, the therapist assists the client to access new resources (both internal and external).

5. The therapist and client continue to practice the skills necessary to participate in the specific purposeful activities that support desired roles and relationships. Through engagement in such activities, the client is able to begin to rebuild an identity based on participation and activities that satisfy general as well as particular interactions in the major life areas of education, work and employment, economic, community, social, and civic life (WHO, 2001).

To facilitate these steps, a therapist can use the motivation techniques delineated by Bandura (1977): performance accomplishments, vicarious experience, verbal persuasion, and stress reduction techniques. For example, a therapist may set up the environmental conditions whereby a client can experience incremental success in performance accomplishments until he or she has attained a specific desired goal, for example, regaining full-time employment in the community after experiencing drug and alcohol abuse problems. The therapist might provide the opportunity for the client to observe, through vicarious experience, how others with whom the client identifies overcame their substance abuse and were able to regain full-time employment and find personally satisfying intimate relationships. Stress reduction techniques may be taught to the client to help him or her deal more effectively with work-related and social stressors or barriers that previously impaired functioning or enabled the client's substance abuse. Verbal persuasion strategies may be used to assist the client in the creation of an internalized repertoire of facilitators that he or she can use to cope with specific stressful events.

Case Scenarios

The following case scenarios illustrate how occupational therapy practitioners can use purposeful activity and occupations to facilitate the resumption of desired roles and

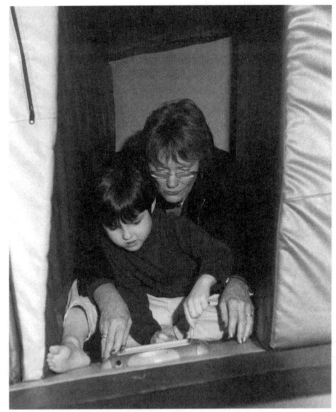

Figure 17.3. A therapist encourages a child to complete an activity in a secure environment.

relationships. The five-step process outlined just previously guides the therapeutic process.

Case Scenario

Tom is a 40-year-old white heterosexual man who sustained a traumatic brain injury (TBI) in an alcohol-related motor vehicle accident at 24 years of age. As a result of his injury, Tom experiences severe short-term memory deficits and sexual disinhibition. Because of these deficits, he requires supportive living services and has spent the past 16 years in four different residential facilities for people with brain injury. At his current residential placement, Tom lives in a community group home that houses four other men with brain injury. Although he possesses the cognitive ability to perform most basic self-care activities with distant supervision (e.g., bathing, toileting, grooming, dressing, household chores), Tom requires close supervision for many IADL (e.g., meal preparation, money management). Further, although he possesses the ability to remember the walking routes around his local community to access shopping, movies, recreational entertainment, and restaurants independently, Tom requires the accompaniment of a staff member in the larger community because of his impulsivity and sexual disinhibition.

Step 1: The identification of roles and relationships disrupted by injury. One of Tom's most disturbing role losses after injury concerns his inability to resume a dating or courtship role. Before his accident, he had enjoyed an active social life that included a series of monogamous sexual relationships with women. His injury occurred to the dorsolateral frontal cortex and hypothalamic neural regions, areas that play a role in regulating sexual desire and response (Miller, 1993). A likely result of neurologic insult to these structures is that Tom became sexually disinhibited and began to exhibit socially inappropriate behaviors with women in public settings. Because of his sexual disinhibition, his placement in TBI residential programs had been problematic, and consequently, Tom experienced a series of admissions and discharges from various residential facilities. Discharges often occurred in response to a specific event in which the facility could no longer tolerate Tom's sexually inappropriate behaviors.

During the first year that Tom resided in his current community group home, a similar situation occurred in which he became sexually and physically aggressive with a female client whom he desired to date. Rather than discharge Tom from the facility, however, his treatment team physically separated him from female clients by moving him to an all-male group home and restricting his community access. When Tom began to receive occupational therapy services in his current residential placement, he identified his desire to engage in dating roles and relationships as his foremost priority.

Step 2: The identification of lost purposeful activities that supported predisability roles and relationships. Tom was able to list the occupations that supported his dating role before injury. Activities that were important included going to dinner; dancing; and attending films, shows, and concerts. However, although he was able to identify some appropriate dating activities, he was not able to articulate or demonstrate the social skills needed to interact appropriately with women. Initially, Tom needed to obtain a repertoire of social skills that will enable him to address a women appropriately, introduce himself, and conduct a conversation without exhibiting sexually disinhibited behaviors. Tom and his therapist compiled a list of the socially inappropriate behaviors that he displays in response to desire to obtain his lost occupation of a monogamous intimate relationship. These dysfunctional behaviors included prolonged staring, violating social norms of personal space, frequently touching others' shoulders and arms, and blurting out sexual propositions. Tom experienced emotional pain when rejected because he exhibited these abrasive behaviors. Intellectually, he understood that he acted in ways that defeated his efforts to find companionship. The therapist and Tom discussed how to replace these behaviors with more socially acceptable ones. To identify appropriate interaction skills with women, Tom and his therapist observed men and women interacting in the larger community environment (e.g., at shopping centers and malls, in restaurants, at the bank). During these observation sessions, appropriate eye contact, respect of another's personal space, and appropriate conversational topics were noted. Tom and the therapist began to role-play use of appropriate interaction skills, first within the safety of the clinic, and then within the actual community setting.

Step 3: The determination of which roles and relationships the client wishes to rebuild and build anew. Although Tom indicated that he wished to reobtain a monogamous sexual relationship with a woman, he recognized that he would be unable to do so without first developing the interaction skills necessary to engage in informal social contact with women. He decided that a casual social role with women he considered as friends would provide the opportunity for him to practice the interaction skills he needed to eventually develop and maintain a more intimate relationship with a woman.

Step 4: The specification of purposeful activities that can support desired roles and relationships. Tom chose to practice social skills with a female friend who also resided at the TBI residential facility. Purposeful activities that Tom chose to participate in included shopping at a local mall, walking in a community park, and dining in a nearby restaurant with his female companion. On these occasions, Tom's therapist was present to cue him when his behaviors deviated from those he had learned in his role-playing sessions. When Tom began to consistently demonstrate socially appropriate behaviors with his female friend, the therapist's level of supervision changed from close to distant observation. For example, as Tom continued to accompany his friend to dinner at a local restaurant, the therapist began to sit at a nearby table, rather than join the couple, in order to offer distant supervision.

As Tom's relationship with his female friend became more intimate, safe-sex practices were reinforced by the occupational therapist and nursing staff so that the couple could engage in the activities of a sexual relationship in the same way that adult couples in the larger society often do.

Step 5: The development of a satisfactory postinjury identity based on desired roles and relationships. Through the desired activities Tom wished to achieve, he was able to rebuild an identity as a dating partner, a role that was inherently related to his concept of himself as a man and enabled him to experience greater satisfaction with male gender roles. Tom's treatment team members had not attempted to offer him social skills training in the context of dating relationships; instead, they attempted to deal with his inappropriate behaviors by restricting his access to women. By allowing Tom to practice interaction skills with women in progressively less supervised settings, he was able to demonstrate that he could assume more socially acceptable behaviors.

Tom's therapist used three of the four motivation techniques described by Bandura (1977): performance accomplishments, vicarious experience, and verbal persuasion. A series of performance accomplishments were achieved by providing the opportunity for Tom to use successfully appropriate social skills in situations that were progressively graded in complexity and activity demands: first in role-playing scenarios with the therapist, then with social activities with a female friend, and finally in establishing a more intimate relationship. The therapist used vicarious experience as a forum for learning by providing Tom with the opportunity to observe the social skills of men and women interacting in the nat-

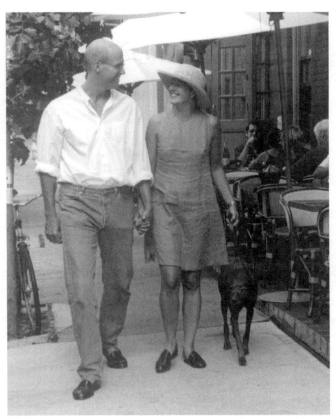

Figure 17.4. Dating is a goal in normal daily activity.

ural community setting. Verbal persuasion was used in the initial role-playing sessions to help Tom to internalize an expanded repertoire of appropriate social skills that he could call on when the therapist was not present.

Through these activities, Tom obtained the skills necessary to engage in dating relationships and fulfilling occupations. Such skills enabled him to feel empowered in his ability to make personal changes in order to achieve a more satisfactory quality of life.

Case Questions:

1. In what other ways could Tom's therapist have used vicarious experience as a learning tool?

2. What other performance accomplishments could Tom have experienced to enhance his social interaction skills with women? How would a therapist set up the environment so that he could experience such performance accomplishments?

3. How did the participation in activity help Tom to reobtain his role as a dating partner?

4. What other activities could Tom participate in to enhance his social skills with women?

5. Describe the process of empowerment that enabled Tom to learn the skills necessary to make positive changes in his quality of life.

Case Scenario

Archie is a 4.9-year-old white boy who lives with his mother, father, and younger brother. His mother reported having an uncomplicated pregnancy with a normal delivery. According to his mother, Archie achieved common developmental milestones by his second year (e.g., walking, talking) but began to lose language skills shortly thereafter and was referred for occupational therapy as part of an early intervention home-based program. Although his parents identified his language delay, they were less concerned about other apparent behavioral issues assessed in clinical evaluations. Archie demonstrated outbursts of temper when required to shift and transition from the performance of one activity to another. He displayed great difficulty with sustained eye contact and could neither tolerate physical touch nor initiate interaction with others in his environment. Archie's play was perseverative, rigid, and limited to two or three specific, favored toys. Additionally, he demonstrated significant sensitivities to visual, tactile, and auditory stimulation.

On his first occupational therapy home visit, Archie ran randomly around his house, avoiding any visual, tactile, or auditory contact. Even when seated in his bedroom with his own selected, preferred toys, he continued to resist overtures initiated by the therapist. The therapist attempted to initiate interaction and build rapport by playing with toys on the floor at Archie's own positional level. Archie fleetingly joined the therapist in a game of peek-a-boo but screamed inconsolably when the therapist attempted to alter the rules of his play.

Step 1: The identification of roles and relationships disrupted by developmental dysfunction. One of the most apparent role impairments was Archie's difficulty in establishing play and social roles typical of a 4-year-old preschooler. Archie demonstrated great difficulty interacting with others and initiating free play. Instead, he often only engaged in solitary play and would typically roll one of his toy cars back and forth until he remained standing still, fixed and motionless with his hand on the car, staring off into space. Archie would remain in this position for minutes at a time, showing signs of distress if disturbed.

Step 2: The identification of lost purposeful activities that supported predisability roles and relationships. Archie's parents were able to identify words and language activities (e.g., singing toddler songs and rhymes) that Archie had previously attained and now appeared to be losing. His parents strongly maintained that as a young infant Archie tolerated holding, eye contact, and sounds and played like most other babies. After the birth of their second child, Archie's mother was more able to identify behavioral differences between her sons.

Archie's family required time to adjust to the presence of therapists in their home. Similarly, the occupational therapist needed to provide time not only for the child but also for Archie's parents. Thus, Archie's parents or babysitter were frequently included in the weekly therapy sessions for the first year of therapy. His parents were provided with information about the types of purposeful activities that could help remediate Archie's developmentally delayed behaviors. It was suggested that complicated and rule-bound activities be excluded from games the parents played with Archie. Instead, games were used that allowed him to exercise his own control and independence. For example, the therapist and Archie built furniture and cubby houses that allowed him to initiate his own entrance and exit. It was important to provide him with multiple safe spaces in which he could relate to and interact with the therapist. Although language was the parents' primary concern, the therapist would not demand syntactical speech. Instead, the therapist would engage in Archie's own language if the theme of his communication was clear. Archie brought one or two of his toys into the cubby house, and the therapist used them to initiate interactive play. Archie's parents extended this type of therapeutic activity and purchased a small tent in which one of the parents would often sit with him and play. Both parents were consistently able to demonstrate pride in Archie's accomplishments. Despite advice from other therapists and a service coordinator, Archie's parents refused to seek an evaluation or treatment from a traditional medical model approach. They did not want a diagnostic category to be assigned, even if it meant a consequent lack of funding to support his occupational therapy. They were adamant about Archie's intervention plan arising from his strengths rather than from a narrow classification of a disease or disorder. The occupational therapist understood their concern. In fact, the parents' view fit with the occupational therapist's use of capacity qualifiers, which are described in the ICF conceptual framework (WHO, 2001) and which encourage practitioners to include prevention, health promotion, and the improvement of participation by removing or mitigating societal hindrances. Further, the framework encourages the provision of social support and facilitators to classify functioning and plan interventions. The occupational therapist considered contextual factors, personal factors, and qualifiers that took into consideration capacity and performance in her occupational profile of Archie.

Step 3: The determination of which roles and relationships the client wishes to rebuild and build anew. Although Archie had learned to function more adaptively in his own home, he felt overwhelmed and frightened when he ventured into larger, unpredictable environments, such as the local playground. Therefore, the therapy sessions more frequently took place in a playground setting to expand Archie's opportunities to interact with other children and build relationships. Initially, he would passively allow himself to be placed in a swing and pushed back and forth until his stimulation level was so diminished that he appeared trance-like. He could not initiate play on novel playground equipment. The therapist used singing and counting activities to help Archie assume a greater control over his arousal level. Games included more active motor planning, such as an expanded game of peek-a-boo and hide and seek. Again, the theme of creating smaller, more manageable spaces within larger settings was used by having him climb into tunnels and playground equipment to rest and talk for rapport building and relationship development.

Step 4: The specification of purposeful activities that can support desired roles and relationships. Archie wanted to learn how to use preschool toys and equipment (e.g., scissors, play dough, puzzles, bats and balls) within the context of his own rules. The therapist began having sessions with Archie at his preschool with small groups of children. His peers quickly included Archie as a center of games because he had become a willing participant in preschool activities by this stage of therapy. His social behavior had advanced from the random running movement and aversion to any close contact with others that the therapist had first observed in the initial home visits. Archie now could initiate social greetings to the therapist—a behavior that carried over to his teachers. In fact, he became very attached to his therapist and teachers. He was able to put his hands on his therapist's chin if he believed he was being ignored; move the therapist's face into his eye contact; and verbalize, "I'm talking to you." This normalization of social responsiveness and adoption of appropriate social roles provided great comfort to Archie's parents, who all along fought the medical categorization of his potential. His ability to move from one activity to another and capacity to use language syntactically and communicatively had begun to catch up to his actual age as his social network expanded.

Step 5: The development of a satisfactory identity based on desired roles and relationships. Archie has moved into an integrated school setting, travels by public transportation to an urban occupational therapy practice, and participates in more challenging activities in which he is required to adapt to the environment rather than adapt his environment. In the occupational therapy practice, he sometimes complains "These are not my toys" but is able to accept the novel toys and interact and play appropriately with other children (in a therapy group) whom he does not see regularly. He currently exercises autonomy with the typical willfulness of a developing 5-year-old. At one particular session, an old friend from his preschool came to the occupational therapy practice at the same time as Archie's session and enthusiastically embraced Archie, covering him with hugs and kisses. Archie not only tolerated such physical contact but also tentatively reciprocated.

Archie's therapist used all four motivation techniques described by Bandura (1977): performance accomplishments, vicarious experience, verbal persuasion, and stress reduction techniques. A series of performance accomplishments was achieved by providing the opportunity for Archie to interact successfully with others in situations in which the activity demands were graded to his abilities, capacities, and performance, first with the occupational therapist in newly created safe spaces within the home (cubby houses), then with the therapist in the larger setting of a local playground, and finally in a preschool setting with other children. The therapist used vicarious experience as a learning forum by providing Archie with the opportunity to observe the play and social skills of other preschoolers in the playground setting, in Archie's preschool classroom, and in therapy group sessions with other children at the occupational therapy practice. The therapist also used verbal persuasion to help Archie attempt interactive play with her and others in his environment. Stress reduction techniques centered on helping Archie to feel a greater sense of control in what he perceived to be unpredictable environments. For example, cubby spaces were created in which Archie was allowed to freely enter and exit as he desired; games were played in which Archie's behaviors were not bound by others' rules; and communication was encouraged that allowed Archie to speak freely without the demand for syntactically correct speech.

Through these occupations, Archie was able to learn interactive play styles and began to build relationships with others in which he was able to demonstrate appropriate eye contact, tolerate physical touching, and initiate and sustain verbal communication. Such social and play skills enabled Archie to feel empowered and in control of his environment and allowed him to build relationships that enriched his emotional life and facilitated greater social and cognitive development.

Case Questions:

1. In what other ways could Archie's therapist have used vicarious experience as a learning tool?

2. What other performance accomplishments could Archie have experienced to enhance his social interaction skills with others? How would a therapist set up the environment so that he could experience such performance accomplishments?

3. How did participation in purposeful activity help Archie to reobtain his role as a member in give-and-take family and school systems?

4. What other purposeful activities could Archie have participated in to enhance his social skills with others?

5. Describe the process of empowerment that enabled Archie to learn the skills necessary to make positive changes in his quality of life.

Summary

This chapter primarily is concerned with issues related to empowerment and how it ties in with occupations and purposeful activity. The fundamental goal is to demonstrate how this quest for personal empowerment leads to a better quality of life.

Empowerment is a combination of skills, competence, self-determination, belonging, and equality. In addition, people who are empowered use their personal qualities and attitudes, allowing them to make changes in their life situations.

Occupational therapy practitioners are impelled to apply knowledge of empowerment as a process to the relationship between disability and disempowerment. When people lose the skills and qualities that are crucial to their sense of selfhood, when the sick role forces them to accept dependency, and when the stigma associated with disability colors how others see them, a therapeutic process is available that can restore the experience of feeling empowered.

The role of the occupational therapy practitioner is to assist those who have lost the ability to assert their selfhood through disability to learn how to facilitate change by developing new skills, by learning from others, and by experiencing the accomplishments that are produced. Allowing clients to traverse this empowerment process involves powers of persuasion and their learning how to deal with added stress.

Occupational therapy practitioners can help clients to accomplish this empowerment by offering many levels of purposeful activity as the means, from ADL through countless activities of leisure and work. Two case studies are presented to illustrate the process and its steps. ■

Acknowledgment

This revised chapter is based on the work of Sharon Gutman, PhD, OTR, "Activities, the Empowerment Process, and Client-Motivated Change," *The Texture of Life*, 2000.

References

American Psychiatric Association. (1994). *Diagnostic and statistical manual of mental disorders* (4th ed.). Washington, DC: Author.

Antonovsky, A. (1992). Can attitudes contribute to health? *Advances: Journal of Mind–Body Health, 8*(4), 33–49.

Bandura, A. (1977). Self-efficacy: Toward a unifying theory of behavioral change. *Psychological Review, 84*, 191–215.

Benner, P. (1984). *From novice to expert: Excellence and power in clinical nursing practice.* Reading, MA: Addison-Wesley.

Benner, P., & Tanner, C. (1987). Clinical judgment: How expert nurses use intuition. *American Journal of Nursing, 87*, 23–31.

Caron, J., & Bergeron, N. (1995). A self-help partnership group for people who have experienced psychiatric hospitalization: An exploratory study. *Canada's Mental Health, 43*(2), 19–28.

Clark, F. A., Parham, D., Carlson, M. E., Frank, G., Jackson, J., Pierce, D., et al. (1991). Occupational science: Academic innovation in the service of occupational therapy's future. *American Journal of Occupational Therapy, 45*, 300–310.

Dunton, W. R., Jr. (1919). *Reconstruction therapy.* Philadelphia: Saunders.

Goffman, E. (1963). *Stigma: Notes on the management of spoiled identity.* New York: Simon & Schuster.

Gutierrez, L. M. (1995). Understanding the empowerment process: Does consciousness make a difference? *Social Work Research, 19*, 229–237.

Gutman, S. A., & Swarbrick, M. (1998). The multiple linkages between women, head injury, alcoholism, and sexual abuse. *Occupational Therapy in Mental Health, 14*(3), 33–65.

Hood, S., Beaudet, M., & Catlin, G. (1996). A healthy outlook. *Health Reports: Statistics Canada, 7*(4), 25–32. (Catalog No. 82-003-XPB)

Horney, K. (1950). *Neurosis and human growth: The struggle toward self-realization.* New York: Norton.

Hutchison, P., Osborne-Way, L., & Lord, J. (1986). *Participating with people who have directly experienced the mental health system.* Toronto, Ontario: Canadian Mental Health Association.

Kielhofner, G. (Ed.). (1995). *A model of human occupation: Theory and application* (2nd ed.). Baltimore: Williams & Wilkins.

Krefting, L. (1991). The culture concept in the everyday practice of occupational and physical therapy. *Physical and Occupational Therapy in Pediatrics, 11*(4), 1–6.

Maslow, A. H. (1968). *Toward a psychology of being* (2nd ed.). New York: Van Nostrand Reinhold.

Mattingly, C., & Fleming, M. H. (1994). *Clinical reasoning: Forms of inquiry in a therapeutic practice.* Philadelphia: F. A. Davis.

Meyer, A. (1922). The philosophy of occupation therapy. *Archives of Occupational Therapy, 1,* 2–3.

Miller, L. (1993). *Psychotherapy of the brain-injured patient: Reclaiming the shattered self.* New York: Norton.

Mosey, A. C. (1986). *Psychosocial components of occupational therapy.* New York: Raven.

Pearlin, L. I., & Schooler, C. (1978). The structure of coping. *Journal of Health and Social Behavior, 19*(1), 2–21.

Reilly, M. (1974). *Play as exploratory learning.* Beverly Hills, CA: Sage.

Smelser, N. J. (1998). The rational and the ambivalent in the social sciences: 1997 presidential address. *American Sociological Review, 63,* 1–16.

Wilson, S. (1996). Consumer empowerment in the mental health field. *Canadian Journal of Community Mental Health, 15*(2), 69–85.

World Health Organization. (2001). *ICF: International classification of functioning, disability, and health, short version.* Geneva, Switzerland: Author.

Wolpe, J. (1958). *Psychotherapy by reciprocal inhibition.* Palo Alto, CA: Stanford University Press.

Wolpe, J. (1981). *Our useless fears.* Boston: Houghton Mifflin.

18

Preparing for the Future:
How Activities Relate to Human
Occupation

Marie-Louise Blount, AM, OT, FAOTA
Shu-Hwa Chen, MA, OTR
Jim Hinojosa, PhD, OT, FAOTA
Paula Kramer, PhD, OTR, FAOTA

This chapter examines the research that supports the therapeutic use of activities, the therapeutic use of occupation, and the implications of this scholarly work on the future of the profession. One of our objectives is to summarize and critique the research related to purposeful activity and occupation. Another is to link this scholarly work with our vision for the profession into the next decade. The profession's valuing of and perspectives on activity and occupation will shape future occupational therapy research and practice.

Before summarizing and critiquing research and scholarly publications, one needs to set a framework for scrutiny and a taxonomy for analysis. These decisions provide a structure for comparing publications that are based on different assumptions and research conducted in multiple paradigms. Some questions we asked to begin this process included the following: Should purposeful activity and occupation be examined as two separate constructs? If so, we would have to have clear and precise definitions. Would it be best to examine activities and occupation as legitimate tools used by practitioners to bring about change, that is, as the means of intervention? Would it be better to examine purposeful activity and occupation from an "ends" perspective as the outcome of intervention? Does examining published research based on research methodology (e.g., quantitative, qualitative, experimental, descriptive) lead to a clear understanding of the findings of the research? Or, should research be examined based on the research question(s) that underlie the study?

Because each of these questions appears to be essential to understanding how activities relate to human occupation, we have used them all to provide a framework for our discussion. We have not made an attempt to critique all the research related to occupational therapy. In fact, we have carefully selected publications to illustrate our line of reasoning and to provide basic information that you can use to develop and refine your own ideas.

Examining Purposeful Activity and Occupation as Distinct Constructs

Although occupational therapy scholars have proposed that purposeful activities and occupation are two distinct constructs, the definitions of the constructs in publications and research studies are not precise. In fact, confusion often is evident when authors claim that the two constructs are similar. For example, in the glossary to the *Occupational Therapy Practice Framework: Domain and Process* (American Occupational Therapy Association [AOTA], 2002) there are the following definitions:

■ *Activity or activities:* "A term that describes a class of human actions that are goal directed" (p. 630).

■ *Purposeful activity:* "An activity used in treatment that is goal directed and that the ...[client] sees as meaningful or purposeful" (p. 633).

■ *Occupation:* "Activities...of everyday life, named, organized, and given value and meaning by individuals and a culture. Occupation is everything people do to occupy themselves, including looking after themselves...enjoying life...and contributing to the social and economic fabric of their communities" (p. 632).

These definitions overlap and do not provide clear distinctions among the constructs. As occupational therapy practitioners, we are ultimately concerned about human occupation. Occupations are grounded in personal meaning, are goal directed, are personally satisfying, and reflect our cultural backgrounds (Hinojosa, Kramer, Royeen, & Luebben, 2003). As practitioners, we must recognize that occupations are made up of activities and tasks. Some activities are purposeful because they are meaningful or have a meaningful outcome for the person engaged in the activity. Other activities occupy time and may not have personal meaning; they just need to be done.

Therefore, we propose that occupational therapy practitioners use the language that is most appropriate for the situation and for what they are trying to communicate. The attachment of the word *occupation* to other concepts does not strengthen our commitment to the construct of occupation. In fact, to the outsider, this attachment may be confusing and limit our ability to communicate effectively.

Purposeful Activity and Occupation as a Means

Many occupational therapy practitioners believe that occupation can be both the means and the end of occupational therapy. These practitioners believe that they can use occupations in their interventions with clients to bring about change. They also believe that the outcome of intervention is the client's ability to engage in their occupations. In this book, we propose that occupations can be defined only by the person who is engaged in them. Occupational synthesis takes place when the client who has received occupational therapy spontaneously and unconsciously engages in activities that are personally meaningful and supports his or her ability to function. From our perspective, occupational therapy practitioners use activities. When possible, the practitioner uses purposeful activities. The goal of intervention and the outcome is that the client integrates these activities into his or her occupations and continues to engage in them as part of everyday life.

When conducting research to examine the efficacy of an intervention, researchers are perplexed about how to study occupation and purposeful activity. Qualitative basic research is beginning to produce a body of theoretical information about occupation. This work should be continued with increased focus on establishing a sound body of theoretical knowledge about the construct of occupation as it relates to people and society.

Establishing the effectiveness of specific occupational therapy interventions requires that we examine the treatment modalities we use within the context of a frame of reference or guidelines for intervention that specify their application. Applied research must examine treatment guidelines within the theoretical rationale that underlies them. Applied research is concerned with practical answers about whether a theoretically based intervention (frame of reference) has the outcome that it predicts. From this perspective, activities are one tool that occupational therapy practitioners use to bring about change. As a tool, activities must be examined within their theoretical context. For example, dressing activities may be used with children to develop body awareness and imaginary play skills. For an adult, dressing may be an activity used to develop socially appropriate self-care skills. When providing occupational therapy, one therapeutic tool is rarely used alone. Most often, based on the theoretical base of the intervention, several tools are used in specified manners as therapeutic media.

Although we suggest examining the use of activities within the context of the frame of reference that is used, much occupational therapy research has focused on establishing the efficacy of using purposeful activity. In these studies, purposeful activities or occupations are the independent or treatment variable (e.g., cause, treatment, controlled factor, manipulated variable). Many of these studies have supported the basic belief that therapeutic activities are more effective if they have personal meaning to the person.

Published Research Based on the Question(s) That Underlie the Study

Many occupational therapy practitioners may believe that they do not need to learn about research because they are only interested in being clinicians. Evidence-based practice, however, demands that all practitioners have a basic understanding of research and its influence on practice. With support from research literature, practitioners can provide better services. When we read published research, it is important for us to first understand the research question(s). Research questions are the foundation for research. Identifying research questions is the first step to conducting useful research. "What exactly do you want to find out?" is the essential question the investigators need to answer before making the selection of appropriate research methods (Punch, 1998). Once the researcher has a clear research question, he or she then determines the kind of data necessary to answer these questions and how the data can be collected and analyzed.

Where do research questions come from? Students often ask this question. As intelligent creatures, we constantly ask questions and search for the answers. Researchers use systematic methods to investigate questions to explain behavior and understand our lives. In fact, finding interesting research questions is not difficult. These questions emerge as we observe our environment and our actions. Questions come from our practice, our everyday observations, and our reading. In this section, only a few examples are presented to illustrate how research is based on research questions.

Occupational therapy practitioners often ask questions related to their daily practice, such as "Are the activities selected effective for achieving the goals?" For example, Paul and Ramsey (1998) asked whether music-making activity as a form of occupationally embedded exercise could improve active shoulder flexion and elbow extension in people with hemiplegia. To improve the quality of services, some may ask "What is the nature of occupations for clients that adds to our understanding about the meaning of occupation for those specific clients?" Lyons, Orozovic, Davis, and Newman (2002) investigated the occupational experiences of people with life-threatening illness while attending a day hospice program. Other researchers have examined the relationships between purposeful activities and performances and behaviors. For example, Yoder, Nelson, and Smith (1989) conducted a randomized group experiment to examine whether differences are elicited by the purposefulness of activities when applied to elderly female nursing home residents by comparing the duration and frequency of rotatory arm movement. These research questions determine what research is done in occupational therapy, and most importantly, they determine what we learn.

Although many occupational therapy researchers have collected much information about the application of purposeful activities and occupations, a great need still exists for more research to substantiate our practice. In 2003, the American Occupational Therapy Foundation (AOTF) and AOTA reaffirmed a list of research priorities, which include questions about

- The effectiveness of intervention in achieving targeted activity and participation outcomes and preventing and reducing secondary conditions;

- The extent of occupation-based intervention to promote learning, adaptation, self-organization, adjustment to life situations, and self-determination across the life span;

- Effectiveness of environmental interventions that support occupation in preventing impairment and promoting participation at the individual, community, and societal levels;

■ Where, when, how, and at what level (body structure and body function, activity, participation, environment) an intervention should occur to maximize activity and participation and the cost-effectiveness of services;

■ Measures and measurement systems to reflect the domain of occupational therapy and the impact of occupational therapy on these factors (body structure and body function, activity, participation, environment);

■ How activity patterns and choices influence health and participation;

■ The impact of activity patterns and choices on society;

■ What conceptual models explain the relationships among body structure and body function, activity, environment, and participation and the role of occupational therapy within these models;

■ What factors contribute to effective partnerships between clients and practitioners that foster and enhance participation; and

■ What factors support practitioners' capacities to maximize the occupational performance of their clients (AOTA & AOTF, 2003).

This list provides directions for researchers to ask questions in different aspects of our practice from specific factors to broad models and from individuals to society.

Just asking questions is not enough. To develop good research questions, occupational therapy researchers need to ask important, relevant, and answerable questions. A research question should be stated clearly and straightforwardly. Occupational therapy practitioners work in many different settings by applying various activities with a wide range of populations. An unlimited potential exists for research. With an increased demand for us to provide evidences and to grow bodies of knowledge supporting our practice, occupational therapy researchers should focus on the investigation of occupational therapy effectiveness and the development of theories about the nature of human occupations and relationships between health and occupation (Gillette, 1991). Once a person has a research question, he or she needs to develop a comprehensive outline that describes the implementation of the study.

Published Research Based on Research Methodology

From earlier emphasis on quantitative research methods to the newly widespread use of qualitative research methods, both qualitative and quantitative research methods are important in occupational therapy research. Choosing to use either a qualitative approach or a quantitative approach does not make research good or bad. It is crucial, however, that a study uses the most appropriate approach to investigate the problem. This is what makes the research valuable or not (Plante, Kiernan, & Betts, 1994).

Specific research questions dictate the best approach, and different research questions will lead to different methods (Plante et al., 1994; Punch, 1998). In this section, our intention is not to educate readers about details of quantitative and qualitative research methods but to provide a few examples of each method to illustrate how both can be used in occupational therapy research.

Quantitative Method

Briefly stated, a quantitative approach focuses on examining preselected variables that have been thought to be pertinent based on either existing theoretical statements or the researcher's own interpretation in order to determine causal and measurable relationships among the variables. The investigators manipulate the numerical data through statistical analysis to seek an explanation of the causes and determinants of the phenomenon (Creswell, 1998; Punch, 1998).

An occupational therapy researcher who uses quantitative designs typically uses experimental, quasi-experimental, or nonexperimental (i.e., correlational, single-subject) designs or identifies and isolates specific variables and uses specific measurement instruments to collect information on these variables. To support and justify therapeutic use of purposeful activities, it has been a great concern for occupational therapy researchers to prove our value to society by presenting the efficacy of occupational therapy intervention. Nelson (1993) believed that with experimental analysis of our practice, occupational therapy practitioners will be led to clear definitions of terms and precise statements about relationships between concepts. In addition, with quantitative research designs, the studies can be replicated to verify the findings and added to our existing knowledge. For example, Lin, Wu, Tickle-Degnen, and Coster (1997) conducted a meta-analysis of 17 quantitative studies to examine the relationship between the purposefulness of the activity and the motor performances. With the presentation of quantitative data, the results reinforce the advantage of activities with added purpose over those with no added purpose.

Furthermore, quantitative research methods have been suggested to provide better communication with other professions in the scientific community. With numerical comparisons, quantitative research findings can strengthen the evidences of the efficacy of occupational therapy intervention. Clark et al. (1997) evaluated the effectiveness of occupational therapy preventive services for well elderly people through a randomized controlled trial. With 361 participants, the authors presented their results in numerical analysis to compare the differences in several outcome measurements elicited by the occupational therapy group, the social activity control group, and the nontreatment control group. Statistically significant findings were found across various domains, providing strong support for documenting the effectiveness of preventive occupational therapy services.

Although it is difficult to manipulate independent variables or obtain a control group, many occupational therapy researchers choose to approach their questions by using descriptive design or one group design. Dolecheck and Schkade (1999) examined six elderly participants' performance in dynamic standing endurance when engaged in different types of tasks. Although the sample size was small, with repeated-measure design, the authors found a statistically significant increase in standing time with personally meaningful activities versus nonmeaningful tasks.

With limited sources of samples, many researchers use single-subject or case study design. Single-subject designs compare each individual's performance across a timeline under different conditions. These designs enable researchers to examine the efficacy of intervention on people with some specific characteristics. With careful inspection of data, it can provide information about why an intervention is effective for one client but not others (Dunn, 1993). Melchert-McKearnan, Deitz, Engel, and White (2000) designed a single-subject, randomized multiple treatment study to compare the effects of two conditions: purposeful activity (play) and rote exercise on performance with two children with burn injuries. The results suggested that the use of a play activity yielded better outcomes than rote exercise. The data, however, implied that there might be a point later in the rehabilitation process when rote exercise may be as effective as play activities in meeting therapeutic goals, and the authors suggested further replication of this study.

Qualitative Method

A researcher chooses to use a qualitative approach when the phenomenon needs to explore and present participant-centered detail holistically within its context. Qualitative research helps the researchers to obtain a better understanding of a social phenomenon from the participants' perspectives (Creswell, 1998). Therefore, qualitative data are useful for developing theories and understanding natural behaviors.

Qualitative research methods can be used to develop theories by generating a systematic knowledge base and understanding about participation in occupations. It also can be used to investigate the effect of occupational therapy intervention on quality of life, health, and wellness. With a focus on participants' perspectives, their experiences, and what these experiences mean to them, qualitative researchers believe that life experience provides the most meaningful data. Furthermore, many researchers believe that qualitative research methods have a goodness-of-fit with searching for viable information about clients' performance in a natural context (Dunn, 1993; Yerxa, 1991).

Many qualitative approaches can be applied in occupational therapy research. They provide new knowledge to the profession by exploring complex, multileveled human qualities (Yerxa, 1991). In a qualitative study, Price-Lackey and Cashman (1996) used a narrative approach with life history interviews to discover the life experience of one woman with a traumatic head injury. This study illustrated the usefulness of gaining clients' perspectives as occupational beings through gathering life histories with a focus on occupation, the importance of collaborative client–therapist goal setting, and the necessity for considering both the doing and the meaning aspects of occupation. It supports the belief that the therapeutic relationship may be enhanced through the use of life history interviewing in practice.

As another example, Perrins-Margalis, Rugletic, Schepis, Stepanski, and Walsh (2000) conducted a qualitative study to investigate the effects of purposeful activity on the performance of people with chronic mental illness. Based on the interpretation of a horticulture experience from the participants' perspective, the authors gained a more in-depth understanding about the effect of horticulture as a group-based activity on quality of life, which was a composition of life satisfaction, well-being, and self-concept.

Future Research on Activities, Purposeful Activities, and Occupation

The health care delivery system and associated reimbursement structures have a direct influence on practitioners' attention to and use of activities, purposeful activities, and occupations. Although we believe that the critical outcome of occupational therapy should be the client's ability to engage in occupations, a wide range of interventions is used successfully by occupational therapists. All the interventions are important and need to be examined for their efficacy and effectiveness in creating environments where clients' performance skills and behaviors positively change. Activity, purposeful activity, and occupation are only three unique therapeutic modalities that practitioners use. Other modalities, beyond the scope of this text, include conscious use of self, use of the nonhuman environment, the teaching–learning process, activity groups, sensory stimulation, and physical agent modalities. Whenever using any of these modalities, the occupational therapy practitioner must keep in mind the central concern—occupation.

Recognizing the importance of activities, purposeful activities, and occupation, it is critical that we understand how and why we must examine these therapeutic tools within the context of occupational therapy. Each is important in its own way.

There are times when occupational therapy practitioners must provide the most cost-effective intervention. In these cases, clients' occupation may take the second place, and the most cost-effective intervention may be activities. At times, if addressing a performance deficit, the occupational therapist may need to provide an activity that must be accomplished or practice a task that needs to be done to complete an activity.

Occupational therapy practitioners find purposeful activities essential because they are the building blocks for occupations—the ultimate target. As occupational therapy practitioners, we learn to select, adapt, modify, grade, and create activities that meet the therapeutic needs of our clients. We understand that if the client understands the purpose of the activity and focuses attention on its completion, his or her performance improves or behaviors change. When this improvement occurs, the client is able to synthesize or incorporate his or her performance and behaviors into daily life occupations.

Occupations need to be studied in the context of the body of knowledge that underlies this fundamental construct. Occupational science leadership identifies the importance of developing a discipline. We cannot afford to ignore the research that is needed to support occupational therapy. Occupational therapy involves the use of a wide range of theoretical approaches and tools to bring about change. Occupational therapy scholars and researchers must provide a body of knowledge that supports the practice of the profession.

Creating Our Future

Many of us are interested in predicting and understanding what the future will hold. The life course itself leads us to speculate about what lies ahead for us as people. And in a larger sense, we would like to know the shape of the future for those close to us, for our professions, even for our nation's interests and for the people on our planet. Some project these interests into the universe and, with more or less information, tie our course to long-term celestial change. For that matter, considerations about the future lead many to speculate about matters of religion and ultimate fates.

Change at the Societal Level

This chapter has a more mundane intent: to look at the future of human activity and how that may affect occupational therapy. We will begin, however, with some notions about change at the societal level to put our thoughts into some context and provide them with some shape.

The future as an area of unknown terrain may seem as inviting as the people, places, and events that may inhabit it and that we are anticipating with joy. Or it may seem fearsome, inhabited by unwanted changes, anticipated losses, and debility. It is clear that our view of future events will vary by age, circumstances, health, and belief systems. We sometimes seek knowledge and understanding in a vain effort to control the future or at least to make it less uncertain.

Media depictions of the future have long been inhabited by sleek, young people wearing body-conforming suits (and never winter coats or umbrellas), standing near glossily curved rocket ships or missile-like automobiles, with ultramodern, uncluttered homes and soaring highways or transit flyovers hurtling through the background of the picture. Some of these elements are to be seen every day in our world. But the world we inhabit is also very different from space-age fantasies. It is the juxtaposition of the startlingly new and strikingly innovative changes with the familiar, expected, tried-and-true, everyday round that we live with.

Exercise 18.1—Personal Reflection

Answer each of the following questions in three sentences or fewer: (a) Who am I? (b) Who would I like to be? (c) What are the similarities between the person I perceive myself to be and the person I would like to be? (d) What are the differences? (e) What conclusions can you draw from this assignment? (Insel & Roth, 1985, p. 74).

It is important to note that we have no way to actually predict what will happen tomorrow, next week, next year, or in 2100. We do, of course, live with certain indicators of direction and possibility. These indicators include knowledge of the past and the present in human affairs, the acceleration of technological change, information about population trends, and calculations about acid rain and global warming. Based on some of these indicators, we therefore will discuss some of the arenas of most significant change and how they are affecting human activity but only as we can see them now, from our vantage point. Sudden, transforming change may be less likely than incremental change, but it too can occur, making all careful study of trends possibly futile.

Media and Modes of Communication

Some of the most rapidly changing aspects of our environment in the mid- to late 20th century were in our modes and means of communication as well as the content of what we communicate. Recent writing (Standage, 1998) suggests that the introduction of telegraphy was, in its day, seen to be as societally transforming as computer technology is perceived today. Since the introduction of the telegraph, however, we have seen the development of all sorts of radio and wireless communication (including wireless telephones in many hands), global print media carried to us by wireless communication and rapid transportation systems, television and video recording in rapidly proliferating forms, and computer technology spawning new applications, wonders, and intrusions every day. The Information Age, indeed, is upon us, and it has already had some interesting effects on the way in which we incorporate activity into our lives.

It is now commonplace for people to have access to television with many channels, a wide range of radio stations of varying types, and online news with chat options. These sources of information and entertainment have transformed people's lives in a very short period of time. Yet, it is still commonplace to hear people say that they are bored or that there is nothing on television or radio. Changes in media and modes of communication also have transformed our activity lives. Just to mention a few of the results for human activity: (a) Many people spend a good part of their workday sitting at a monitor and keyboard; (b) television watching and little physical activity fill the leisure hours of many, perhaps the same, people; and (c) knowing which buttons to push and when operates not only the stereo, VCR, and DVD but also many household appliances, cars, and jet aircraft. The use of exercise equipment is one mode of balancing human activity. Contemporary lives have overall become much more sedentary. A current hot topic is widespread obesity. It is related to activity pattern as well as to the importance of food in our lives, as discussed in Chapter 3.

The ways in which we use our hands to accomplish tasks also have radically changed. Technology has freed us from many old-style manual tasks. Instead of writing letters and going to the post office to mail them, we send e-mails or instant messages. In some cases, however, technological changes have created the need for more complex fine motor skills. There are now programs that allow one to talk into the computer rather than typing. The trends just described are likely to continue through the coming decades.

OTHER TECHNOLOGICAL CHANGES

Although communication technology has a primary effect on our lives, it can be seen even from the previous discussion here, that technological change affects many aspects of our existence. These changes are primarily affecting the lives of people in the so-called developed world. Places still exist where it would be difficult to find a telephone, where many people cannot read, and where hand tools are the principal means of influencing the home, leisure, and work environments. How technological changes will move to new populations in the future is, in itself, a challenging topic to ponder.

With rapidly developing and available technological devices and equipment, people have developed new ways of interacting with the devices and with each other. Today, many people must have special skills to operate the stereo and VCR, the digital satellite television, and many household appliances. Special skills and knowledge are needed to operate modern cars. Even more expertise and experience are needed to control the advanced equipment that is an essential aspect of flying a jet or for information processing.

For most of us now and in the future, changing technology will affect every aspect of our lives, from high-powered toothbrushes to food processors (Hafner, 1999), to color copiers, to magnetic resonance imaging, to robotics, to mood- and activity-enhancing drugs, just to name a few. Technological change and new products will affect not only our knowledge and interaction but also our bodies, how and why we move, and what we think and desire. "We have always been empowered—yet oddly constrained—by the vocabulary of the moment" (Hall, 1999, p. 128). All of this will lead to some transformations in our daily activities, and for occupational therapy practitioners, there will be an increased need to understand and analyze these changes and the new activity patterns that are formed. It will be critical to explore them with our clients, whose own lives will have altered activity patterns, emerging interests, and restructured circumstances. These changes will have occurred even before we take into account the influence of disability and possible new limitations in the lives of these clients.

Technological change will add to the resources available in the rehabilitation process and may like other societal changes affect the need for and the way our services are offered. These changes affect the way in which we carry out our daily activities, the way in which we feel about the things we do, and the tools we use.

CHANGES IN HEALTH AND ILLNESS

In the developed world, increasing attention paid to the maintenance and promotion of health concerns about personal habits (e.g., smoking) and environmental effects (e.g., food additives) have led to changes in practices for some people and to legislation and social restriction in other cases. How people will define healthy practice and healthy living in the future remains to be seen, but occupational therapy practitioners and other health care practitioners are likely to continue giving attention to prevention and health promotion activities.

Other recent health and illness trends that will probably extend into the future include the realization that newer, frequently more virulent communicable diseases could spread rapidly around the world because of increased international travel. The notion that a disease might be restricted to one community, one region, one nation, or even one continent is probably an illusion. Along with greater concern about the spread of such diseases, more attention probably will be paid to international public health measures.

In the United States, another notable health trend likely to extend into the future is the increasing use of pharmaceuticals as the major remedy of traditional medicine. This development has already had a significant impact on the health care system. How the growth of pharmaceutical treatments will influence the future structure and practice of health care is still a matter for speculation, but there is no doubt that it will have an effect on how health care is delivered.

CHANGING RESOURCES

Recent history has indicated that the way in which money, goods, and other resources are generated, traded, and expended in the world has changed. We can be sure that such change will continue. We can be fairly sure that economic troughs and booms and consequent adjustments will occur in all quarters of society. We will later note how some recent changes have influenced the delivery of health care. Fluctuating resources and, in the United States, no guaranteed health care coverage for all suggest that any type of health care may not be available to some portion of society. Any economic uncertainty and resulting shortages of services will lead to segments of society being unable to fulfill their personal goals for well-being, to consequent social unrest and to anomie. In good times, more possibilities for addressing social ills and shortages exist, but the choices that are made will never address all of the social inequities that exist. People seeking to improve their life chances and to find solutions for their own personal dilemmas will have difficulties doing so when the economy is faltering and will have more opportunities to meet their goals in prosperous times.

Occupational therapy practitioners will have to take issues of resources and their effects on people's lives into consideration when planning intervention, perhaps even more so than they do currently. Creativity and ingenuity particularly will be called for with clients who have fewer resources and pressing needs. But at the same time, perhaps knowledge of how to access online investing and the latest sophisticated adapted equipment may be required for other clients. Thus, as we need to be prepared to work in a world where types and knowledge of technology will be ever changing and continually more demanding, we also will need to pay more attention to our own adaptive skills, our knowledge of the simplest and most rudimentary ways to solve problems of living and doing, and our willingness to offer our services *pro bono* when required to provide those services in a somewhat equitable fashion.

Tradition: The Pull of the Familiar

The "X Files" world of sleek mystery and intellect is not the one we live in every day, and it may not be the one in which we live in the future. Most of us would not be satisfied with form-fitting spacesuits and barren landscapes filled only with objects constructed by people, objects that emphasize efficiency above other features. Within most of us stirs a desire for the asymmetric, the familiar, even the traditional. As one of the authors was writing these words, she was influenced by the landscape surrounding her. She observed that she was distracted by the goldfinches and the wildflowers as she sat outdoors and wrote. The natural beauty all around her reinforced the obverse of the electronic world that was at her fingertips. Yes, electricity, telephones, and a computer were nearby, but her world, as well as all of our worlds, is shaped also by family, expected behaviors, familiar foods, joys of work, and beautiful objects.

Most of us enjoy a world that combines the new and startling with the established and familiar (Friedman, 1999). Sociologists have called the fireplaces in our homes, the oatmeal we eat for breakfast, and the flowers in our window boxes "rural survivals." We have every reason to believe that the good and bad of our past and present activity lives will follow us in some form into the future. Occupational therapy practitioners who emphasize the importance of arts and crafts in our quiver of purposeful activities are reminding us that our knowledge of how to make things with our hands, of how to shape beauty, are human impulses that will not be lost to us or our clients in the future.

Consequences of Change

Looking at our daily activities and even those activities that are special or unusual, it is clear that adaptation to change is a requirement of the human condition. This is true for each of us just as it is true for the little child trying to overcome difficulties of movement, the young adult trying to cope with a devastating injury, or the 85-year-old dealing with even modest physical and mental changes caused by aging. Human beings hold some aspects of their futures in their heads and hands. As stated earlier, some aspects of the future have already been laid out by past actions and happenstance. We can foresee some of these developments by careful reading of current trends. Most people make choices that shape their futures. Nations also plan educational, transportation, communication systems, and relationships with other nations that influence the future, the environment, and the ability to deal with one another.

Much of what occurs in our lives and in the larger world, however, is unplanned by human beings and, indeed, unplannable. Furthermore, all of our actions have unintended consequences. At one point in time, no knowledge existed of a link between tobacco smoking and lung cancer. There are discernible but unintended connections among World Wars I and II and developments in the Balkans. The history of European relationships with the people of the Middle East has led to some of the upheavals we see in the world today. Our efforts to lead healthy lives do not invariably lead us to the outcomes that we anticipated. Serendipity and tragedy are always available to surprise and shock us. These observations only serve to remind us that a good future is always uncharted and that the best treatment plans need reconsideration.

The Life Course

One scientific genre that provides us with reports from time to time is the approach to human development that promotes the extension of the healthy human life span. A world that over the past several centuries has become cleaner for many of us and provided better nutrition, safer childbirth, fewer children per family, and the diminution of some diseases has permitted and extended the life spans of many human beings. A conscious plan and intent by some to move further in that direction holds out tantalizing notions of even longer, more successful lives.

Nonetheless, as occupational therapy practitioners, a major concern of our emphasis on normal and therapeutic activity must currently and in the future be on enhancing and fulfilling an already-extended life course. We must continue to attend to all the issues of human development, both healthy and deleterious, that we have made our focus. In the future, the promises and consequences of human development and aging and how they intersect with purposeful activities and occupation will continue to be a central theme for us. In doing so, we should not over- or underemphasize either end of the life cycle, nor should we neglect adolescence, young adulthood, or middle adulthood—no matter what chronological ages these periods encompass or, for that matter, whatever they may be called. The transitions of life and aging as a usual and inexorable process always will color our activities and interests and, therefore, the way in which we apply activities therapeutically.

Belief Systems and Human Actions

Predictions of the future and generalizations about outcomes cannot fail to take into account how ideology, convictions, and political actions affect human behavior. Neat plans become messy not only because of unintended consequences but also because the choices we make are outcomes of our interpretations of the world based sometimes on fervently held beliefs, religious traditions, political leanings, or ideological conditioning. A portion of what makes the future unpredictable are these very belief systems that lead people to make war, demand conformity with the tenets of their religion, promote new educational systems, fear change, and engage in new individual or shared activities, just to name a few possibilities. Therefore, we truly cannot know what the future will hold for occupational therapy, even as it is our responsibility as practitioners to stand for, promulgate, and adapt the tenets of our profession in the climate of the belief systems that develop. Furthermore, those of us who have been engaged in this process must pave the way for you, the occupational therapy practitioners of the future, to draw from the knowledge and achievements of the past, to avoid the pitfalls that experience has shown us, and to learn from the indicators that people have provided, about where purposeful activities are moving and changing and how their positive attributes can be applied by occupational therapy practitioners in assisting clients to lead fuller and more satisfying lives.

Genetic Engineering

In efforts to assess the scope of the future and how it will affect human activity, one area of knowledge that is bound to influence our very beings is the burgeoning science of genetics and efforts to understand how the genetic map works. Work to increase knowledge in this area has been and will continue to be wildly successful. Alterations to the gene pool, to treat illnesses and disabilities, to promote fertility, or to vary heritability are highly likely to affect the practice of our profession and even who our clients will be. For example, future practice will no doubt embrace more twins and triplets. More complex multiple pregnancies and low birthweights will produce children in need of intervention. In the future, our profession will continue to see a changing human landscape resulting from increased knowledge of and success with various methods of enhancing fertility. Changes in the field of fertility intervention already are coming to our attention, but some commentators believe that they will affect a relatively small proportion of the population. Nonetheless, occupational therapy practitioners specializing in pediatrics will probably see many representatives of this portion of the population.

Cloning, efforts to modify genetic impairment, and even selective eugenics will be discussed and used by some to control reproduction, reproductive choices, and heritable disease. As with other predictions for the future, one can be sure that some of these creations will have unintended consequences. Possibilities for new and as yet unimagined developments in the areas of genetics and reproductive technology are probably among the most revolutionary changes that will affect our notions about family, our definitions of human beings and relationships, and occupational therapy practice.

Future Practice

As the chapters in this book have described, occupational therapy practice is based in the use of purposeful activities with the ultimate goal that clients can engage in occupations. As occupational therapy practitioners, we believe in the importance of activities and occupations. In the real world, however, many practitioners often are unable, unwilling, or reluctant to use purposeful activities as part of their daily interventions. Why do some occupational therapy practitioners not use purposeful activities? Frequently, when practitioners are asked what they do in practice, they often answer by describing specific intervention strategies or techniques. Many often describe specific hands-on manipulations or exercises that are done during the treatment sessions. Some state or infer that devising an activity with a client takes more time than just giving that client an exercise to do. The focus is on the result of the exercise rather than on the meaningfulness of the activity. These kinds of answers reinforce the belief that the techniques for the treatments are more important than the performance of the specific activity itself, when the ability to perform the activity may be the goal that the client is trying to achieve. Occupational therapy practitioners are ultimately concerned with the client's ability to engage in occupations. Engagement in occupations requires that clients be able to perform the many purposeful activities that are the foundations to the specific occupations of their lives. Therefore, as occupational therapy practitioners, we should be comfortable explaining the outcomes of intervention in terms of the clients' abilities to engage in occupations. *Activities are used in treatment because they are the foundations for engaging in occupations. Thus, our measures of success are really the clients' abilities to perform the specific activities so that they can ultimately engage in occupations. As occupational therapy practitioners, we need to reaffirm the importance of the person's ability to perform occupations.*

The future of occupational therapy is rich as society focuses on function, the person's ability to engage in meaningful tasks. The challenge to occupational therapy practitioners is to move forward and yet be true to their roots. We have to value personal needs and desires and what is meaningful to our clients. We have to put aside our expectations of the client and focus on the client's expectations for him- or herself. We need to learn about the cultures of our clients and work together with clients to identify meaningful activities and occupations that are consistent with their values and their heritage. This is the art of our practice, focusing on the will of the client and not on the desires of the practitioner. Once we have mastered artful practice that is true to our profession, we have to move forward in the world of science. The world of science involves documenting what we do and explaining how valuable it is to the person. Once the importance of occupation to the person is recognized, the value to society becomes immediately apparent. Through the effective use of occupational therapy, society can count on people who are willing and able to engage in meaningful occupation.

Occupational therapy's concern with a person's ability to perform purposeful activities and occupations is grounded in functional outcomes. In the therapeutic process, the therapist first establishes functional goals. These goals are meaningful to the client and will assist the client to perform activities and occupations successfully. To determine whether the intervention has been effective, occupational therapists need to have clearly identified functional outcomes. Inherent in functional outcomes is the client's ability to perform purposeful activities so that he or she can engage in occupations. Functional performance implies that a person is able to perform specific activities that allow him or her to perform occupations and, thus, be a more functional human being. What could be more functional than dressing oneself, feeding oneself, or being able to take care of one's children? From our view, occupational therapy is based on a concern for developing optimal and independent function. The foci of future practice will be the measurement of the success of the intervention through the demonstration of functional outcomes and the refinement of our theoretical base through the determination of which frames of reference or types of interventions are most efficacious for our clients. Further, by highlighting the importance of the person's ability to do something valued as a measure of the success of our interventions, our value to society will be demonstrated.

Our concern for the person needs to be broadened to involve the context of his or her life. We can no longer focus only on the person's needs and physical environment. Activities occur in a broader framework. Meaningful activities for a person often relate to others. Family, social, and community contexts have to be included in interventions. Currently, we do this in a limited manner. Children are treated with family-centered care. On inpatient units, there is a push to involve the families of clients. As a broad base, however, our focus is still on the individual without concern for the broader context of his or her life. This conceptual expansion will bring interventions out of a clinical setting, making the activity more meaningful to the client and other significant people in his or her life. It brings the practice of occupational therapy into contact with a larger population and demonstrates our value to a broader public.

Another possible change in our practice will be attending to groups as well as to individuals. We use groups in intervention; however, there is great potential in the broader conceptualization of groups as populations. Currently, we treat people with repetitive motion injuries. In the future, we may direct more of our attention to the prevention of such injuries by intervening with groups who may be prone to such problems. We might be involved in changing the environment, or we might try to change the way specific activities are done. Prevention is just a small part of our practice today but should become more significant in the future. Our increasing aging population will demand our attention to help them to adapt their activities so that they can continue to be vitally involved in their chosen occupations. The adaptation of activities on a broader scale will become an essential component of practice.

Reflecting on future practice, we realize that the future is always unpredictable, sometimes exciting, and often threatening. Although we cannot predict what the future actually holds, we can reflect on whether there is a sound foundation upon which the future can evolve. Today, occupational therapy has the potential of being a prominent profession in the 21st century. This potential will become a reality if occupational therapy practitioners continue to provide interventions that are responsive to societal change. Shifts in the sites of practice and service delivery models also are evident in all areas of practice. Since the 1990s, occupational therapy services have shifted from "clinic" settings to more integrated community, classroom, and home settings.

The strength of occupational therapy has always been its practitioners' willingness and abilities to adapt and change in response to society. If occupational therapy is to continue to be viable, however, practitioners must continually examine their interventions in the light of a changing society. We must examine society to set our intervention priorities and to select the most appropriate tools for interventions. What activities do people value? What activities do people desire and need to engage in? How can occupational therapy practitioners use activities therapeutically if they do not know what activities in a society are foundational to its occupations? Additionally, occupational therapy practitioners need to have an expanded appreciation of society that includes understanding needs of people who are minorities, poor, chronically ill, or elderly. Whether and how occupational therapy addresses these issues may determine how viable occupational therapy will be in the next decade. Occupational therapy practitioners must become familiar with changes in the health care and education systems as they evolve. They cannot afford to continue to watch passively and attempt to respond to changes; occupational therapy practitioners must become active in the shaping of newly emerging systems. Moving beyond direct services, practitioners must advocate for the concerns of the individual client within managed services. They must begin to create new service delivery models that ensure quality care in natural environments.

Education: Purposeful Activities and Occupation

As previously mentioned in this chapter, many things in the world go in cycles. Ideas come in and out of fashion like skirt lengths. As professions grow and develop over time, they too experience a fluctuation of ideas. They respond to societal changes or else they become obsolete. When the profession of occupational therapy was founded, its basis was called occupation and it stressed the importance of engaging in occupation for a healthy productive life. People may have used the term *occupation* differently then, but they clearly recognized its importance to daily life.

Over the years, the centrality of the term *occupation* to occupational therapy changed. During the 1940s, the term *occupation* became much less crucial to the profession. We focused more on activities and activity analysis, moving away from the importance of occupation to the client. The intent was to match the activity with the client's diagnosed condition. Our practice became somewhat mechanistic, focusing on the goals of the therapist rather than on the needs of the client. We worked within a medical model and followed many medical procedures and dictates. Therapeutic modalities became crafts, exercises, and the use of machinery. We also attempted to move toward a concentration on science or what was perceived at that time to be science. The profession wanted to be closely allied with medicine and, therefore, to be viewed as more scientific within that perspective. At this time, educational programs were jointly accredited by the AOTA and the American Medical Association. Educational programs became more science oriented as well, introducing more basic sciences into the curriculum and decreasing the emphasis on crafts. The relationship of arts and crafts to the profession became less clear, and the relevance of crafts to practice was questioned. The term *occupation* is almost nonexistent in the literature written during this time frame. Much of what was generally considered to be part of our domain of concern was absorbed by other professions, some traditional and others that were just developing at this time. In retrospect, it seems that we were less aware of the value of what we do than others were.

War efforts changed the focus of life. During World War II, occupational therapists were an essential part of the rehabilitation team. The focus of intervention was activities of daily living, work, and exercise. Medicine devalued the active involvement of the patient in care and the use of crafts by occupational therapists, and a view of the patient as actively involved in his or her own treatment did not fit well with this perspective. Although therapists continued to use crafts, their use was frequently questioned. From this period through the 1960s, therapeutic intervention was minimally involved with the positive aspects of activities and occupation and concentrated on function. Education during this period centered even more heavily on the sciences, with a strong emphasis on the motor system. Activities were still included in curricula but were quite prescriptive. Activities were matched to the person's deficit areas, not to the person's interests or values.

During the late 1970s, occupational therapy literature began exploring the importance of returning to the roots of the profession. There was an increase in theory building and discussion of the importance of research. Some of the literature focused on trying to view occupational therapy as a basic science, with concepts that were easily measured, whereas other writings focused on the concept of occupation. The terms *activities, purposeful activities,* and *occupation* were used interchangeably and thought to be synonymous. In treatment, therapists moved away from using diversional activities, and interventions flowed from theoretical information. Frames of reference became more prominent in practice. The profession began to debate its philosophical base, finally adopting *The Philosophical Base of Occupational Therapy* (AOTA, 1979). The terms *occupation* and *purposeful activities* were indicated to be synonymous.

Education made a dramatic change during the 1970s. Theories of occupational therapy were introduced into curricula. Several authors articulated models of practice for the profession. Various degree levels emerged, as did postprofessional education. Students were taught to relate their activities for clients to theory. This evolution continued through the 1980s with the development of more theories and frames of reference. Clearer relationships were drawn between theory and practice.

During the past decade, our profession has learned that science is not necessarily synonymous with the basic sciences and can include the social and behavioral sciences and the concept of scientific inquiry. We have experienced a renewed emphasis on scholarship and research but from a broader perspective, including both quantitative and qualitative methodologies. A renewed focus on occupation has emerged.

The change in our perspective also can be seen in the changes in educational standards as well. The 1983 and 1991 *Essentials and Guidelines for an Accredited Educational Program for the Occupational Therapist* (AOTA, 1983a, 1991a) and the *Essentials and Guidelines for an Accredited Educational Program for the Occupational Therapy Assistant* (AOTA, 1983b, 1991b) do not even use the word *occupation*. Instead, the terms are *activity* and *purposeful activities*. In the most recent educational standards, *Standards for an Accredited Educational Program for the Occupational Therapist* (Accreditation Council for Occupational Therapy Education [ACOTE], 1998a), and *Standards for an Accredited Educational Program for the Occupational Therapy Assistant* (ACOTE, 1998b), *occupation, activity,* and *purposeful activities* are all used, with the focus being most heavily on occupation.

Exercise 18.2—Standards

Review the *Standards for an Accredited Educational Program for the Occupational Therapist* and the *Standards for Accredited Educational Program for the Occupational Therapy Assistant* (ACOTE, 1998a, 1998b). Answer each of the following questions: (a) Do the definitions in the glossary of *activity, purposeful activity,* and *occupation* give you a clear picture of the relationship among these terms? What is that relationship? (b) Identify the relationship between purposeful activities and occupation in your own life. Think of three examples. (c) Keeping these three examples in mind, look closely at Section B 2.0, "The Basic Tenets of Occupational Therapy." In your educational experience to this point, how have the differences among these terms been exemplified?

Although little agreement exists among scholars on the definitions of occupation and purposeful activities, they do agree that these concepts are basic to occupational therapy. The profession adopted a hierarchy (AOTA, 1997) with *occupation* as the umbrella term and *purposeful activities* being an important component under that umbrella. The newest educational standards also suggest a hierarchy, although it is somewhat different. It is critical that our profession continue to explore these terms, define them, and debate their relationship to one another and to the practice of occupational therapy.

The challenge to education for the future is to encourage the exploration of these concepts, to debate their meanings, and to identify how they relate to practice. Students need to think about the relationship among activity, purposeful activity, and occupation and how these concepts apply to intervention and to the profession as a whole. These concepts are the cornerstone of our profession and need our attention. Although our profession has grown extensively, it has also come full circle, moving closer to its roots. It is critical that we clarify the meaning and importance of occupation and purposeful activities and through this, explain and describe what we do and its importance to society.

Summary

In 1961, Mary Reilly claimed that "occupational therapy can be one of the greatest ideas of 20th-century medicine" (Reilly, 1962, p. 1). As we move into the 21st century, despite changes in society and technology, occupational therapy continues to provide a very valuable service to people and society. We have changed and grown, just as society has changed and grown, and yet we still provide a fundamental and meaningful service to people by helping them to maintain control of their lives through participation in occupations and activities that are meaningful to them. The future will provide the practice of occupational therapy with many challenges, yet behind each challenge lies an opportunity to promote the importance of human activity and occupation. ■

References

Accreditation Council for Occupational Therapy Education. (1998a). Standards for an accredited educational program for the occupational therapist. *American Journal of Occupational Therapy, 53,* 575–582.

Accreditation Council for Occupational Therapy Education. (1998b). Standards for an accredited educational program for the occupational therapy assistant. *American Journal of Occupational Therapy, 53,* 583–589.

American Occupational Therapy Association. (1979). The philosophical base of occupational therapy. *American Journal of Occupational Therapy, 33,* 785.

American Occupational Therapy Association. (1983a). Essentials of an accredited educational program for the occupational therapist. *American Journal of Occupational Therapy, 37,* 817–823.

American Occupational Therapy Association (1983b). Essentials of an accredited educational program for the occupational therapy assistant. *American Journal of Occupational Therapy, 37,* 824–830.

American Occupational Therapy Association. (1991a). Essentials and guidelines for an accredited educational program for the occupational therapist. *American Journal of Occupational Therapy, 45,* 1077–1084.

American Occupational Therapy Association. (1991b). Essentials and guidelines for an accredited educational program for the occupational therapy assistant. *American Journal of Occupational Therapy, 45,* 1085–1092.

American Occupational Therapy Association. (1997). Statement: Fundamental concepts of occupational therapy: Occupation, purposeful activity, and function. *American Journal of Occupational Therapy, 51,* 864–866.

American Occupational Therapy Association. (2002). Occupational therapy practice framework: Domain and process. *American Journal of Occupational Therapy, 56,* 609–639.

American Occupational Therapy Association & American Occupational Therapy Foundation. (2003). *Research priorities and parameters of practice for occupational therapy.* Retrieved December 20, 2003, from http://www.aotf.org/html/priorities.html.

Clark, F., Azen, S. P., Zemke, R., Jackson, J., Carlson, M., Mandel, D., et al. (1997). Occupational therapy for independent-living older adults: A randomized controlled trial. *Journal of the American Medical Association, 278,* 1321–1326.

Creswell, J. (1998). *Qualitative inquiry and research design choosing among five traditions.* Thousand Oaks, CA: Sage.

Dolecheck, J. R., & Schkade, J. K. (1999). The extent dynamic standing endurance is affected when CVA subjects perform personally meaningful activities rather than nonmeaningful tasks. *Occupational Therapy Journal of Research, 19,* 40–54.

Dunn, W. (1993, June). Useful research strategies for studying service provision in real-life contexts. *Developmental Disabilities Special Interest Section Newsletter, 16,* 1–3.

Friedman, T. L. (1999). *The Lexus and the olive tree: Understanding globalization.* New York: Farrar, Straus & Giroux.

Gillette, N. (1991). The Issue Is—The challenge of research in occupational therapy. *American Journal of Occupational Therapy, 45,* 660–662.

Hafner, K. (1999, May 27). Honey, I programmed the blanket: The omnipresent chip has invaded everything from dishwashers to dogs. *The New York Times,* p. G125.

Hall, S. S. (1999, June 6). Journey to the center of my mind. *The New York Times Magazine,* 122–128.

Hinojosa, J., Kramer, P., Royeen, C. B., & Luebben, A. (2003). The core concept of occupation. In P. Kramer, J. Hinojosa, & C. B. Royeen (Eds.), *Perspectives in human occupation: Participation in life* (pp. 1–17). Philadelphia: Lippincott, Williams & Wilkins.

Insel, G. M., & Roth, W. T. (1985). *Core concepts in health* (4th ed.). Palo Alto, CA: Mayfield.

Lin, K., Wu, C., Tickle-Degnen, L., & Coster, W. (1997). Enhancing occupational performance through occupationally embedded exercise: A meta-analytic review. *Occupational Therapy Journal of Research, 17,* 25–47.

Lyons, M., Orozovic, N., Davis, J., & Newman, J. (2002). Doing–being–becoming: Occupational experiences of persons with life-threatening illnesses. *American Journal of Occupational Therapy, 56,* 285–295.

Melchert-McKearnan, K., Deitz, J., Engel, J. M., & White, O. (2000). Children with burn injuries: Purposeful activity versus rote exercise. *American Journal of Occupational Therapy, 54,* 381–390.

Nelson, D. L. (1993, June). The experimental analysis of therapeutic occupation. *Developmental Disabilities Special Interest Section Newsletter, 16,* 7–8.

Paul, S., & Ramsey, D. (1998). The effects of electronic music-making as a therapeutic activity for improving upper extremity active range of motion. *Occupational Therapy International, 5,* 223–237.

Perrins-Margalis, N. M., Rugletic, J., Schepis, N. M., Stepanski, H. R., & Walsh, M. A. (2000). The immediate effects of a group-based horticulture experience on the quality of life of persons with chronic mental illness. *Occupational Therapy in Mental Health, 16*(1), 15–32.

Plante, E., Kiernan, B., & Betts, J. D. (1994). Method or methodology: The qualitative–quantitative debate. *Language Speech and Hearing Services in Schools, 25*(1), 52–54.

Price-Lackey, P., & Cashman, J. (1996). Jenny's story: Reinventing oneself through occupation and narrative configuration. *American Journal of Occupational Therapy, 50,* 306–314.

Punch, K. F. (1998). *Introduction to social research: Quantitative and qualitative approaches.* Thousand Oaks, CA: Sage.

Reilly, M. (1962). Occupational therapy can be one of the greatest ideas of 20th-century medicine, 1961 Eleanor Clarke Slagle Lecture. *American Journal of Occupational Therapy, 16,* 1–9.

Standage, T. (1998). *The Victorian Internet: The remarkable story of the telegraph and the nineteenth century's on-line pioneers.* New York: Walker.

Yerxa, E. J. (1991). Nationally Speaking—Seeking a relevant, ethical, and realistic way of knowing for occupational therapy. *American Journal of Occupational Therapy, 45,* 199–204.

Yoder, R. M., Nelson, D. L., & Smith, D. A. (1989). Added-purpose versus rote exercise in female nursing home residents. *American Journal of Occupational Therapy, 43,* 581–586.

Index

About the Editors

Jim Hinojosa, PhD, OT, FAOTA, is professor and chair of the Department of Occupational Therapy at New York University. He earned a doctorate in occupational therapy at New York University; a master's degree in special education from Teacher's College, Columbia University; and a bachelor's degree in occupational therapy from Colorado State University. Dr. Hinojosa's extensive publishing record includes more than 90 articles and chapters and 6 textbooks. He has served as chairperson of the Commission on Practice of the American Occupational Therapy Association (AOTA), on the AOTA Executive Board, and on the Board of Directors of the American Occupational Therapy Foundation. Currently, Dr. Hinojosa is member-at-large on AOTA's Commission on Continuing Competence and Professional Development. In recognition of his leadership, AOTA presented him with their highest honor, the Award of Merit, in 1994.

Marie-Louise Blount, AM, OT, FAOTA, is clinical professor and director of the professional-level master's program in occupational therapy at New York University. She earned a master's degree in sociology at Boston University in 1964 and a bachelor's degree in education (occupational therapy) at Tufts University–Boston School of Occupational Therapy in 1957. She is the coeditor of the quarterly journal *Occupational Therapy in Mental Health*. Professor Blount was formerly chair of the Occupational Therapy Department at Towson State University in Maryland and prior to that position also served on the occupational therapy faculties at Howard University and Tufts University.